Emergency-Room Care

Emergency - Room

EDITED BY

BY 26 AUTHORS

Care SECOND EDITION

Charles Eckert, **M.D.** *Professor and Chairman, Department of Surgery, The Albany Medical College of Union University, Albany, New York*

ITTLE, BROWN AND COMPANY • BOSTON

Copyright © 1967, 1971
by Little, Brown and Company (Inc.)

Second Edition

Library of Congress catalog card No. 70–146335

ISBN 0–316–20867 (C)

ISBN 0–316–20869 (P)

4317–20]2–M10/71 (C)

4321–20I2–M10/71 (P)

Published in Great Britain
by Churchill/Livingstone, Edinburgh and London

Printed in the United States of America

Contributing Authors

All are affiliated with The Albany Medical College of Union University, Albany, New York, unless otherwise designated.

RALPH D. ALLEY, M.D.
Clinical Professor of Thoracic Surgery

JOHN A. BALINT, B.A., M.B., B.Chir.
Professor of Medicine; Head, Subdepartment of Gastroenterology

HARVEY R. BERNARD, M.D.
Professor of Surgery

JOHN H. CARTER, M.D.
Associate Professor of Surgery; Chairman, Emergency-Room Policy Committee

JOSEPH T. DOYLE, M.D.
Professor of Medicine; Head, Subdepartment of Cardiovascular Disease

CHARLES ECKERT, M.D.
Professor and Chairman, Department of Surgery

DUMONT F. ELMENDORF, JR., M.D.
Assistant Clinical Professor of Medicine

WALTER J. FRIEDLANDER, M.D.
Professor and Chairman, Department of Neurology, University of Nebraska College of Medicine

ALICE E. FRUEHAN, M.D.
Assistant Professor of Medicine

JOHN E. GAINOR, M.D.
Clinical Professor of Pediatrics

FLOYD B. GOFFIN, M.D.
Professor of Otolaryngology; Head, Subdepartment of Otolaryngology

JULES S. GOLDEN, M.D.
Professor of Psychiatry, The Albany Medical College of Union University; Professor and Head, Department of Psychiatry, Nairobi University, Kenya

DONALD B. KETTELKAMP, M.D.
Associate Professor of Orthopedic Surgery, University of Iowa College of Medicine

RICHARD A. LENDE, M.D.
Professor of Neurological Surgery

W. BRANDON MACOMBER, M.D.
Clinical Professor of Plastic Surgery

A. M. MARCHIONNE, Ph.D.
Associate Professor of Psychiatry

HAROLD E. MARDEN, JR., M.D.
Assistant Clinical Professor of Urology

THOMAS M. OLDER, M.D.
Assistant Clinical Professor of Surgery

PAUL R. PATTERSON, M.D.
Professor and Chairman, Department of Pediatrics

MANUEL J. PEARL, M.D.
Associate Professor of Obstetrics and Gynecology

WILLIAM A. PETERSEN, M.D.
Assistant Clinical Professor of Pediatrics

SAMUEL R. POWERS, JR., M.D.
Professor of Surgery

ROBERT D. REINECKE, M.D.
Professor and Chairman, Department of Ophthalmology

MAKIS J. TSAPOGAS, M.D.
Professor of Surgery

MARK K. WANG, M.D.
Associate Clinical Professor of Plastic Surgery

HAROLD F. WELCH, M.D.
Associate Professor of Surgery

Preface to the Second Edition

Emergency departments of general hospitals have assumed positions of increasing importance in the delivery of medical care in this country since the first edition of this book was written. The need to provide increased medical service has resulted in expanded facilities and led in many hospitals to the appointment of a corps of full-time physicians in an effort to meet these requirements. No specific educational program has yet been evolved to provide a background adequate to carrying out satisfactorily the functions of an emergency-room physician. For this reason we believed it important to revise this book, as well as to correct deficiencies present in the first edition and to bring it up to date. Several chapters have been entirely re-written and a new chapter on drug abuse has been added for obvious reasons.

Albany, New York   C. E.

Preface to the First Edition

This manual has been prepared for the use of professional personnel working in the emergency rooms of general hospitals. It may also prove to be of some value to hospital administrators. In it we have attempted to provide a guide to current emergency-room practice, using as a model experience with the care of patients in the emergency room of The Albany Medical Center Hospital. It is believed that this experience is reasonably typical of that in most general hospitals throughout the country, since our institution serves a dual function: as university teaching hospital and as community hospital. Furthermore, the community has no city- or county-supported hospital.

The authors have chosen for the most part to avoid lengthy discussions of alternative methods of management in the belief that by simply giving the particular method preferred in our own institution they will increase the value of the book as a ready reference source. However, we acknowledge a priori that valid differences of opinion may exist.

Much of the material contained in this book has received practical trial by our own house officers. We are grateful for the suggestions offered by these critical young men. We are also grateful to Mr. Fred Belliveau of Little, Brown and Company for the helpful advice he has given in the book's planning and preparation.

Albany, New York   C. E.

Contents

Contributing Authors   v

Preface to the Second Edition   ix

Preface to the First Edition   xi

Introduction   I
CHARLES ECKERT

1. Planning and Operation of the Emergency Room   5
JOHN H. CARTER

2. The Severely Injured Patient   23
SAMUEL R. POWERS, JR.

3. Thoracic Emergencies   33
RALPH D. ALLEY and THOMAS M. OLDER

4. Cardiac Emergencies   63
JOSEPH T. DOYLE

5. Neurosurgical Emergencies   87
RICHARD A. LENDE

6. The Unconscious Patient   99
ALICE E. FRUEHAN

xiii

7. *Vascular Emergencies*   107
    MAKIS J. TSAPOGAS

8. *Abdominal Emergencies*   121
    HAROLD F. WELCH

9. *Urological Emergencies*   135
    HAROLD E. MARDEN, JR.

10. *Obstetrical and Gynecological Emergencies*   145
    MANUEL J. PEARL

11. *General Principles in the Management of Wounds*   171
    CHARLES ECKERT

12. *Orthopedic Injuries*   183
    DONALD B. KETTLEKAMP

13. *The Hand*   221
    MARK K. WANG, W. BRANDON MACOMBER,
    DONALD B. KETTLEKAMP, and CHARLES ECKERT

14. *Maxillofacial Injuries*   251
    MARK K. WANG and W. BRANDON MACOMBER

15. *Burns*   265
    MARK K. WANG and W. BRANDON MACOMBER

16. *Ocular Emergencies*   277
    ROBERT D. REINECKE

17. *Otorhinolaryngological Emergencies*   289
    FLOYD B. GOFFIN

18. *Poisoning*   299
    PAUL R. PATTERSON

19. *Gastrointestinal Emergencies*   315
    JOHN A. BALINT

20. *Infectious Disease*   329
    HARVEY R. BERNARD and DUMONT F. ELMENDORF, JR.

21. *Neurological Emergencies* 337

WALTER J. FRIEDLANDER

22. *Pediatric Emergencies* 351

WILLIAM A. PETERSEN

23. *Psychiatric Emergencies* 371

JULES S. GOLDEN and A. M. MARCHIONNE

24. *Drug Abuse* 393

JOHN E. GAINOR

Index 409

Emergency-Room Care

Introduction

CHARLES ECKERT

Public demand for care in emergency departments of general hospitals has increased tremendously in recent years. A number of factors are responsible for this; among these are: the shortage of physicians in family practice, increased awareness on the part of the public of the possibility of obtaining medical care in emergency rooms when a family physician is not available, and a population increase with no lag in the accident rate.

Many patients presenting in the emergency room have problems of chronic disease or trivial illness. The former, after careful screening to exclude urgent problems, should be given an early appointment in the outpatient department, while the latter should be given appropriate medical advice and sent home. Surprisingly, despite an increase in the above categories, the number of patients requiring immediate admission to the hospital also continues to rise. In many hospitals this has resulted in a shortage of beds available for elective admission. In teaching hospitals this disproportion can have deleterious effects on the educational program. It can also have a harmful effect on public relations.

The increased number of patients to be seen may make it impossible to render adequate service without the expansion of both personnel and physical facilities. A lag periodically occurs between the increased demand for service and ability to provide it. In the case of the emergency room, such a lag is likely to be disastrous because of

I

reduced efficiency of patient care and subsequent criticism by the public of the institution as a whole. Perhaps in no other area of hospital operation is the interface between the hospital and the public so thin. Prolonged waiting, delays in obtaining roentgenograms, or the impression that another patient has been improperly treated is likely to create a poor image. Realizing that the voluntary hospitals in this country up to the present time have been largely dependent upon the goodwill of the public for many phases of their funding, we feel it is particularly important for hospital administration to interpret correctly the changing trends in order to reduce the periodic "lag phases" to a minimum.

In hospitals that are departmentalized, the increase in nonsurgical cases seen in the emergency room has brought about a reorganization with involvement of all departments in the responsibility for the full operation of the emergency room. Insofar as possible, this has been coordinated with the outpatient department for the study of those patients needing investigation that can be conducted on an ambulatory basis. It is to be emphasized that no patient who comes to the emergency room seeking medical attention is referred to either the outpatient department or his private physician without a careful screening examination in the emergency room, including studies deemed necessary on an emergency basis.

The distinction between private, semiprivate, and ward patients is rapidly disappearing with increased government involvement in medical care. We maintain a panel of staff members from all departments who are willing to care for those eligible patients who request a private physician but do not have one who is a member of our staff. Patients eligible for private medical care who do not wish a private physician are assigned to the member of the staff currently consulting on the teaching service in the specialty in which the patient falls. They are thereafter treated as teaching patients, with the staff physician having final responsibility for their care, a situation in no way different from the management of other patients in the teaching environment.

Although the increased utilization of emergency-room facilities is due to a great extent to the increase in patients with medical illness, there has been a constant rise in surgical patients as well. The frequency of serious accident cases, involving multiple organ systems in particular, is greater with each passing year. The trend toward specialization in surgical practice creates a situation in which the patient with multiple injuries is likely to have multiple physicians, each caring for his special area of interest without assuming overall responsibility for the patient. The priorities for definitive treatment are determined by the comparative threat to the patient's life, and as such should be well defined. Our solution to this problem is to assign patients with multiple injuries to the general surgical service or to a private practitioner of general surgery, as the case may be. Either assumes responsibility for requesting consultations, assigning priorities, and for the overall care of the patient. With this system problems seldom arise. In this manual, reference to the securing of consultation with representative specialists has been intentionally omitted for the most part, but the reader will understand that in each instance consultation is obtained as necessary. The securing of multiple consultations, unless they are immediately available, which is seldom the case, sometimes causes undue delays in the initiation of treatment or disposition of the patient. These delays are avoidable by the assumption of responsibility for decision on the part of the senior resident staff physician or the physician in charge of the emergency room.

On occasion, patients are seen in the emergency room who have been transferred from the emergency rooms of other hospitals. When this is done, proper notification of the transfer should be given. It is also essential that a record accompany the patient, containing pertinent information concerning the previously obtained history and physical examination, laboratory reports, and any medication or other treatment which may have been given. If roentgenograms were obtained, the actual films should accompany the patient with the understanding that they will be returned as soon as they are no longer of use.

A final word is necessary concerning the advice and instruction given to patients by the emergency-room physician. Complete explanations in nontechnical language, preferably in words of one syllable, should be given. The physician should never assume, on the basis of a patient's education, work in a scientific field allied to medicine, or seeming comprehension, that any detail will be logical and obvious to him. It is in just such patients that the possibility of misinterpretation or illogical behavior is greatest. All instructions should be clearly explained and set down on paper as well, and in readable script. A copy of the instructions should be placed in the record.

Planning and Operation of the Emergency Room 1

JOHN H. CARTER

Two great mistakes are made in the organization and management of emergency rooms. The first is attempting to do too little, and the second is attempting to do too much. To chart a safe middle path it is important that fundamental decisions be made early to define the scope of activities of a given emergency room. These decisions will depend to some extent on the size and type of hospital involved, the available hospital personnel, the type of community (metropolitan, urban, or rural), other available medical facilities, and medical personnel in the community. To avoid doing too little, an emergency room must be capable of managing at all times such true emergencies as cardiac arrest, airway obstruction, crush injuries of the chest, life-threatening external blood loss, shock, and so forth. The greater problem for emergency rooms today is to avoid trying to do too much. Strict regulations *prohibiting* the use of the emergency room for minor elective surgical procedures, or for emergency surgical procedures which require general anesthesia, or for elective medical, pediatric, or psychiatric work will do much to alleviate the problem. The most effective way to avoid overuse of the emergency room is to provide outpatient clinics elsewhere in the hospital to handle the increasing number of patients presenting themselves in emergency rooms throughout the nation who, in fact, are not true emergencies but come to hospital emergency rooms for lack of other medical facilities.

Delays in the management and disposition of patients are the main targets of criticism of emergency rooms by the public. To avoid this it is important that the emergency facility be adequate in size and sufficiently well staffed to cope with a variable patient load. Efficiency also requires that, once primary care has been given, the patient be rapidly referred for prompt hospital admission, transfer, or discharge.

PHYSICAL PLANT

Location

The emergency room should be centrally located within the hospital with ready access to the street, x-ray, blood bank, laboratories, operating rooms, morgue, obstetrical unit, general hospital wards, and record room.

Emergency-Room Entrance

The entrance should be well marked and easily visible from the street. Although the approach to the emergency room should be adequate, it is a mistake to make it too large. When a great deal of space is available, relatives' cars, police cars, press cars, and ambulances tend to clutter up the ambulance port and reduce efficiency. A smaller port discourages people from parking near it and forces police, ambulance drivers, and others to discharge their duties and then move their vehicles. The ambulance port should be covered for protection in inclement weather.

Size and Shape

An expansive emergency room is an efficient emergency room. Everything should be large: the doors between rooms, the booths, the corridors, the storerooms, the cabinets, and the sinks. This means generous floor space. Wide open spaces enable personnel to move beds, x-ray machines, stretchers, and heavy equipment easily and quickly; they add immeasurably to efficient patient care. For example, a serious impediment to efficient operation of an emergency room will be created if someone carelessly forgets to plan doors large enough to accommodate a hospital bed.

In general, the emergency room should be round or square, with the nursing station in the center of the area. This enables the doctors and nurses to have easy visible and physical access to any part of the facility on a moment's notice. The central nursing station should be of sufficient size to accommodate both nurses and doctors and should provide adequate areas for charts and desk space for paper work. Multiple telephones are essential.

Examining Areas

Although partitioned booths are necessary, elaborate separate closed-off booths or examining rooms are dangerous and inefficient and should be avoided. Despite modern electronic devices, confused, unattended, unseen patients in closed booths can get into serious, unrecognized, and even fatal difficulties. The examining rooms should be at least 8 × 10 feet in size and consist of partitioned booths with a simple sliding curtain across the front of the booth to provide adequate privacy and maximum efficiency.

In addition to a portable examining stretcher, each booth should contain a stool, chair, small desk with appropriate stationery, Mayo stand, intravenous pole, tape, gooseneck lamp, stethoscope, flashlight, tongue blades, blood pressure apparatus, sterile rubber gloves, lubricants, emesis basins, tissue paper, appropriate linen, restraints, suction catheters, and, most important, wall oxygen and wall suction.

Surgical Suite

The surgical suite should be a large separate area or room, well lighted and readily visible from the nursing station. It should be a self-contained unit adequate not only for minor surgery but for more major surgical emergencies such as closed thoracostomy, open cardiac massage, tracheostomy, control of massive external hemorrhage, and emergency deliveries.

The area should be free of partitions so that stretchers, beds, and equipment can be moved about easily and more than one seriously injured individual can be handled by a minimum number of personnel at one time. It should contain several versatile stretchers that can be used as operating tables. Standard operating tables are inefficient, impractical, and expensive, and should not be used. Overhead lighting should be similar to that used in standard operating rooms.

The surgical suite should contain the same equipment as the general examining booths plus mobile floor spotlights, arm boards, caps, masks, scrub sinks, appropriate equipment for shaving and preparing the skin, sterile dressings, a wide selection of suture materials, surgical instruments, sterile surgical packs, sterile delivery set, closed thoracostomy set, and tracheostomy set. Most, if not all, of this equipment should be kept in wall cabinets around the periphery of the surgical suite so that floor space is not wasted and improvisations can be made quickly as the situation demands.

Air conditioning in this area is very desirable. Wall suction and oxygen, as in the examining booths, are indispensable.

Fracture Room

Although the surgical suite may double as a fracture room, if possible it is most desirable to have a separate fracture room. Certainly any emergency room with an annual number of patient visits in excess of 15,000 should have a separate fracture room. For convenience, the fracture room should be adjacent to the emergency department.

Visibility from the central nursing station and proximity to radiographic facilities are important aspects of the planning of the fracture room. In general, the fracture room should be equipped in the same way as the surgical suite but in addition should contain an orthopedic table, traction apparatus, splints, plaster, electric cast cutters, crutches, felt, sheet wadding, dressings, a large sink equipped with a plaster trap, and wall-type x-ray view boxes.

Radiology Unit

About one-third of the patients seen in an average emergency room have roentgenograms of some type taken while there. Making these studies constitutes the greatest bottleneck and is the single largest factor conducive to inefficiency in most emergency rooms. It is essential, therefore, that the emergency room be easily accessible to the radiology unit. In fact, any emergency room with an annual number of patient visits in excess of 15,000 should have a separate x-ray unit with assigned technicians, an available radiologist, and automatic film-developing devices.

Regardless of the accessibility of the radiology unit, a portable x-ray machine should be kept in the emergency room for use with patients who are too ill to be moved to an x-ray table. Of course, appropriate view boxes are essential.

Laboratory

A small, well-equipped, well-lighted laboratory with microscopes, centrifuges, Bunsen burner, dyes, testing papers and solutions, slides, applicators, and filter paper should be adjacent to the emergency room. Use of such a laboratory should be confined to physicians working in the emergency room, and examinations should be limited to blood counts, urinalyses, sputum stains, examination of urethral and vaginal discharges, stool examinations, and examinations of cerebral spinal fluid.

Waiting Area

An attractive, comfortable waiting room with adjacent toilet facilities near the emergency room will help keep relatives, friends, police, and press out of the emergency-room area and thereby increase efficiency. Telephone booths and vending machines should be provided.

Patient Observation Area

Although not essential, a small semiprivate ward of four to six beds, which is adjacent to the emergency room and manageable by emergency-room nursing personnel, is helpful in resolving problem cases. By eliminating the need for observation in the emergency room, it is kept clear of "doubtful cases." Strict rules should be enforced limiting the time a patient may stay in the observation area. If this is not done, within a short time the demand for hospital beds will destroy the purpose of the unit.

Professional Quarters

Comfortable quarters with beds and showers should be adjacent to the emergency room for use by doctors on duty in the emergency room during slack periods.

Business Office

Emergency rooms are primarily concerned with patient care, but they are also places of business. A branch of the business office within the emergency room greatly increases efficiency by expediting admissions to the hospital and discharges from the emergency room. This station should be manned on a 24-hour basis.

Closed Psychiatric Area

Although we strongly recommend open booths for the emergency room in general, it is desirable to have one closed, soundproof "padded cell"-like area in which agitated alcoholic patients or severely disturbed psychotic patients can be temporarily placed and kept from interfering with the operation of the emergency room. Such a room also provides a quiet area where psychiatrists can interview and evaluate less severe psychiatric emergencies in privacy.

The room should have no equipment other than a bed or stretcher and several chairs. It is desirable that it also have a large window of unbreakable glass to allow observation of patients from the nursing station, if constant attendance is impossible.

Contagious Disease and Poison-Control Area

This is another exception to the open-booth policy. At times it becomes necessary to use the emergency room for evaluating patients suspected of having a contagious disease. If contagious disease is proved, it becomes necessary to decontaminate the area. A separate room where such cases can be evaluated will minimize the problem of contamination. The room should be equipped with wall cabinets for storage of supplies. These cabinets can be closed during evaluation of patients in order to reduce possible contamination.

In modern practice a room for contagious disease will be used infrequently. Therefore, for purposes of economy it can also be used as a poison-control center. A poison treatment cabinet containing appropriate antidotes and lavage equipment must be provided. The use of a separate room will take agitated children and distraught parents from the mainstream of the emergency room.

Library

A small reference library is desirable. Ours includes the hospital "Policy Book," the *Physicians' Desk Reference,* the hospital formulary, a medical dictionary, and a copy of this book, in addition to books separately requested by different departments.

To summarize: By the very nature of the work involved, an emergency room requires open, large, and well-lighted areas. Since the work load of an emergency room cannot easily be controlled or compartmentalized, all space should be planned so it can serve multifunctional purposes. Shortages of nurses and physicians also demand a physical plant that provides personnel with maximum opportunity to see and take care of a large number of patients with a minimum of effort. Having a large open ward, although aesthetically undesirable, is still the most efficient way to run a hospital; the same holds for an emergency room, regardless of hospital size.

EQUIPMENT

Examining Tables

One never knows when a patient comes into the emergency room and is placed on a stretcher whether he will need cardiac resuscitation, pelvic examination, suture of a laceration, transportation to another part of the hospital, and so forth. Therefore, *all* stretchers in the emergency room should be alike and should conform to the following specifications: mobility, durability, easy operation and design, versatility so that the patient may be easily placed in Fowler's or Trendelenburg's position or placed in stirrups for pelvic examination, attached straps for restraints, adaptable side rails as additional protection, a crank for raising and lowering the table, and adequate brakes so that the stretcher can be "locked" to the floor when necessary.

Elaborate stretchers that require extra equipment or complicated operating maneuvers should be avoided, for they will interfere with efficient patient management. For example, special stretchers for radiography are not in order because they cannot be used to change the patient's position, and unless all the stretchers in the emergency room are equipped for radiography the litter that is so equipped is usually occupied by someone else when it is needed most or stands off in a corner waiting to be used. In general, patients can be positioned well enough on more versatile stretchers so that cassettes can be safely and easily placed under injured parts.

With proper stretchers, as previously emphasized, there is no need for operating tables in the emergency room.

Conventional Supplies

Conventional items include culture tubes, appropriate bottles for blood chemistry, blood counting, the typing and cross matching of blood; urine specimen cups; syringes and needles; and catheters, nasogastric tubes, and intravenous tubing. It is better to keep these supplies in one centrally located place than to try to equip each examining booth separately.

Sterile Supplies and Special Equipment

It is better to store previously sterilized individual basic surgical sets than to attempt to assemble separate pieces of equipment each time a surgical procedure is performed. The basic set should contain as a minimum: a needle holder, suture scissors, dissecting scissors, toothed and plain forceps, scalpel handles, hemostatic clamps, sterile medicine glasses, and sterile towels. In general, it is better that preparation and sterilization of equipment be done in the central supply room rather than that the burden of sterilizing and cleansing equipment be placed on the nursing staff of the emergency room. More specialized instruments—for example, small self-retaining retractors, small drills, bone cutters, and rongeurs—can be stored separately to be used as needed.

Special therapeutic and diagnostic equipment should be sterilized and ready for use in a centrally located area rather than being included in each examining booth. Such special equipment will include trays for neurological examination, lumbar puncture, closed thoracentesis, and tracheostomy, including all sizes of adult and pediatric tracheostomy tubes; endotracheal tubes of all types and sizes; proctoscopes; vaginal specula; myringotomy knives; splinter forceps; rectal biopsy forceps; electrocardiograph machine; external cardiac defibrillation equipment; and cutdown sets.

A list of routine or special equipment applicable to all hospital emergency rooms is impractical. In any given hospital it is good policy for those in charge of the emergency room to consult the head of each hospital department and subdepartment to learn what that department considers essential in the emergency room. Experience will demonstrate the need for supplementation from time to time.

Drugs

A list of drugs needed in the emergency room is also important. There should be an abundant and easily accessible supply of those drugs and intravenous fluids considered necessary by each department in the hospital. The hospital pharmacist should actively participate in the planning and management of the supply and storage of drugs. A refrigerator should be available for perishable drugs. In general, drugs stored in the emergency room should be limited to tried and true preparations—for example, phenobarbital rather than a dozen types of tranquilizers. Plasma expanders and a variety of intravenous fluids are to be included in this list.

Patient Records

Good emergency-room records not only reflect the quality of patient care but are essential for compensation cases and for medicolegal purposes. The emergency record should be designed in such a way as to encourage the examining physician to record systematically and accurately history, physical examination, diagnosis, diagnostic procedures, and instituted therapy. The form must also contain a great deal of socioeconomic information. Sample forms used at the Albany Medical Center Hospital are shown in Figures 1-1 and 1-2. The original form should be kept with the patient's record if he is admitted to the hospital, or sent to the hospital record room if he is discharged from the emergency room. Carbon copies should be available for distribution to the business office, compensation boards, insurance companies, and so forth.

EMERGENCY-ROOM STAFF

All medical disciplines are deeply involved in emergency-room care. The most important single step that can be taken in starting a new emergency room or in improving an old one is the formation of a policy committee for the emergency room. The policy committee should consist of representatives of each of the major medical disci-

NO. 22707

ALBANY MEDICAL CENTER HOSPITAL

EMERGENCY ROOM RECORD

MED. RECORD NO. _____

NAME _____ AGE ____ SEX ____ DATE OF ADMISSION _____

CHIEF COMPLAINT: _____

HISTORY: _____

PHYSICAL FINDINGS: T_____ P_____ R_____ BP _____
CHECK ALL SIGNIFICANT NORMAL AND ABNORMAL FINDINGS.

| 1 SKIN & SCALP | 2 LYMPH NODES | 3 EENT | 4 NECK | 5 CHEST | 6 CARDIOVASCULAR | 7 BREASTS |
| 8 ABDOMEN | 9 GENITAL | 10 RECTAL | 11 PELVIS | 12 MUSCULO-SKELETAL | 13 MENTAL | 14 NEUROLOGICAL |

SPECIAL EXAMS: _____

X – RAY: _____

DIAGNOSIS

1. (_____) _____
2. (_____) _____
3. (_____) _____
4. (_____) _____
5. (_____) _____

DRUGS	NAME	DOSE	FREQUENCY	DURATION
1.				
2.				
3.				
4.				

TETANUS TOXOID: YES_____ NO _____   TETANUS ANTITOXIN: DOSE _____

OTHER TREATMENT _____

DISPOSITION _____

PHYSICIAN'S SIGNATURE _____

MEDICAL RECORD

AH-39A MED. RECORD

Fig. 1-1. Sample emergency-room record to be completed by the physician in attendance.

No. 22707

ALBANY MEDICAL CENTER HOSPITAL

EMERGENCY ROOM RECORD

MED. RECORD NO. _____

DATE PREVIOUS ADMISSION _____

NAME ON PREVIOUS ADMISSION _____

ADMITTED TO: HOSP. ☐ CLINIC ☐ ER ☐

DATE OF E.R. VISIT

MO.	DAY	YR.

PATIENT ACCOUNT NO.

LAST NAME _____ FIRST & MID. INIT. _____

PT. ADDRESS

NUMBER AND STREET	CITY	STATE

AGE MO. YR.

DATE OF BIRTH

MO.	DAY	YR.

TELEPHONE NO. _____

SEX _____ RACE _____ RELIGION _____

MARITAL STATUS

| S | M | W | D | Sep. |

DATE AND TIME OF INJURY _____ VETERAN ☐ NO ☐ YES INJURED AT WORK ☐ NO ☐ YES

AM   AM   AM

TIME OF ARRIVAL _____ PM TIME SEEN BY HOUSE DOCTOR _____ PM TIME SEEN BY CONSULTANT _____ PM

BROUGHT IN BY _____ ADDRESS _____

POLICE NOTIFIED	OFFICER'S NAME
☐ NO ☐ YES ☐ LOCAL ☐ STATE	

TREATED BY _____ REFERRED TO DR. _____

ADMITTED ☐ NO ☐ YES LOCATION _____ DOCTOR – SERVICE _____

CLOTHES TO	VALUABLES TO	APPOINTMENT TO	TIME	MO.	DAY	YR.
			AM PM			

PATIENT – OCCUPATION _____ EMPLOYER NAME _____

EMPLOYER ADDRESS _____

TELEPHONE NO. _____

NEXT OF KIN, NAME _____ RELATIONSHIP _____

ADDRESS _____

PAYER NAME _____ PHONE NO: _____

ADDRESS _____

HOSPITAL INSURANCE – CODE OF BENEFITS

EXCEPTIONS

DEDUCTIBLE

INDEMNITY

NAME OF SUBSCRIBER OR POLICY HOLDER _____

CONTRACT OR POLICY NO. _____ GROUP NO. _____

NAME OF INSURANCE CO. _____ ADDRESS _____

MAIL COMPLETED FORMS TO: NAME _____

ADDRESS _____

MEDICAL RELEASE SIGNED BY _____

ASSIGNMENT – SIGNED BY _____

CLERK

E.R.	X – RAY	EKG	SUTURES NO.	TOXOID	PENICILLIN	MEDICATION	OTHER
$							

I. V. SOLUTIONS				LEVINE TUBE		CATHETERS	
G/S	G/W	SALINE	RINGERS	REGULAR	RUBBER	FOLEY	DESERETS

BANDAGES			GAUZE ROLL	CRUTCHES	WALKING HEEL	FINGER SPLINT
ACE 3"	ACE 4"	KLING	NO.			

SURG. PROCEDURE	OPERATING ROOM	RESUSCITATION	EEG	ROCHESTER NEEDLES
MINUTES	MINUTES			

MEDICAL RECORD

AH-39 ADM. RECORD

Fig. 1-2. Sample emergency-room record to be completed by the emergency-room clerk.

plines and the hospital administration. Thus each department is aware of emergency-room problems, and improvements can be made with dispatch and minimum controversy.

Professional Staff

MEDICAL STAFF. Providing professional coverage in the emergency room is the responsibility of the medical staff. Appropriate lists of private physicians and surgeons on call in all of the medical disciplines should be kept in the emergency room. The names of such physicians should be given to those emergency-room patients requesting private care but without a specific physician or surgeon to call upon. Similar lists should be kept for compensation cases. A physician or surgeon who is habitually negligent or tardy in discharging his responsibilities in the emergency room should be withdrawn from the emergency-room panel. Any physician who is a member of a given hospital staff is presumably qualified to be on the hospital's emergency-room panel. In a large institution there may be enough volunteers from among the members of the attending staff to provide adequate coverage. In smaller hospitals it may be necessary to require participation on the emergency-room panel so that the hospital can fulfill its community obligation.

The actual on-the-spot professional coverage of an emergency room depends on the type of hospital involved.

Since surgical patients represent only about 25 percent of emergency-room admissions and since the emergency room is an invaluable teaching experience for all house officers, staffing of the emergency room should not be limited to surgical residents and interns.

One function of the emergency-room policy committee is to brief house officers on their responsibilities prior to the house officers' tour of duty in the emergency room. It is particularly important for them to understand that on difficult medical or administrative problems they should consult senior members of the house staff or attending staff, and the actual chain of command should be clearly delineated.

Regardless of his competence, a house officer who does not easily understand and speak English should either be kept out of the emergency room or be very closely supervised, since misunderstandings due to a language barrier can be embarrassing or lead to avoidable complications.

All house officers should be instructed to cooperate with the police and other authorized public officials. They should also be cautioned against making or expressing verbally or in writing anything other than medical statements and should refer any medicolegal problems to the hospital administration or the emergency-room policy committee.

Lack of a house staff does not release a hospital from the obligation of providing adequate professional coverage of its emergency room. In general, voluntary systems of coverage are unsatisfactory. There has been a healthy trend in recent years for smaller hospitals to pay physicians to run the emergency room or to allow a group of physicians to form a semiprivate corporation to operate the emergency room under contract with the hospital. Coverage is thus assured. Under these circumstances there should be conspicuously displayed in the emergency room a notice that, since the physician treating the patient is doing so as a private contractor, the patient, in addition to a hospital fee, must also pay a specified fee to the physician.

In this arrangement for emergency-room coverage it is best to keep the private practices of the contract physicians entirely separate from the operation of the emergency room. Like all policy decisions in the emergency room, this one must be made by the administration of the hospital in consultation with the employed physicians.

NURSING STAFF. The staffing of the emergency room by nurses should be given priority over the staffing of any other part of a hospital, not only in terms of numbers, but in terms of quality. The nurses selected for emergency-room work should be screened for intelligence, ability, reliability, flexibility, and an expressed desire to work in the emergency room rather than in more routine areas of the hospital. In general, younger nurses tend to meet all of these diverse requirements better than do older nurses. Nurses in the emergency room must be given authority in keeping with their nursing responsibilities. However, they must recognize that it is ethically and legally improper for a nurse to make diagnoses or institute therapy. The number of nurses in the emergency room at any given time will, of course, depend on the patient load and the supply of nurses. Since peak loads in the emergency rooms occur during the 8 A.M. to 8 P.M. period, staffing should be planned accordingly. A nurse from the emergency room, preferably the head nurse, should sit as a member of the emergency-room policy committee.

Auxiliary Personnel

FLOOR CLERK. A full-time floor clerk to help the nurses and physicians with the necessary paper, administrative, and communication work in the emergency room is very important. The responsibilities of this position should include filing, recording, handling phone calls, making out requisitions, filling out forms for the doctor's or nurse's signature, running errands, keeping inventories, and performing innumerable other small but necessary nonmedical tasks which would otherwise fall to a nurse or a physician. The floor clerk by preference should be well educated, but a well-motivated high school graduate can be trained to fill the position admirably.

NURSE'S AIDES AND ORDERLIES. The emergency room can quickly become littered with patients awaiting transport as well as with equipment, clothing, and body wastes. Since it is essential that the area be kept as functional as possible, sufficient personnel to cope with these factors leading to disorder must be available. It is important to have a liberal number of aides and orderlies in the emergency room at all times without assignment to avoid multiple conflicting responsibilities.

Summary

The chain of command should be somewhat as follows:

1. The emergency-room policy committee should have representatives of all major departments in the hospital and should make overall policy decisions.
2. Physicians in the emergency room should make all on-the-spot professional decisions and should have authority to call consultants when needed in accordance with hospital policy.
3. Nurses should have authority to carry out necessary nursing procedures without prior physician authorization.

MEDICOLEGAL PROBLEMS

Although they differ in details from hospital to hospital, the medicolegal problems involving emergency rooms are fundamentally alike. They center around negligence, consent, compensation, and special situations such as rape.

Negligence

It is obvious from recent court decisions handed down in this country that a hospital today is responsible not only for its administrative acts but for the acts of its employees as well. *Employees* is a broad term covering resident physicians, interns, nurses, and paramedical and domestic personnel who work in the emergency room. Therefore, only the most competent available personnel in all categories should be assigned to the emergency room.

The manner in which patients are handled in the emergency room is very important. A patient (or his relatives and friends) in an emergency room is usually frightened, anxious, and "sensitized." Things he may overlook under normal circumstances now irritate and antagonize him. Although the doctors and nurses in the emergency room may not be impressed with his problem, *he is!* Therefore, empathy and consideration on the part of all personnel are major factors in minimizing complaints. One of the tasks of the emergency-room policy committee should be periodic "spot checks" of the attitude and competence of the personnel in the emergency room.

Consent

In an emergency room consent may be implied from the circumstances. Nevertheless, it is mandatory to make every effort to secure written consent from each patient or his next of kin, particularly if the patient is a minor, is unconscious, or is essentially incompetent.

In a life-and-death situation a note on the emergency-room chart outlining the facts of the situation and signed by the physician responsible for the case will usually suffice.

If there is no life-and-death urgency but delay in treatment may jeopardize the end result of proposed therapy, the hospital administrator in charge, not a professional employee, should make the final decision to institute appropriate diagnostic and therapeutic procedures.

Usually the permission sheet used in the hospital proper will suffice in the emergency room, but this matter should be cleared in any given hospital with the legal advisers to that hospital.

Special Situations

In some situations, including rape, suicide, homicide, intoxication, child abuse, and such matters as drawing blood alcohol levels for the police, the procedure to be followed cannot be left up to the individual working in the emergency room at the time. The hospital must formulate very precise steps to be followed, the details of which should be readily available in the emergency room. These procedures must, of course, conform to local, state, and federal ordinances.

It should be impressed on individuals working in the emergency room that they must avoid, in conversation and in writing, any opinions beyond those of a strictly medical nature. For example, an intern may record that a patient's breath has the odor of alcohol; he should not say, "The patient is drunk." He may comment that a woman's perineum is bruised and that there are sperm in the vagina; he should not say, "The patient was raped." These matters should be left to the courts.

Compensation

Although in most states compensation laws require that elective care be rendered to patients by physicians with a compensation board rating, emergency care can be administered by any physician, including interns. Nevertheless, lists should be kept in the emergency room of hospital staff members with their various compensation board specialty ratings for less urgent cases. Similar lists should be kept of local industrial plant physicians.

When a private physician renders care in a compensation case, he is responsible for filling out the appropriate compensation forms. When a physician employed by the hospital renders treatment, the hospital administration should take care of the paper work. Usually it is necessary for the head of a given department to sign and be responsible for such cases even though he receives no payment and usually does not even see the patient.

While the compensation laws of the states are variable, in New York State compensation cases receiving primary care in the emergency room may not return for follow-up care but must be referred to a private physician.

DISASTER PLANNING

Every hospital disaster plan should make provision for such essentials as staff physician and house staff physician assignments, arrangements to set aside certain areas of the hospital for the increased patient load, maintenance of adequate supplies in these areas at all times, and a prearranged mechanism for communication and cooperation with other hospitals in the area, the local police, fire, and health departments, ambulance services, and civil defense officials.

As far as the emergency room proper is concerned, several principles should be kept in mind.

1. The emergency room should be used as a triage area and not for treatment except in such lifesaving situations as control of cardiac arrest, tracheostomy, control of severe external hemorrhage, or closed thoracostomy. Patients should not be allowed to accumulate in the emergency room. Emergency medical tags should be available for identification of each patient, with space for including, in addition to the patient's name, the tentative diagnosis and treatment (if any is given) in the emergency room.

2. The emergency room should serve as a center of communications, receiving and coordinating all information from outside and from within the hospital.

3. In a disaster the emergency room should be in the charge of a senior surgeon with several surgical assistants responsible to him to serve as triage officers. These are the most important people in any plan and should be as experienced as possible. They should not be asked to assume duties elsewhere in the hospital until the crisis is under control.

4. Disaster planning is the proper function of the emergency-room policy committee.

The Severely Injured Patient

2

SAMUEL R. POWERS, JR.

The initial treatment of a severely injured patient may well determine whether the patient will survive. The time of initial treatment also provides the best opportunity for prophylaxis of the late complications of trauma. In assessing the order of priority for management of multiple injuries, it is useful to consider injuries in terms of (1) those that may result in the death of the patient within minutes, (2) those that may result in the death of the patient within hours, and (3) those that may result in the death of the patient within days. It is apparent from this classification that the first order of priority involves assessment of conditions which may result in the immediate death of the patient, and these are almost invariably associated with respiratory or cardiac dysfunction.

INJURIES WHICH MAY RESULT IN DEATH WITHIN MINUTES

Recognition and therapy of immediately life-threatening situations usually do not require elaborate equipment. The basic principle of all emergency treatment is to detect and correct any inadequacy of oxygen delivery to the tissues. Adequate oxygen delivery necessitates an adequate exchange of oxygen by the lungs, transfer of oxygen across the pulmonary membranes into the bloodstream, and satisfactorily functioning circulation to deliver the oxygenated blood to the tissues.

Ventilation: The Transfer of Oxygen into the Lung

The cardinal signs of inadequate ventilation are dyspnea and cyanosis. The depth of cyanosis is not an accurate reflection of the severity of the ventilatory insufficiency. Clinical cyanosis results when approximately 4 gm of reduced hemoglobin per 100 ml of blood is present. The severely injured patient usually has a total hemoglobin level of less than 10 gm. Cyanosis will be apparent only when the oxygen saturation is around 50 percent, a value incompatible with prolonged survival. Therefore: cyanosis, or its absence, is not a useful clinical guide. The most common and most easily correctable form of ventilatory insufficiency is that which is due to obstruction of the airway, the inlet for oxygen into the tracheobronchial tree. The majority of airway obstructions are within reach of the forefinger and can be removed by merely opening the patient's mouth and feeling for the source of the obstruction. If this is not immediately ascertained, a laryngoscope should be used to visualize the space between the vocal chords, and the area should be carefully and thoroughly cleansed by suction catheter. Airway obstruction due to the presence of vomited food particles or clotted blood may be easily corrected with this maneuver. If a completely free airway cannot be immediately obtained, an endotracheal tube should be passed. The use of an endotracheal tube is vastly preferable to an emergency tracheostomy, since it can be carried out rapidly and without the danger of adding to the patient's injuries. It is surprising that most surgeons are more familiar with the technique of tracheostomy than that of intubation with an endotracheal tube, and probably for this reason tracheostomy is frequently carried out when it is unnecessary and under conditions in which it may result in serious complications. Once the endotracheal tube is in place, the decision can be made as to whether a tracheostomy will be necessary. If so, it can be carried out in a leisurely fashion, under sterile conditions, without the urgency of the situation in which a patient is rapidly dying.

When an adequate airway has been established and there is still evidence of cyanosis or dyspnea, it must be assumed that there is a mechanical interference with the operation of the bellows mechanism. This can be caused by the presence of fluid or air in the chest, multiple fractures of ribs producing a flail (or stove-in) chest, or central nervous system depression. Following insertion of an endotracheal tube, artificial ventilation should be begun by a bag and valve assembly until a mechanical respirator can be procured.

Physical examination should readily reveal the presence of either air or blood in the thorax and whether there is an open chest wound or fractured ribs. These problems can usually be adequately controlled in an emergency situation by the use of such simple techniques as intercostal drainage with underwater seal, and the covering of sucking wounds with a petroleum jelly gauze pack. These measures are not intended to be definitive therapy but may be lifesaving in an emergency situation.

A special situation which requires immediate attention in order to prevent the rapid deterioration and death of the patient is that due to tension pneumothorax. The situation is usually associated with fractured ribs; an air leak permits air to accumulate under increasingly positive pressure in the pleural space. As this occurs, the mediastinal structures are pushed to the opposite side with progressive angulation of the great vessels as they enter the heart. Thus a picture of ventilatory insufficiency as indicated by cyanosis is associated with evidence of inadequate cardiac filling as judged by falling blood pressure and disappearance of peripheral pulse. The diagnosis is readily made from the physical signs of air under pressure in one hemithorax, concomitant with a mediastinal shift which is best recognized by percussion of the cardiac border. The location of the trachea may be misleading, since people with chronic pulmonary disease may have deviation of the trachea in the absence of an acute process. Shift of the mediastinum is a reliable guide and is indicative that immediate measures should be taken. It is an easy procedure to insert a needle into the chest and allow the air pressure in the thorax to come to atmospheric levels. As soon as this has occurred, the mediastinal shift will begin to correct itself and relief from cyanosis and rapid improvement in blood pressure will occur. It will be recalled that a pneumothorax without tension is well tolerated, and therefore the emergency treatment does not require the use of a catheter or underwater seal. An 18 gauge needle inserted into the second interspace anteriorly will provide immediate and dramatic relief of this condition.

While the foregoing measures are being completed, it is essential to obtain an arterial blood sample for determination of pH, pCO_2, and pO_2. Only if these are within the normal range should ventilation be considered adequate. Clinical judgment is a **poor** guide in this situation and should be supplemented by repeated blood gas determinations.

Transfer of Oxygen from the Lungs into the Bloodstream

The transfer of oxygen will be seriously limited if the tracheobronchial tree contains aspirated vomitus or blood. Once an endotracheal tube has been put in place, careful suctioning of the tracheal tree can be carried out. Although this will usually not be necessary in the conscious patient with an intact cough reflex, it may be lifesaving in the unconscious patient. Likewise, any injury to the chest wall which interferes with the coughing mechanism may permit the development of a traumatic "wet lung" from which the patient may literally drown in his own secretions. Frequent tracheal aspiration is necessary in order to permit adequate diffusion of oxygen across the pulmonary capillary membrane.

Transport of Oxygen to the Tissues by the Bloodstream

When ventilation has been restored so that a normal amount of oxygen is being transported into the lung, and this oxygen is diffusing adequately in the bloodstream, cyanosis will usually disappear. It is important to realize that this does not necessarily mean an adequate quantity of blood is being delivered to the tissues. It merely signifies that whatever quantity is being delivered does contain an adequate amount of oxygen. Failure of the circulation to deliver an adequate quantity of well-oxygenated blood will result in tissue hypoxia. Sudden failure of the circulation as evidenced by disappearance of heart sounds and peripheral pulses is usually due to either cardiac tamponade or cardiac arrest. Auscultation over the heart and inspection of the neck veins should provide an immediate differential diagnosis between cessation of circulation due to cardiac standstill and that due to cardiac tamponade. With blood in the pericardial sac, the neck veins are markedly distended and usually pulsating. There is also an absence of peripheral pulses and heart sounds because the latter have been muffled by the presence of blood in the pericardium.

With cardiac arrest, the absence of peripheral pulses and heart sounds is associated with collapse of the neck veins and the absence of venous pulsations. Under the latter circumstances, closed-chest massage should be promptly begun as soon as an endotracheal tube is in place and mechanical or artificial ventilation is in progress. It is clearly of no value to perfuse blood through the tissues if the blood contains no oxygen.

The basis of closed-chest cardiac massage is the forceful compression of the lower end of the sternum against the vertebral column. Thus the patient must be on a firm surface such as a metal stretcher; if this is not available, the patient should be placed on the floor. Adequacy of the massage is readily detected by feeling for a peripheral pulse which is palpable while massage is being carried out. Most patients who are capable of resuscitation will show a prompt restitution of heartbeat within a short period of time. If this does not happen, the intracardiac injection of epinephrine, 2 to 3 ml of a 1:10,000 dilution, may be of help. It should be noted that the force necessary to produce adequate compression of the heart between the sternum and the vertebral bodies is not as great as one might expect. Undue compression will result in unnecessary fractures of ribs; therefore, continuous monitoring of the peripheral pulse should be carried out and only sufficient force used to produce a palpable pulse. More vigorous efforts are of no avail and may well be dangerous.

If closed-chest massage fails to reinstitute a prompt ventricular contraction, the physician is frequently tempted to open the chest so that direct cardiac massage can be carried out. It has been repeatedly demonstrated that direct cardiac massage is less effective than closed-chest massage and, further, that open cardiac massage is never effective where closed massage has failed.

If massage does not produce a palpable peripheral pulse, it may be because ventricular fibrillation has developed. This can be ascertained by an electrocardiograph, which should be coupled to the patient as soon as massage begins. Ventricular fibrillation can usually be corrected by a closed-chest or external defibrillator. Experience has shown that in order for this technique to be successful the patient must have been given a period of adequate massage associated with adequate ventilation so that the myocardium is well oxygenated. Defibrillation is carried out by a standard commercially available machine which every emergency room should have. The electrodes are applied to the chest wall, one over the apex of the heart, the other over the base, with sufficient electrolyte paste to make certain that good contact is obtained and the skin will not be burned. A single shock of 440 volts for a quarter of a second will usually be effective, but it may be necessary to increase it to as high as 750 volts. Failure of these measures to reinstitute an adequate cardiac beat probably indicates extensive myocardial necrosis, generally from a myocardial infarction (see also Chapter 4, Cardiac Emergencies).

In the event that the diagnosis of cardiac tamponade has been made, quick and dramatic relief can be obtained by inserting a needle into the pericardial sac. This is best done using a spinal needle placed just at the tip of the xiphoid process directed upward at an angle of approximately 45 degrees to the chest wall. If blood is encountered, the removal of even as small an amount as 30 to 40 ml will result in immediate improvement of the patient, with the appearance of peripheral pulses, disappearance of cyanosis, and collapse of the neck veins. If there is any question as to whether cardiac tamponade is present, a needle introduced in the manner just described carries little risk and may be lifesaving.

Mental Check List for Conditions Which May
Result in Death Within Minutes

1. Presence of dyspnea and cyanosis.
2. Signs of air and/or fluid in the pleural cavity as evidenced by tympany or dullness to percussion, distant or absent breath sounds, mediastinal shift.
3. Signs of cardiac tamponade (distension of neck veins, muffling of heart sounds, feeble peripheral pulses).
4. Inability of patient to cough, presence of paradoxical motion of the chest wall, and presence of fractured ribs.
5. Signs of cardiac arrest (no audible heartbeat, absent respiration, no peripheral pulse, dilated pupils).

INJURIES WHICH MAY RESULT IN DEATH WITHIN HOURS

Dealing with injuries which may result in death within hours consists almost entirely in the recognition and management of shock, whether due to blood loss, myocardial failure, or sepsis. The differential diagnosis between these various forms of shock is generally obvious, but sometimes it is obscure and cannot be ascertained on the grounds of clinical judgment alone. Recent advances in the knowledge of the physiology of shock as well as its therapy have emphasized the need for a systematic protocol to be followed when any patient is admitted with a suspicion of shock from any cause.

Shock is best defined as an abnormal state in which there is inadequate perfusion of the tissues. This definition implies that measures to improve tissue perfusion must be undertaken rapidly and that clinical and laboratory signs of improved tissue perfusion must be continuously observed and monitored. Low tissue perfusion can be recognized clinically by the following criteria: state of consciousness, appearance of the skin and mucous membranes, rate of capillary filling of the nail beds, degree of filling of peripheral veins, rate and quality of the pulse and respiration, and volume of urine output. You will notice that hypotension is not mentioned, since this may be a late sign of shock, occasionally evident only after irreversibility has occurred. Severe shock, as indicated by marked reduction in tissue perfusion, may be present when the blood pressure is apparently normal.

The clinical observations should be supplemented by measurement of central venous pressure and urine output. The measurement of central venous pressure is an extremely useful guide to the adequacy of venous return to the right side of the heart. Since the normal heart will respond to increases in venous return by an increase in stroke volume, it is clearly to the advantage of the patient to maintain venous return at an optimum level. When the rate of return exceeds the ability of the pump, heart failure ensues and the pressure in the central venous system increases. This pressure is conveniently measured by inserting a catheter by means of an antecubital vein or by inserting a plastic needle in the external jugular vein directed downward toward the thorax. In either case, the catheter should be within the confines of the thoracic cage, and its end should then be connected to a suitable pressure-measuring device. The simplest form of the latter is a spinal fluid manometer which may be taped to an intravenous pole. The base of the manometer should be adjusted to the level of the right auricle, which is usually midway between the anterior chest and the patient's back, corresponding to the midaxillary line in a patient who is supine. Normal values for central venous pressure are between 7 and 15 cm of water, and therapy is directed toward maintaining central venous pressure within this range.

At the time the central venous pressure catheter is inserted, a separate large-diameter plastic needle should be inserted in a peripheral vein for the administration of fluid or blood as necessary. The needle should be of at least 15 gauge and preferably inserted at the level of the antecubital space or above.

The adequacy of tissue perfusion to the visceral organs is well demonstrated by the production of urine by the kidneys. If renal perfusion is adequate, a urine volume of between 40 and 60 ml per hour should occur; any value less than this should be taken as evidence of inadequate renal, and probably also other visceral organ perfusion.

While these three tubes are being inserted in the patient (central venous pressure, intravenous fluids, urinary bladder), a sample of blood should have been sent for cross matching and some type of fluid replacement commenced. There is no unanimity of opinion as to the best plasma expander to be used while waiting for blood to be available, but recent work would suggest that a balanced electrolyte solution such as lactated Ringer's solution is entirely adequate. This fluid should be administered at a sufficient rate to maintain the central venous pressure between 7 and 15 cm of water and to maintain a urine volume of around 40 ml per hour.

It is important that these measures be instituted immediately when the patient enters the emergency room, since with progression of shock there may be collapse of the peripheral veins causing further delay in the institution of replacement therapy.

Failure of the patient to respond to the administration of intravenous fluids as evidenced by an improvement in central venous pressure, an improvement in capillary perfusion, and restoration of a urine output must be taken as indicative of continuing concealed hemorrhage. The response to therapy is probably the most accurate clinical guide to the presence of continuing blood loss, and failure to respond must never be interpreted as being due to such nonspecifics as the effects of crush injury or nervous shock. Concealed hemorrhage of sufficient magnitude to produce a state of shock can occur in only a very few areas of the body without being immediately and readily detected. These areas are the abdominal cavity, the retroperitoneal area, and the lower extremities. Failure to respond or even a worsening of the patient's condition following the rapid intravenous administration of fluids demands the rapid transfer of the patient to an operating room where prompt and secure hemostasis can be obtained.

Inspection for sites of external bleeding can be carried out at the same time that these measures are being taken and requires that the patient's clothing be completely removed. It is impossible to carry out an adequate examination of an injured patient when any clothing remains upon him. The inspection must be done carefully and gently so as not to disturb the patient, but if it is not done, obvious external injuries may be overlooked. Once these initial measures have been accomplished, the patient can then be safely transferred to another part of the hospital for definitive treatment of the injured parts.

*Mental Check List for Conditions Which May
Result in Death Within Hours*

1. Clinical signs of low perfusion (coldness, clamminess, poor capillary filling, rapid pulse and respiration, absence of urine output).
2. Level of central venous pressure and urine volume measured in milliliters per 15-minute period (central venous pressure between 7 and 15 cm of water, and urine volume between 40 and 60 ml per hour).
3. Evidence of continuing concealed hemorrhage (failure of central venous pressure to rise, failure of clinical signs of shock to improve, absence of urinary response).

CONDITIONS WHICH MAY RESULT IN DEATH WITHIN DAYS

Emergency-room treatment should consist of prophylaxis against infection and acute renal failure. This should include routine prophylaxis against tetanus and, if there is any evidence of external injury, the institution of antibiotics, usually in the form of relatively large doses of aqueous penicillin administered in the intravenous solutions. The prevention of renal failure will best be carried out if adequate fluid replacement results in a normal venous pressure and a normal urine output. Failure of urine output to increase when there is a normal or slightly elevated venous pressure is an indication for the use of an osmotic diuretic such as mannitol, which can be added to the intravenous program as a 10% solution. This solution is given in the amount necessary to institute urine flow in the range of 40 to 60 ml per hour. Once that range is achieved, the mannitol solution should be replaced by other solutions.

It should be emphasized that large volumes of blood do not have to be given in this period since the erythrocyte mass can be restored at a later date. Adequate filling of the vascular and extracellular space with a balanced electrolyte solution is an effective method for restoration of the failing circulation until blood is available. The use of unmatched blood is to be deprecated as unnecessary and potentially dangerous.

Treatment of specific injured organs or portions of the body need not and should not be deferred while the above-mentioned emergency measures are being carried out. A rapid assessment of the probable associated injuries should result in prompt request for consultative services in the specialty areas involved. The emergency treatment of specific organs frequently determines whether function of an organ will be preserved and the degree of disability which may ensue. It is the responsibility of the physician who administers the initial emergency care to see to it that the activities of other physicians are coordinated in the overall best interest of the patient. Each specialist will tend to concentrate on his own field of interest, and one individual must therefore have charge of determining the order of priority and the relative urgency of treatment of various injuries. The function of the specialist consultant at this early stage is not only to provide emergency treatment of injuries which fall within his field of competence but also to inform the coordinating physician as to the probable consequences of each particular injury and the relative urgency of definitive treatment.

Mental Check List for Conditions Which May Result in Death Within Days

1. Prophylaxis of infection (tetanus prophylaxis, initial management of open wounds, use of antibiotics).
2. Prevention of acute renal failure (adequate fluid intake, use of mannitol, maintenance of a normal urine output).
3. Careful examination of the entire patient (look carefully for multiple injuries, obtain adequate consultative services, arrange for priority of treatment of specific organs or areas of the body depending upon urgency for both short- and long-term function of those parts).

Thoracic Emergencies 3

RALPH D. ALLEY
THOMAS M. OLDER

Immediate correction of disordered pulmonary function must take precedence over all else in the treatment of the acutely injured, for oxygenation is the proximate need of all bodily functions. Correction of disordered physiological states must precede the delineation and correction of anatomical injury.

In this chapter the emphasis will be on clinical observation and therapeutic technique in acute thoracic injuries. Emergency measures will be discussed first, followed by the treatment of penetrating and nonpenetrating wounds, and finally, the indications for emergency thoracostomy. A knowledge of the elements of pathological physiology of the cardiopulmonary apparatus is assumed.

Success in treatment of acutely injured patients rests upon an orderly systematic approach to their management. The initial examining physician begins his appraisal of the patient's general condition at the first glance, but he immediately focuses his attention on the respiratory and circulatory impairment and takes action accordingly. What he does will also take into account the nature and implications of the responsible injury.

In order of their priority the emergency measures are:

1. Restoration of adequate respiration.
2. Control of hemorrhage.
3. Treatment of actual or impending shock.
4. Dressing of all open wounds to prevent further contamination.

EMERGENCY MEASURES IN THORACIC INJURIES

In patients with thoracic injuries, emergency measure number one, restoration of adequate respiration, is the crux of therapy. It is accomplished by: (1) relief of airway obstruction and artificial ventilation, (2) splinting of the unstable chest wall, (3) sealing of an open pneumothorax, (4) relief of pulmonary compression, (5) relief of cardiac compression. The techniques required for achieving these objectives follow.

1. Relief of Airway Obstruction and Artificial Ventilation

There is no single method of treatment. Foreign bodies, including blood clots, must be removed from the mouth and pharynx. A retrolapsed tongue obstructing the airway must be pulled forward. It may be sufficient to grasp the angles of the jaw and push the chin forward simultaneously with dorsiflexion of the head (Fig. 3-1). If this does not suffice, the tongue may be pulled forward with an instrument. When the jaw can be opened, the introduction of an oral pharyngeal airway is preferable (Fig. 3-2). When the jaw cannot be

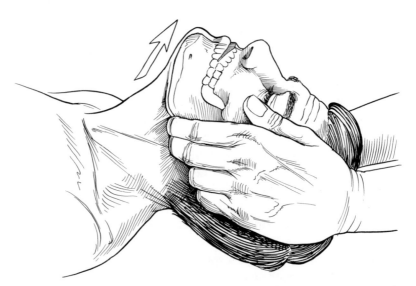

Fig. 3-1. Clearing the airway. Dorsiflexion of the head and forceful elevation of the jaw will open the hypopharynx blocked by a retrolapsed tongue.

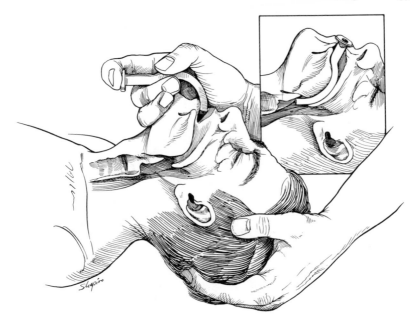

Fig. 3-2. Insertion of an oropharyngeal airway. Extension of the head loosens the jaw and permits introduction of a metal or plastic airway into the hypopharynx. This will facilitate suctioning and prevent the tongue from blocking the pharynx by falling backward.

opened, nasotracheal intubation can be carried out, but this may be difficult in the disoriented, wildly obstreperous patient. An emergency tracheostomy may be the only alternative in this situation.

When is it necessary to assist ventilation in addition to clearing the airway, mouth-to-mouth respiration is effective. The use of a resuscitube, an oral pharyngeal airway with an integral connector, is more efficient than mouth-to-mouth breathing and safer for the operator (Fig. 3-3). An Ambu bag or similar hand-operated bellows ventilator is an invaluable aid to assisting ventilation in all stages of resuscitation or transport of the patient (Fig. 3-4). It may be used initially with the anesthesia face mask attached, and preferably with an oral pharyngeal airway in place. Later, if the patient is intubated or has a tracheostomy performed, the bellows unit is separated from the face mask and connected to the endotracheal or tracheostomy tube, with standard anesthetic connectors. Oxygen can be attached to the unit when desired and respiratory pressure and rate are varied manually as needed. When long-term respiratory assistance is required the patient is attached to a suitable respirator.

Use of laryngoscopy and oral tracheal intubation with a cuffed

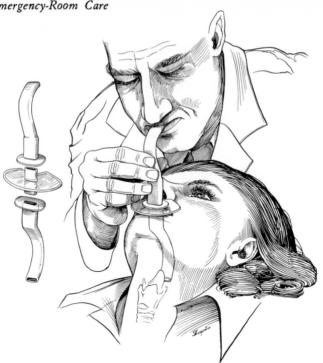

Fig. 3-3.   Resuscitube airway. A child-size and an adult-size airway are joined by a connector. The end of the appropriate size serves as an airway and the other end as a mouthpiece, permitting more efficient and safer ventilation than mouth-to-mouth breathing. The connector is held firmly against the mouth, and the nose is occluded with the left hand (not shown) to prevent loss of air from the mouth or nose.

endotracheal tube is the most direct and effective method of establishing and controlling the airway. Ventilation can be controlled, and retained or reaccumulating secretions can be aspirated from the lower respiratory tract. In the uncooperative patient a muscular relaxant may be used to facilitate intubation but should be avoided by operators not skilled in the art of intubation.

BRONCHOSCOPY.   Emergency bronchoscopy is seldom necessary to clear the lower air passages, since endotracheal suctioning can be carried out effectively with a nasotracheal catheter. If the patient's head is extended and the tongue pulled forward, this catheter can generally be passed expeditiously. Turning the patient's head alternately from right to left will permit differential aspiration and irrigation of each main bronchus. Patients who have vomited and aspirated

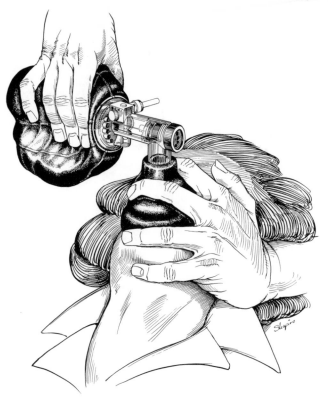

Fig. 3-4. Artificial ventilation. A hand-operated bellows attached to a mask or an endotracheal tube is an indispensable aid to emergency artificial ventilation. Note that the mask is pressed firmly against the face and the head is kept extended. An airway is in place.

should have bronchoscopy and a thorough bronchial lavage employing 0.85% saline solution.

TRACHEOSTOMY. Certain patients with associated maxillofacial injuries, unconscious patients, and many patients with serious chest injuries will require a temporary tracheostomy. Control of the airway by preliminary oral tracheal intubation permits the leisurely and precise execution of tracheostomy. The procedure should be carried out in the operating room whenever possible. Since it may be necessary to accomplish it in the emergency room, in some instances, the following description is given.

The patient is positioned supine, with a padded lift beneath the shoulders to bring the trachea forward. For cosmetic reasons a trans-

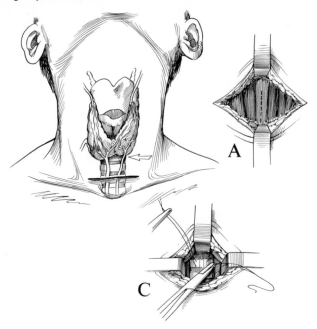

Fig. 3-5. Tracheostomy. (A) A transverse incision is made through the skin and platysma 2 finger-breadths above the suprasternal notch. (B) The strap muscles and middle cervical fascia are incised in the midline and retracted. (C) The thyroid gland is retracted cephalad and stay sutures are placed in the 3d tracheal ring. (D) A small portion of the 3d ring is excised, and when a cuffed tube is used, the 4th ring is cut in the midline. (E) Traction is applied to the stay sutures. The tube is inserted into the stoma at a right angle to the trachea and then rotated into alignment with the trachea as it passes downward. The stay sutures are kept in place to facilitate exposure for reinsertion of the cannula, if necessary, in the early postoperative period.

verse incision is preferred. After separation of the strap muscles, the isthmus of the thyroid is retracted cephalad and exposing the trachea (Fig. 3-5). A small piece of the third cartilaginous ring (0.5 cm or less) is excised, and the fourth ring is cut in the midline if necessary. In infants and children, two, or if necessary, three rings are cut longitudinally but no cartilage is removed. Care is taken to place the tracheostomy stoma accurately. It must be in the midline for the cannula to lie properly without angulation. If the stoma is too high, subglottic edema will make removal of the tracheostomy tube difficult, and if the stoma is too low, massive hemorrhage from erosion of the innominate artery may occur. Before the endotracheal tube is removed and the tracheostomy cannula inserted, the lateral edges of

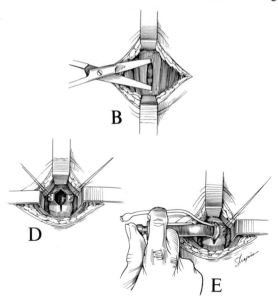

the opening in the trachea are caught up with traction sutures of 000 chromic catgut. These sutures are left long and strapped to the anterior chest wall to be used later to facilitate reinsertion of the cannula, should it inadvertently slip out of the trachea. The traction sutures are particularly useful during the first few days postoperatively, before a firm sinus tract leading to the tracheal opening has been formed. The skin incision should be left open to permit easy exit of air coughed out around the cannula; otherwise, massive subcutaneous emphysema can result. A cannula of adequate length should be selected. Cannula straps should be prestretched and then tied firmly when the neck is in the flexed position. This is particularly important in infants who have a marked range of mobility of the clavicle, which can become impinged behind the flange of the tracheostomy cannula, and the cannula thereby thrust out if it is not securely tied. In adults, the tracheostomy tube should have an inflatable cuff on it to permit ventilatory assistance with a respirator. The cuff may also be useful in preventing aspiration of vomitus and oral pharyngeal secretions in obtunded patients.

2. Splinting of the Unstable Chest Wall

A flail chest is the result of multiple fractured ribs which leave a segment of chest wall unsupported. When the patient inspires, this segment is sucked in by the negative intrapleural pressure and interferes with inflation of the lung. This paradoxical motion of the chest wall is easily missed on casual inspection of the chest, especially when subcutaneous emphysema, hematoma, or other soft-tissue injury is present. It is important to inspect and palpate the chest carefully from different positions, searching for an area of false motion. Even small amounts of paradox can significantly cripple the bellows action of the chest, leading to insidious hypoxia, particularly in patients with preexisting lung disease.

The most expeditious and effective treatment of a flail chest is intubation of the trachea and positive-pressure ventilation, the so-called "internal stabilization" of the chest wall. In less severe cases the paradoxical area can be stabilized externally by strapping it with adhesive or by placing sand bags on the unstable area. Long-term management will be discussed later in this chapter.

3. Sealing of an Open Pneumothorax

A chest-wall injury with an opening into the pleural space should be treated by immediate application of petrolatum gauze or other airtight bandage to seal the hole and prevent air from sucking in and blowing out. When feasible, this is applied at the end of forceful expiration to expel as much air as possible from the chest before it is sealed. Thoracostomy tube drainage may also be necessary to release trapped air in the thorax prior to more definitive wound care.

4. Relief of Pulmonary Compression

Failure of respiratory distress or shock to be corrected by relief of airway obstruction, ventilation, support of the flail chest, and closure of open pneumothorax raises the possibility of pneumothorax, hemothorax, or occult bleeding at other sites. This is generally suggested by the nature of the injuries and a high index of suspicion. Physical examination is diagnostic in most cases but bilateral injuries or subcutaneous emphysema may confuse physical signs (a hyper-resonant percussion note is elicited over even small amounts of subcutaneous emphysema). When time or circumstances permit, a chest roentgenogram (preferably erect or semierect) is valuable to confirm a hemothorax or pneumothorax. If the patient's condition is too poor to warrant the necessary delay, the roentgenogram is not taken, and diagnostic thoracentesis is carried out immediately to confirm the presence and location of fluid or air, followed by thoracostomy tube drainage if appropriate. The techniques of thoracentesis and thoracostomy tube drainage follow.

THORACENTESIS. Thoracentesis is primarily a diagnostic procedure, but is also useful in therapy when only episodic aspiration from the pleural space is required. It may be performed with or without infiltration of local anesthesia, depending on the urgency of the situation and the level of consciousness of the patient.

A number of factors must be taken into account in selecting the appropriate site for thoracentesis. The commonest error is to insert the needle too low. When done on the right side, under the mistaken notion that a hemothorax is being aspirated, this error can lead to the aspiration of large quantities of blood from the liver. On the left side, the spleen, the colon, or the stomach can be punctured, with the potentially disastrous consequences of hemorrhage or infection. This error is the logical result of being conditioned to the interpretation of standard roentgenograms of the chest, which are customarily taken with the patient standing in an upright position in full inspiration. In the nonemphysematous patient with a chest injury, with respirations splinted by pain, the dome of the diaphragm may be elevated to the

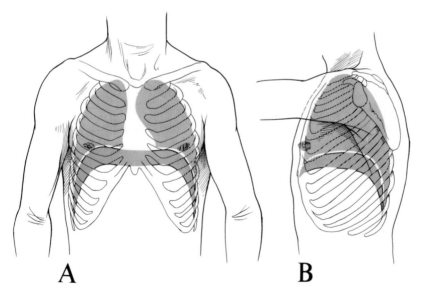

A   B

Fig. 3-6. Diaphragmatic excursion (A). Note that in expiration (B) the diaphragm rises to the anterior 4th interspace, producing a narrow costophrenic angle that is difficult to tap.

level of the 4th anterior rib (Fig. 3-6). Elevation of the diaphragm is also greater in the obese. With the patient in the supine posture, the weight of the abdominal viscera is responsible for elevation of the diaphragm; in the stooped sitting posture, the thrust of the thighs elevates the abdominal contents. Loculations of fluid or air are localized by topographical study of frontal and lateral roentgenograms. In the usual case, the pleural space is free of adhesions, and fluid and air are distributed about the lung in a shell which is determined by gravity. Therefore, air is most effectively aspirated from an anterior-superior approach, and fluid from a posterior-inferior approach, as determined by the position of the patient. To avoid penetrating the heavier shoulder girdle muscle masses, a site just beneath the pectoral fold in the anterior axillary line is selected for the aspiration of air, but the more inferior site in the posterior axillary line is best for the aspiration of fluid.

In a formal thoracentesis the site selected is prepared, draped, and infiltrated with procaine anesthesia. A 14 to 18 gauge needle or trocar catheter is inserted through the lower portion of the interspace to avoid injury to intercostal vessels (Fig. 3-7). The upper border of the rib below serves as a warning that the pleura is about to be traversed, so that penetration sufficiently deep to injure the underlying lung should be avoided. With a three-way stopcock interposed, the contents of the pleural space can be aspirated by a syringe or a vacuum system. In cases with severe hemorrhage in which blood for transfusion is not immediately available, a hemothorax may be evacuated by citrated donor bottles with a view to retransfusion of the patient's own blood. If a pneumothorax due to a small air leak is the problem, a trocar catheter may be left in place and connected to an underwater seal or suction system. An indwelling needle should not be used for this purpose because, with pulmonary reexpansion, the lung will be punctured repeatedly by the protruding needle point.

THORACOSTOMY TUBE. Traumatic pneumothorax and hemothorax usually require thoracostomy tube drainage. The drainage tube provides instant relief of pulmonary compression, prevents recurrence, and affords a means for monitoring continuing air leak or intrapleural hemorrhage.

The procedure for thoracostomy tube drainage follows the general principles outlined for thoracentesis. The usual sites are over the 3d rib (2d intercostal space) in the midclavicular line anteriorly for air, and over the 6th rib (5th intercostal space) in the posterior axil-

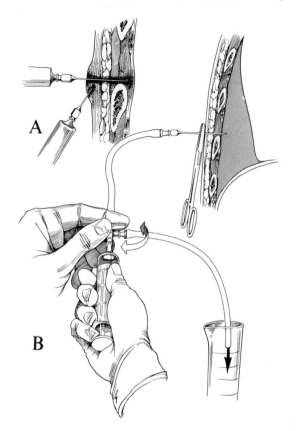

Fig. 3-7. Thoracentesis. (A) A subcutaneous wheal is raised with local anesthesia, then an additional injection is given over the rib, avoiding the neurovascular bundle. The pleura is entered with the needle to confirm the presence
of fluid or air. (B) A large-bore (14 to 18 gauge) needle is then inserted
into the space and the needle is fixed with a clamp to avoid deeper penetration.
With the use of a three-way stop cock, the fluid is removed aseptically.

lary line for fluid. The suitability of the site selected is confirmed
following procaine infiltration by needle aspiration of the pleural
space. A stab wound is made, deep enough to incise the subcutaneous
fascia, and a large-bore catheter (No. 28 French for adults) is introduced into the pleural space by one of several methods. Preferred
methods are the use of the trocar catheter designed for the purpose
(Fig. 3-8) and, alternatively, introduction of a catheter through a
Babcock trocar (Fig. 3-9). In the absence of suitable equipment, a
sinus track can be established with a Kelly clamp, and the clamp
used as an inserter. Though crude and traumatic, this method is

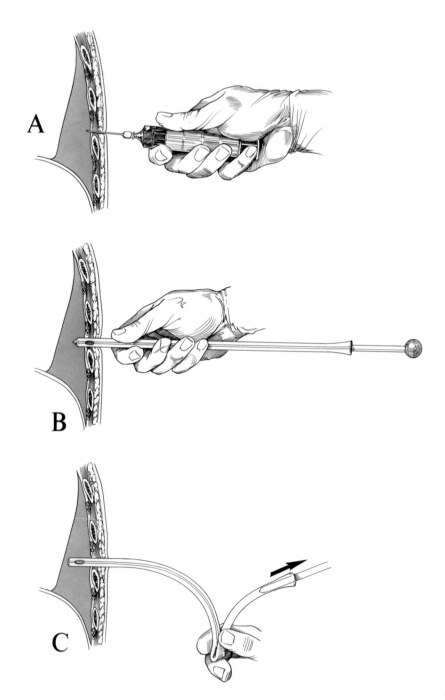

effective. If possible, introduction of a drainage catheter through the back, where the patient will have to lie upon it, should be avoided. The introduction of a catheter into an interlobar fissure should also be avoided. Following placement, the catheter is connected to underwater seal or suction drainage. The drainage system should provide for a calibrated collecting receptacle to permit monitoring of blood loss.

5. Relief of Cardiac Compression

Any penetrating injury, but especially a puncture or stab wound, of the chest or upper abdomen may have entered a cardiac chamber or lacerated a coronary vessel. The heart is compressed as blood fills the unyielding pericardial sac, causing hypotension, diminished heart sounds, distended neck veins (high central venous pressure), and paradoxical pulse. A paradoxical pulse in association with shock is diagnostic of cardiac tamponade. It may be detected as a dampening of the pulse amplitude during inspiration, or, more clearly, by noting a definite drop in systolic pressure at the end of inspiration.

When tamponade is present, a large-bore spinal needle (14 to 16 gauge) is inserted subcostally to the left of the xiphoid and directed toward the medial border of the right scapular spine until the diaphragmatic pericardium is punctured (Fig. 3-10). This is signified by a slight but definite resistance, followed by a sense of moving through a definite structure. The rhythmic grating of the epicardium against the needle point confirms that the needle tip is in the pericardium, but the grating may not be felt when the needle is first introduced because of restricted cardiac activity. The stylette is removed from the needle and a small amount of blood spurts out. Further aspiration with a syringe will yield an additional small amount of blood. Great care must be taken to keep the needle tip in the thin pericardial space and not advance it into the right ventricle. Aspiration of large amounts of dark blood suggests that the needle is in the

Fig. 3-8. Thoracostomy tube drainage with a trocar catheter. (A) After injection of a local anesthetic agent, the pleural space is explored with a needle to confirm the presence of fluid or air. (B) After an incision is made in the skin, the underlying fascia is cut with a scissors, the trocar catheter is pushed into the space, and the catheter is advanced on the stationary trocar to the desired depth. (C) As the trocar is withdrawn, the tube is kinked to prevent the entry of air into the pleura until the tube is attached to an underwater seal. The trocar also serves as a measuring device to estimate the depth to which the catheter has been inserted.

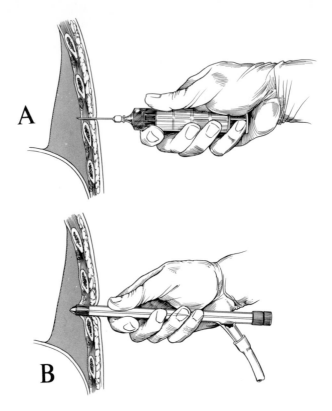

Fig. 3-9. Thoracostomy tube drainage with a Babcock trocar. (A) The pleural space is explored with a needle to confirm the presence of fluid or air. (B) The trocar is introduced through a skin incision in the chest wall into the pleural space. (C) The trocar is removed. (D) A clamped chest catheter is inserted through the barrel. (E) As the trocar is removed over the chest catheter, the clamp is advanced in preparation for connection to an underwater seal.

right ventricle. Successful relief of tamponade is clearly evident in the response of the patient: immediate rise of blood pressure, decrease in neck-vein distension, loss of paradoxical pulse, louder heart sounds, and diminished restlessness. The needle should be removed when the tamponade is relieved to avoid injury to the heart. When active bleeding persists from the heart or a coronary vessel, repeated aspiration may be necessary en route to the operating room. Repeated pericardicenteses are preferable to the introduction of a small-bore indwelling catheter, because between aspirations the catheter will become occluded by clot.

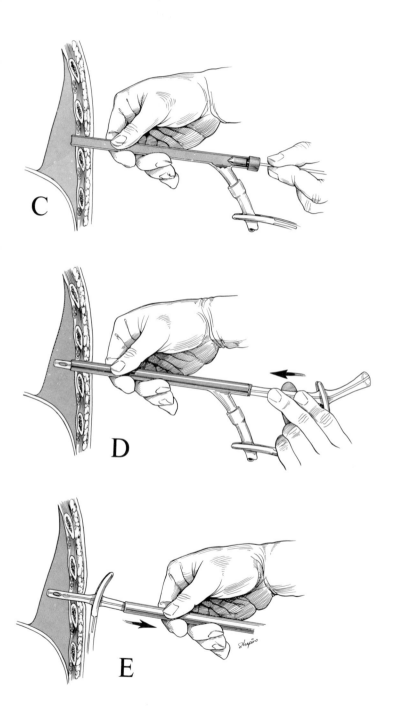

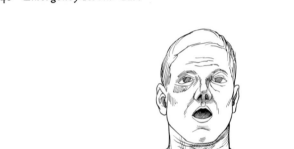

Fig. 3-10. Pericardicentesis. A large-bore needle with a stylette is introduced into the pericardium by inserting it through the skin to the left of the xyphoid process, and directing it at a 45° angle to the patient, toward the border of the right scapula. A syringe is attached for aspiration.

ROENTGENOGRAPHY IN THORACIC INJURIES

In general, roentgenographic evaluation of the acutely injured should precede manipulative procedures such as thoracentesis and closed thoracostomy tube drainage, unless the attendant delay will jeopardize the patient's life. Physical findings alone have inherent limitations, are often misleading, and occasionally invite disaster in consequence of erroneously applied therapy. A classic example is traumatic rupture of the left hemidiaphragm, with gaseous distension of an intrathoracic stomach. On the basis of physical findings, a mistaken diagnosis of tension pneumothorax has led to closed thoracostomy tube drainage with immediate outpouring of gastric contents into the pleural space and the necessity for correction by emergency thoracotomy. If unrecognized, this error may result in death of the patient.

Frontal and appropriate lateral thoracic roentgenograms should be taken, with the patient in an erect or semierect position if his condition will permit. Films taken in the supine position are conducive to erroneous diagnosis. A hemothorax may appear larger or smaller than it is, and pneumothorax may be overlooked. Other pitfalls in the interpretation of roentgenograms of the acutely injured are the characteristically "bad" x-rays—often portable films, which do not measure up to the usual standard studies because of a shorter tube–patient distance and varying degrees of ability on the part of the patient to cooperate. The typical result is a partially lordotic view exhibiting the magnified distortion of a short focal distance, blurred by motion, and displaying an uncertain degree of inspiration. It is important, therefore, to develop skills in interpreting bad x-ray films, for there is scant reference material on the subject.

Since the postinjury state is dynamic, serial roentgenographic study may be indicated. Initial studies may be nondiagnostic or retrospectively diagnostic, as serial films display widening of the mediastinum, developing pneumothorax or hemothorax, or the emergency of gas-filled bowel through a diaphragmatic rent initially plugged by omentum. Supine and erect, frontal and lateral abdominal films, when indicated, may show free intraperitoneal air or hematoma. Delineation of hematoma due to ruptured spleen is often aided by temporary insufflation of air through a nasogastric tube.

Most commonly the value of roentgenograms lies in the detection and determination of the degree of pneumothorax or hemothorax. Roentgenograms compensate for possible errors in physical examination invited by subcutaneous emphysema (see Subcutaneous and Mediastinal Emphysema, in the second section of this chapter). They also aid in the recognition of pulmonary contusion and distinguish extrapleural from intrapleural hematoma, and they invite attention to injury to midline structures which might otherwise escape critical notice. Finally, especially in unconscious patients, they may offer the only clue to preexisting intrathoracic disease or to previous injury.

WOUNDS

Nonpenetrating Wounds

CONTUSIONS. Contusions of the chest are injuries unaccompanied by fractured bones. The absence of fractures may prove deceptive and cause the examiner to overlook serious associated internal injuries. This is more apt to occur in children and young adults, whose ribs are resilient. Hence, a careful history of the circumstances of the injury is perhaps more important with this group than with any other. Traumatic rupture of the aorta due to decceleration contusion of the thorax, rupture of the diaphragm due to faulty application of a seat belt, ruptured spleen, ruptured bronchus with mediastinal emphysema or pneumothorax, hemothorax, myocardial contusion, and hemopericardium are among the lesions which are associated with contusions and which are often overlooked clinically. An inventory of these considerations should be reviewed in the light of the circumstances of the patient's injury before the judgment is rendered that the patient has a trivial contusion and may be discharged home for outpatient surveillance.

SIMPLE FRACTURES OF THE RIB. Simple rib fractures may occur from a direct blow, from contrecoup crushing forces that originate elsewhere in the thoracic cage, or from a suppressed cough. In the last case the fractures are characteristically in relation to the diaphragmatic costal margins. The diagnosis rests on localized pain, aggravated by respiration and coughing, and point tenderness and crepitation over the fracture site. Most fractures of the bony rib can be demonstrated by roentgenography, but diagnosis of fractures of the costal cartilages and costochondral separations must be made by physical examination.

Treatment is symptomatic. The time-honored practice of chest strapping should be avoided, for it limits respiratory movements if efficiently applied, obscures physical signs and subsequent roentgenograms, impedes subsequent treatments such as thoracentesis, and is painful to remove.

MULTIPLE RIB FRACTURES—THE FLAIL CHEST (STOVE-IN CHEST). A note of warning from Barrett [1] should serve to sharpen the wits and dispel complacency and indecision in the recognition and therapy of the flail or stove-in chest:

Patients with multiple injuries, including a "stove-in chest" often die without obvious cause. Hemorrhage has been stemmed, transfusions have been given to correct shock, and ample morphine has relieved the sharp edge of pain. The sedated patient lies quietly in bed and his shallow paradoxical movements escape critical notice; but death steps in suddenly, peacefully, naturally—and unnecessarily. . . . If an injured patient reaches the hospital alive, respiratory failure should still be reversible; but minutes count.

The flail chest is the result of an injury in which multiple ribs have been broken in more than one place. It is practically always associated with serious intrathoracic or intra-abdominal visceral injuries. Diagnosis of flail chest is apparent on inspection of and palpation of the unstable area of the chest wall. Lacking structural stability, the flail area reflects rather than activates the ventilatory changes in intrapleural pressure. The resulting paradoxical motion cripples respiration and cough in a manner comparable to open pneumothorax, leading to hypoxia, hypercapnia, and retained secretions.

Localized and unilateral areas of instability and paradox can be controlled by local padding and immobilization of the flail area by strapping. More aggressive forms of therapy may be indicated in patients with diminished respiratory reserve stemming from respiratory disease unrelated to the injury. The flail chest is descriptive of massive injury with multiple, bilateral rib fractures accompanied by one or more fractures of the sternum. Pulverized chest is descriptive of the most severe form, which is usually the result of being caught between moving machine parts in an industrial accident. Therapy consists of immediate restoration of adequate ventilation and stabilization of the flail areas. As an emergency temporary expedient, both of these objectives can be accomplished by intubating the patient with a cuffed endotracheal tube and providing controlled positive-pressure ventilation. This ensures maximum respiratory efficiency of noncontused lung, and the paradoxical motion of the chest wall is eliminated by "internal pneumatic stabilization."

During resuscitation, a plan for further therapy appropriate to the case is selected. Usually a tracheostomy will be needed. If the flail area involves only the sternum, and the lateral anterior ribs are stable, fixation can be achieved by one or more Kirschner wires passed transversely beneath the sternum. In this instance tracheostomy may not be necessary. Where lateral stability is lacking, traction applied to multiple towel clips fastened through the outer cortex of various unstable costal and sternal elements will serve to correct the deformity and overcome paradoxical motion (Fig. 3-11). If towel clips are used, a large size must be selected and the stab wounds for introducing the points must be made in such a way that skin is not compressed between the shanks of the clip when the instrument is closed. Otherwise, unnecessary pressure and necrosis of skin will occur and the risk of infection will be increased. All patients immobilized with overhead towel clip traction should have a tracheostomy, and the tracheostomy should be retained until traction is discontinued. The most severely injured and those with preexisting diminished respiratory reserve should be treated by "internal pneumatic stabilization" employing a cuffed tracheostomy tube connected to a respirator using controlled hyperventilation. The resulting alkalosis has a sedative effect which decreases the resistance of automatic cycling of the machine.

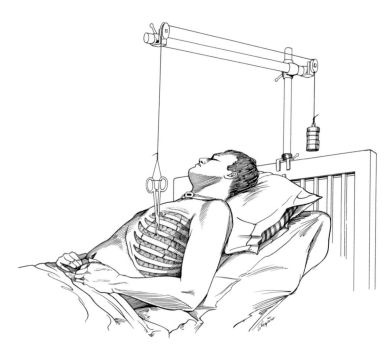

Fig. 3-11. External stabilization of the chest wall. One or more towel clips are carefully placed around the rib, with care to avoid the intercostal vessels, at the center of the flail segment. The clamp is then suspended with enough weight to stop the paradox. A tracheostomy is done.

SUBCUTANEOUS AND MEDIASTINAL EMPHYSEMA. Subcutaneous emphysema is usually the result of the escape of air from a small laceration of the lung into the tissue of the chest wall through a tear in the parietal pleura due to rib fracture. The movements of ventilation, coughing, and straining aggravate the condition. Pneumothorax is usually present but not in patients with prior pleural symphysis due to previous disease or injury. Prior pleural symphysis abets the rapidity with which massive subcutaneous emphysema may develop because pneumothorax cannot occur to compress the leaking lung and the openings in the lung and parietal chest wall are held in apposition.

Subcutaneous emphysema is never caused by air sucked into the chest wall from a superficial wound. Hence, its presence demands accurate diagnosis of internal injury.

The superficial tissues are swollen, nontender, cool, and finely crepitant on palpation. In extensive emphysema the body from head to feet may be massively involved. Usually the legs escape, however, because of the firm attachments of Scarpa's fascia inferiorly.

Since even mild degrees of subcutaneous emphysema will impart resonance to the percussion note and increasing degrees of emphysema proportionately dampen the transmission of sounds from underlying structures, physical findings may be misleading.

Mediastinal emphysema occurs as a result of an intrapulmonary tear with centripetal tracking of air along the bronchi, rupture of the trachea or major bronchi, or rupture of the esophagus. When sufficient tension has developed, mediastinal emphysema will rupture into one or both pleural cavities, giving rise to secondary pneumothorax. Mediastinal emphysema under tension may embarrass the airway and impede circulation by pressure upon the great veins. It is quickly allayed by tracheostomy.

Though massive subcutaneous emphysema may be uncomfortable, no primary therapy is required. Therapy is directed to the source of the air leak.

EXTRAPLEURAL HEMATOMA. Extrapleural hematoma is fairly common but seldom diagnosed. It is often seen in patients with pleural symphysis. The blood that escapes from a ruptured chest wall vessel collects in the plane of the endothoracic fascia. Roentgenograms show a parietal opacity having a sharp, rounded, or scalloped medial margin and based upon the chest wall. Aspiration or catheter drainage is unsatisfactory because the blood is always clotted. Resolution is spontaneous without fibrothorax.

PNEUMOTHORAX. Pneumothorax is usually due to the escape of air from a laceration of the underlying lung. Though external trauma plays a predominant role, spontaneous pneumothorax is commonly seen in males, usually in their third decade. Classically, during modest exertion or coughing the patient suddenly develops chest pain on the affected side and then becomes short of breath. Although in a minority the pneumothorax complicates a specific lung disease, in most instances it stems from rupture of an emphysematous bleb. (Infrequently, spontaneous pneumothorax is complicated by hemothorax secondary to associated tearing of adhesions or lung, and the hemorrhage may be serious, for a bronchial artery which bleeds under systemic artery pressure is at fault.)

Pneumothorax that occupies less than 20 percent of the pleural space can be treated expectantly providing the patient is under close surveillance. Pneumothorax greater than 20 percent, and life-threatening tension pneumothorax must be treated by thoracostomy tube drainage leading to an underwater seal or valved suction drainage system. In a critical situation initial relief of tension pneumothorax can be achieved by insertion of a 15 gauge needle into the pleural space and aspiration of air in phase with the patient's respiratory efforts. For obvious reasons, repeated thoracentesis is not a satisfactory method for treating pneumothorax due to persistent air leak.

HEMOTHORAX. Hemothorax or hemopneumothorax is usually indicative of a more serious injury than pneumothorax alone. Discounting the cause and source of bleeding, the primary objective of treatment of hemothorax is pulmonary expansion and obliteration of the pleural space. In the majority of instances, repeated thoracentesis or thoracostomy tube drainage will suffice. Thoracostomy tube drainage should always be employed in intrathoracic hemorrhage of a magnitude requiring monitoring for blood replacement. Patients with intrathoracic hemorrhage are also candidates for control of hemorrhage by thoracotomy (see Emergency Thoracotomy, in a later section of this chapter).

GASTRIC DILATATION. Acute gastric dilatation due to swallowed air as a result of hyperventilation frequently follows chest injury.

Gastric dilatation is abetted by the reflex paralytic ileus, which accompanies thoracic trauma and is actively increased by positive-pressure ventilation without a cuffed endotracheal tube. The consequent increase in intra-abdominal pressure impairs ventilation and venous return, and unless promptly relieved by the passage of a nasogastric tube invites the additional hazard of vomiting and aspiration. Undue prominence of the upper abdomen and a wide area of tympany extending above the left costal margin suggest the diagnosis. Too often the diagnosis is not considered until it appears on the roentgenogram as a startling advertisement of oversight.

In the practical management of most serious chest injury cases the passage of a nasogastric tube should be part of the resuscitative phase of therapy. This ensures early decompression of the stomach, is a safeguard against the aspiration of vomitus, and prevents delayed gastric dilatation.

TRAUMATIC ASPHYXIA. Traumatic asphyxia is an uncommon but dramatic complication of severe compression injuries of the thorax. The area drained by the superior vena cava, predominantly the face, neck, and upper chest, is dark blue, and the conjunctivae are scarlet and edematous. These changes are due to a combination of stagnation of blood in the venules of the skin and petechial hemorrhages. Of itself, traumatic asphyxia is usually not serious, but all such patients should be admitted to the hospital for a period of observation and treated by elevation of the head of the bed to promote resolution. Occasionally, as a result of prolonged compression, petechial hemorrhages (including involvement of the brain) will dominate the picture. In this case therapy demands safeguards against the development of cerebral edema, including the avoidance of overhydration.

Penetrating Wounds

In the emergency care of a patient with one or more penetrating wounds of the thorax, it must be determined whether the injury will respond to first aid alone or whether major surgery will be required. The decision rests in part on the response to resuscitative measures and in part upon the nature of the injury.

With stab wounds, knowledge of the type and length of weapon used is important. Since the axis of penetration follows the direction of the thrust, information about the circumstances and the assailant is also useful. Women tend to stab in an overhand manner using household implements such as kitchen knives; in neighborhoods without refrigerators, ice picks may be used. Men usually thrust upward with pocket knives, switchblades, and hunting knives.

In the evaluation of gunshot wounds the type of weapon and distance from the victim are important. The blast injury adjacent to the track of the bullet is in proportion to the velocity of the missile. Hence, a rifle shot is more injurious than a pistol shot. Since in self-inflicted gunshot wounds the heart is usually the intended target, a knowledge of the dominant hand of the patient may be useful; left-handed persons are more likely to be successful, for right-handed persons usually extend the wrist while pulling the trigger. (The instinctive difference in manipulating objects is exemplified by the inverted manner in which most left-handed individuals hold a pencil in writing.)

The site of peneration and sites of perforation of missiles and weapons are valuable topographical reference points for projecting the course through the underlying regional anatomy. Contrary to popular belief, bullets seldom ricochet off bony structures, and the skin site of entry and exit or final roentgenographic position of the bullet defines its path in the majority of instances—that is, providing the posture of the patient at the time he was shot is known, for the mobility of the skin about the shoulder girdle and pectoral area, for example, is great. This is also why a sucking wound of the chest may become apparent only after the position of the arm has been changed. Thoracic wounds over the mediastinum or suprasternal wounds inflicted by a downward thrust suggest great-vessel or cardiac injury. Parasternal wounds, even though relatively superficial, may cause serious bleeding from the internal mammary vessels. The latter vessels are anatomically unique in that they are anchored to fibroperiosteal structures at intercostal space intervals by at least four short branches. These points of fixation prevent the elastic recoil, which is one of nature's hemostatic mechanisms in combating hemorrhage from the ends of a divided vessel.

Bleeding is more serious from an injured systemic artery than from a pulmonary artery branch, reflecting the marked differential in pressure between the two systems. Bleeding from injury to the lung seldom requires operation, not only because the pulmonary artery pressure is one-sixth the systemic artery pressure, but also because the rapidly developing associated hemopneumothorax has a compressive effect on the underlying injured lung with a consequent tendency to self-sealing. The potential of diaphragmatic penetration and perforation of subdiaphragmatic structures is great when the level of the site of penetration is below the fourth anterior rib. Similarly, upper abdominal sites of entry invite the possibility of associated injury to intrathoracic structures.

The therapy of simple pneumothorax and hemothorax due to penetrating wounds is the same as described above when they are due to nonpenetrating wounds.

For more serious injuries demanding thoracotomy, the reader is referred to the following section.

EMERGENCY THORACOTOMY

The majority of patients who sustain thoracic trauma requiring hospitalization will respond to emergency measures short of thoracotomy. For a minority the emergency room is a receiving station for evaluation, resuscitation, other emergency treatment, and continuous reappraisal; behind the scenes preparation for surgery must proceed simultaneously. Timing is important and will vary with the case. Sometimes operation cannot await resuscitation but is necessary for resuscitation. Sometimes surgery is semiurgent and the patient may benefit by transitional hospital bed admission, freeing the emergency room for other cases. The indications for operative intervention must be clearly in mind. They are as follows:

Continued or recurrent intrathoracic hemorrhage
Ruptured thoracic aorta and arch branches
Continued or recurrent pericardial tamponade
Rupture of larynx, trachea, and bronchi
Compound rib fracture and major chest wall defect
Thoraco-abdominal wounds
Ruptured diaphragm
Esophageal perforation
Intrathoracic foreign bodies

Continued or Recurrent Intrathoracic Hemorrhage

Massive hemothorax is not per se an indication for emergency thoracotomy unless a large clotted hemothorax must be evacuated to restore respiration. Continuing or recurrent intrathoracic hemorrhage is often an indication for operative control of bleeding. Factors which bear on the decision are (1) estimate of the source of the hemorrhage as judged from the nature of the injury and the color of the blood, (2) rate of blood loss through the intercostal drainage tube, and (3) response of the patient to blood replacement. Continuing blood loss in excess of 200 ml per hour and absence of a diminishing trend after restoration of blood volume are relative indications for surgery. Observation should include monitoring of the central venous pressure and urinary output, and the efficacy of pleural space drainage should be repeatedly checked by thoracic roentgenograms with the patient in an erect position when his condition permits.

Ruptured Thoracic Aorta and Arch Branches

Characteristically, patients who survive rupture of the thoracic aorta sufficiently long to be admitted to the hospital are young (late teens and early twenties), often do not appear seriously injured, and frequently have no rib fractures. The injury is the result of an abrupt deceleration and almost invariably involves the first portion of the descending aorta. A widened mediastinum due to hematoma should alert the examiner to the possibility. Physical findings are usually scant. A soft murmur over the area, front or back, and hypertension in the upper extremities due to partial aortic obstruction, evidence of cervical hematoma, and a paralyzed left vocal cord are occasionally present. Once suspected in the acute injury patient, the diagnosis should be confirmed by aortography and emergency reparative surgery carried out, for fatal hemorrhage frequently occurs during the first 48 hours after injury.

The second most common site for aortic rupture is the ascending aorta at the level of the aortic sinuses. Injury here is almost invariably fatal, owing to rupture into the pericardial sac.

Injury to the arch branches and innominate or subclavian veins is much less common than rupture of the aortic isthmus, and is usually secondary to skeletal injury about the thoracic inlet. The nature of the vascular injury can be surmised from physical examination confirmed by angiography, and emergency surgery is indicated by the findings. It is important to avoid attempts at manipulative reduction of skeletal injuries such as posterior sternoclavicular dislocation, however, because serious internal hemorrhage may result. Manipulative reductions must await thoracotomy repair of the injured vessel.

Continued or Recurrent Pericardial Tamponade

The presence of hemopericardium with tamponade, whether due to blunt trauma or the more common penetrating wound, should sound the alarm for probable thoracotomy. The diagnosis is suspected by the findings of distended neck veins, elevated central venous pressure, muffled heart sounds, and paradoxical pulse in the absence of other signs of congestive heart failure. The diagnosis is established and therapy initiated by pericardicentesis. This is best done by threading a plastic catheter into the pericardium through a 14 or 16 gauge needle. The needle is introduced through the skin over the left xiphocostal notch and directed toward the medial border of the right scapular spine until the diaphragmatic pericardium is punctured (see Fig. 3-10). The needle is removed and the catheter used for continuous aspiration of the pericardial sac.

The majority of stab wounds will require urgent cardiorrhaphy, and the intrapericardial catheter will serve only to relieve tamponade during a hurried trip to the operating room. Since the ventricular myocardium has a tendency to be self-sealing, if the weapon causing the injury was of small diameter (such as an ice pick), cardiorrhaphy may occasionally be avoided. Conservatism in the management of penetrating wounds of the heart, however, favors early operation. Care should be exercised in positive-pressure ventilation because in the presence of tamponade compromised venous return may be further impeded.

Rupture of Larynx, Trachea, and Bronchi

Such injuries may occur from a direct blow or as a result of penetrating wounds. The injuries to the undivided airway produce immediate massive emphysema of the visceral compartment of the neck and mediastinum, with progression to involve the trunk and head. Emergency tracheostomy to relieve airway compression may be necessary. There is little correlation between the size of the airway injury and the degree of emphysema. Major injuries, such as traumatic separation between the cricoid cartilage and the trachea, require urgent operation to prevent stenosis.

Rupture of a lobar or main-stem bronchus is manifested by mediastinal emphysema usually accompanied by tension pneumothorax. Suspicion of a major bronchial rupture is aroused by continuing massive air leak through the thoracostomy drain and the rapid development of intractable atelectasis in the lobe or lung affected. To prevent infection and stricture, confirmation by emergency bronchoscopy should be followed at once by surgical repair.

Compound Rib Fracture and Major Chest Wall Defect

Compound rib fracture due to penetrating foreign bodies and large chest wall defects due to industrial accidents, goring by a bull, or a shotgun blast at close range require operating-room care. The immediate necessity is to prevent air from being sucked into and pumped out of the pleural cavity as the patient breathes. Respiratory dynamics are restored by sealing the chest wall with a firmly applied tampon of petroleum jelly gauze, and the development of a closed tension hemopneumothorax from injury to the deeper structures is prevented by closed thoracostomy tube water-sealed drainage. Definitive surgical treatment, including debridement, removal of foreign bodies and bone fragments, and repair of the lung and other intrathoracic structures, is in the province of the operating room.

Thoraco-abdominal Wounds

Thoraco-abdominal wounds involving the left hemidiaphragm are an absolute indication for abdominal exploration. Wounds penetrating the right hemidiaphragm and liver are a relative indication. First-aid treatment in preparation for operation should include (1) nasogastric tube decompression of the stomach and (2) treatment of pneumothorax by thoracostomy tube drainage to forestall tension pneumothorax in consequence of positive-pressure anesthesia.

Ruptured Diaphragm

Though crushing injuries of the chest may cause rupture of the diaphragm, in the majority of instances the injury is secondary to a compressive blow to the abdomen. Consequently, rib fractures or other superficial evidence of thoracic injury is usually absent. Symptoms of moderate chest pain and severe cardiopulmonary distress in consequence of gaseous distension of intrathoracic stomach and bowel may be preceded by an interval of relative well-being. In most instances the left hemidiaphragm, which is unprotected by the liver, is affected. Associate rupture of the spleen is surprisingly uncommon but when present increases the urgency of surgical intervention. Moreover, hemorrhage into the thorax from the ruptured spleen may obscure the true diagnosis and invite the serious error of inserting a thoracostomy tube into intrathoracic bowel.

Usually the diagnosis is obvious and relief of respiratory distress is promptly obtained by passage of a nasogastric tube to decompress the intrathoracic stomach. Occasionally angulation of the stomach at the gastroesophageal junction will prevent passage of the tube. Rupture of the right hemidiaphragm and rupture of the left hemidiaphragm plugged by protruding omentum may be difficult to detect but roent-genographic findings of slight elevation and irregularity of the dia-phragmatic contour and obliteration of the costophrenic sinus are suggestive. Though usually not an indication for urgent operation, detection is important and elective operation indicated because chest discomfort will persist indefinitely if the defect is left unrepaired.

Esophageal Perforation

Injury to the esophagus due to crushing or penetrating wounds is uncommon because of this structure's relatively protected prever-tebral position. Early detection offers a rare opportunity for primary repair, and failure of detection invites a fatal mediastinitis. Perfora-tion of the esophagus due to diagnostic instruments or swallowed foreign bodies typically occurs at the proximal, middle, or distal level of the normal anatomical narrowing of the esophagus. Associated mediastinitis is usually well advanced when the patient presents for diagnosis, and mediastinotomy drainage is imperative.

The cervical esophagus is the usual site of perforation due to penetrating wounds. Comparable wounds of the thoracic esophagus are more often fatal because of associated injury to adjacent vital structures. Rupture of the esophagus and traumatic tracheo-esophageal fistula are usually due to a crushing injury which at the moment of impact compresses these structures between the sternum and spine. Almost invariably the upper thoracic esophagus is the site of rupture; survivors of such injury are young people.

The first symptoms are pain and dysphagia, and the first physical sign is cervical emphysema. Until proved otherwise, interstitial em-physema which seems confined to the neck is due to airway or esophageal injury. Roentgenograms will show mediastinal emphy-sema initially and progressive widening of the mediastinum with a prevertebral air-fluid level on later films, as swallowed saliva escapes through the rupture site setting the stage for infection. The diagnosis and site of perforation should be promptly established by swallowed contrast material.

Intrathoracic Foreign Bodies

The mere presence of an intrathoracic foreign body is not an in-dication for urgent operation. Metallic foreign bodies less than 1 cm in size which do not impinge upon vital structures can probably be observed indefinitely. Impalement by knives, spears, and other objects calls for immediate operation. The object should not be removed until operative control of the region penetrated has been achieved.

REFERENCE

1. Barrett, N. R.   Early treatment of stove-in chest. *Lancet* 1:294, 1960.

SUGGESTED READING

Hughes, R. K.   Thoracic trauma: A collective review. *Ann. Thorac. Surg.* 1:778, 1965.

Cardiac Emergencies

JOSEPH T. DOYLE

THE SIMPLE FAINT

Of all cardiovascular emergencies the most common one is the simple faint, and it is also the most spectacular. Under appropriate conditions no one is immune to this form of syncope. Factors contributing to fainting are anxiety, fatigue, hunger, dehydration, blood loss, sedation, antihypertensive drugs, excessive heat, pain, or prolonged standing—indeed, virtually any noxious stimuli. It is a usual occurrence in any emergency room, since the patient and his friends and relatives are all potential fainters.

The mechanism of the faint is thought to be a massive vagal discharge with inappropriate peripheral vasodilatation. Typically, the fainter becomes visibly anxious and uneasy; his skin pales and he breaks out into a clammy sweat; he may yawn; there are gastrointestinal rumblings and perhaps the passage of flatus. Finally, abruptly, consciousness is lost. The appearance of the fainter is frighteningly deathlike. The pulse is strikingly slow and the blood pressure very low. There may be mild anoxic convulsive movements. Unless he is restrained from falling, collapse is self-restorative by bringing heart and brain to a common level. Indeed, every effort should be made to lower the fainter to the floor or to some flat surface. Maintenance of the upright posture could conceivably result in anoxic brain damage.

In recumbency, consciousness soon returns, but it is likely to be lost again if the fainter tries immediately to stand.

Treatment is mostly preventive. No patient should be required to stand longer than is essential to management. His sensibilities should not be violated more than is absolutely necessary by the sights, sounds, and smells of his environment. Judicious reassurance and sedation work wonders. The free use of aromatic spirits of ammonia is warmly commended. Friends and relatives should be politely but firmly ushered to the waiting room.

ACUTE MYOCARDIAL INFARCTION

The diagnosis of acute myocardial infarction is usually obvious from the history of crushing chest pain associated with sweating, profound weakness, shortness of breath, and fear of imminent death. The true state of the patient may be masked by shock, acute pulmonary edema, or a cardiac dysrhythmia. Very occasionally the presenting picture will be that of a cerebrovascular accident due to cerebral embolization from a left ventricular mural thrombus overlying a recent and usually unrecognized infarction. The differential diagnosis of acute myocardial infarction includes acute anxiety states, often with hyperventilation; acute pericarditis; dissecting hematoma of the aorta, with or without encroachment on the coronary ostia; pulmonary embolism; acute pneumonitis; pneumothorax; and, rarely, an intra-abdominal catastrophe.

The diagnosis of acute myocardial infarction should, if possible, be documented electrocardiographically. The patient must be considered to have an infarction if the clinical evidence is strong, despite a normal electrocardiogram. Of the so-called cardiac enzymes, creatine phosphokinase (CPK) may be expected to show a diagnostic rise within 12 hours. Any patient who has sustained a recent stroke should routinely have an electrocardiogram. If at all possible, a base line roentgenogram of the chest should be done, since other diagnostic possibilities may later require consideration. A worthwhile precaution is to start a slow intravenous infusion in the event that parenteral therapy later becomes an urgent necessity. In view of the very high mortality of acute myocardial infarction during the first 72 hours, continuous electrocardiographic monitoring for at least this period should, whenever possible, be carried on for every patient with a proved or strongly suspected infarction. This recommendation is predicated on the assumption that a professional staff fully knowledgeable in cardioresuscitative techniques is in continuous attendance.

The emergency treatment of acute myocardial infarction includes the relief of *pain,* the control of *shock,* and the management of hazardous *dysrhythmias.*

Morphine sulfate, 8 to 10 mg, is the most effective means of relieving *pain* and *anxiety.* The subcutaneous route is usually satisfactory. Hypotension and intense cutaneous vasoconstriction may hinder prompt absorption from subcutaneous depots, and under these circumstances morphine should be given intravenously. On theoretical grounds, the vagotonia commonly associated with inferior wall infarction and manifested by bradycardia and impaired atrioventricular conduction, is a relative contraindication to morphine. In these instances meperidine (Demerol) or, possibly, heroin may be preferable analgesics.

Cardiogenic *shock* is caused by feeble performance of the left ventricle due to deletion of contractile elements and, probably, to ill-defined vasodepressor reflexes. The peripheral arterial blood pressure may be a poor index of aortic root pressure. The single most useful gauge of the adequacy of cardiac output and perfusion pressure is the maintenance of a reasonable urinary output. Transient hypotension occurs almost invariably with large myocardial infarctions and requires no treatment. True shock, if rigorously defined by the manifestation of oliguria or anuria, is probably untreatable by present methods except, perhaps, the still experimental technique of extracorporeal support of the circulation. The sympathomimetic pressor amines have been widely endorsed for the treatment of cardiogenic shock. The following have been reported at one time or another to be particularly effective: levarterenol (Levophed), metaraminol (Aramine), mephentermine (Wyamine), methoxamine (Vasoxyl), ephedrine, and methamphetamine (Methedrine). On theoretical grounds, reduction of cardiac work by ganglionic blockade effected by trimethaphan camsylate (Arfonad) or guanethidine (Ismelin) merits consideration.

All varieties of tachysystolic *dysrhythmia* may complicate acute myocardial infarction. So long as circulatory compensation is maintained, it is probably wise to withhold energetic treatment. Supraventricular tachycardia often subsides spontaneously. If dysrhythmia is clearly responsible for a life-threatening fall in cardiac output, cardioversion should be employed. The technique is described elsewhere. Otherwise the dysrhythmias can usually be promptly controlled by rapid intravenous digitalization with lanatoside C, digoxin, or digitoxin. It is essential first to ascertain whether the patient has been receiving digitalis. Reasonable caution should be exercised in calculating the dosage, for the damaged heart may be especially sensitive to the toxic effects of digitalis. Ventricular tachycardia is always of ominous portent since deterioration into immediately fatal ventricular fibrillation may occur unpredictably. The management of these complications is discussed elsewhere. Even a single ventricular premature contraction may precipitate ventricular dysrhythmia, while the occurrence of several ventricular premature contractions per minute should be taken as an augury of impending ventricular tachycardia or fibrillation. Runs of three or more ventricular premature contractions technically constitute ventricular tachycardia. The experience of coronary intensive care units amply justifies the prompt and aggressive treatment of ectopic ventricular activity with lidocaine (Xylocaine). This drug is given as an intravenous bolus, 50 to 100 mg, or 1 mg per kilogram of body weight, which can be immediately repeated two or three times. Suppressive therapy is maintained by titrating the rate of delivery of 1000 mg lidocaine dissolved in 500 mg glucose 5% in water at an average rate of 2 to 5 mg per minute so as to maintain a stable cardiac mechanism. Intravenous quinidine and procaine amide are less desirable antidysrhythmic agents because of their greater hypotensive effects, although they continue to be useful by the oral route for prophylaxis. In cases unresponsive to these measures, capture and overdrive of the right ventricle by a catheter electrode should be considered when facilities are available. A fall in cardiac output caused by depression of the rate of sinus node discharge to 50 beats or less per minute may often be effectively combatted by the intravenous administration of atropine sulfate, 1 to 3 mg. Bladder paralysis and acute glaucoma should be anticipated as possible complications of vagal blockade.

Impaired atrioventricular conduction becomes significant only if it progresses to complete heart-block with an unacceptably slow idioventricular rhythm. The treatment of this complication is considered later. Transient atrioventricular dissociation usually with a ventricular rate in the low-normal range, arising from a nodal pacemaker, occurs fairly commonly with inferior wall infarctions and is associated with a substantially increased mortality. Atropine sulfate, 1 to 3 mg by vein, may be given. If this maneuver is ineffective, a transvenous pacing catheter should promptly be inserted. This procedure is described on page 83.

ACUTE PULMONARY EDEMA

Impairment of left ventricular function by arterial hypertension; aortic or mitral valvar disease; myocardial damage due to deficient coronary blood flow, infarction, or cardiomyopathy; and excessive abbreviation of the diastolic filling period by tachycardia are all characterized by a rise in left ventricular end-diastolic filling pressure and in left atrial pressure. Increased left atrial pressure necessitates a corresponding rise in pressure in the pulmonary veins and in the capillary bed of the lung. Above a pressure of 35 to 40 mm Hg, a highly proteinized fluid transudes from the pulmonary capillaries into the alveoli and may quickly cause death by asphyxiation. A very similar picture occurs in tight mitral stenosis or when the left atrial return is impeded by pulmonary embolization, thrombotic or tumorous obstruction of the pulmonary veins or left atrium, or high-altitude pulmonary edema.

Acute left ventricular failure may occur with catastrophic suddenness. More commonly it is manifested first by paroxysmal nocturnal dyspnea as left ventricular function gradually deteriorates. In the latter instance, orthostatic salt and water retention have occurred during the day and cause occult dependent edema. In recumbency, the edema fluid is no longer sequestered by gravity and reenters the circulation. The augmented blood volume overloads the weakened left ventricle. Typically, the patient is awakened a few hours after he has gone to sleep by anxiety, heaviness in the chest, and increasing breathlessness. He may at first get relief by sitting up, but as the paroxysms worsen he may rush to the window and gasp for air. Breathing becomes faster and more labored as the lungs stiffen and engorge. The patient complains that air does not seem to reach his lungs, which indeed it does not because of obstructing edema fluid in the alveoli. All accessory muscles of respiration are brought into play. The air passages fill with tenacious, foamy, and often blood-tinged edema fluid, which is ineffectually expectorated. The chest is filled with loud bubbling and musical rales and rhonchi. Bronchospasm may occur. The resultant wheezing respirations are properly termed cardiac asthma. The neck veins are distended. The nail beds are cyanotic. There is a copious cold sweat. A dreadful apprehension and mental clarity persist until death.

The emergency treatment of acute pulmonary edema is directed toward rapid lowering of the excessively high pulmonary capillary pressure. The single most effective measure is the administration of *morphine,* preferably by vein, since absorption from a subcutaneous injection may be slow and erratic because of intense vasoconstriction. The mechanism of action of morphine is complex and incompletely understood. Anxiety is relieved; lung-stretch reflexes are desensitized and the respiratory center is obtunded; and there is a direct action on the myocardium. *Oxygen* is helpful, although ventilation may be impeded by the foamy, sticky edema fluid. Intravenous aminophylline, 1.0 gm, delivered very slowly, is a time-honored therapeutic gambit which often relieves the bronchospastic element of acute pulmonary edema. *Intermittent positive-pressure* breathing may be highly effective in providing counterpressure against the increased hydrostatic pressure in the pulmonary capillaries. In desperate situations, tracheal intubation and continuous positive-pressure breathing may save the patient from drowning. It should be appreciated that the resultant increase in intrapleural pressure obstructs venous return to the right side of the heart and may critically reduce cardiac output. To a lesser extent the same liability accompanies the partial sequestration of the venous return by rotating *tourniquets.* This maneuver disencumbers the engorged lungs and gives the disabled left ventricle a chance to pump out the excessive central blood volume. Blood pressure cuffs are applied high on the arms, and specially lengthened cuffs are applied as high as possible on the thighs. Cuff pressure on three extremities is maintained at 80 mm Hg or at three-quarters of systolic pressures below 100 mm Hg. The venous return from the fourth extremity is not obstructed. Every 15 minutes, in rotation, the fourth extremity is obstructed, and the circulation is allowed to return to normal in one congested limb. Once the patient's condition improves, a single tourniquet is removed every 15 minutes so that the myocardium is not overwhelmed by an abrupt increase in the circulating blood volume. *Phlebotomy* is rarely indicated. If it is done, the blood should be removed under sterile precautions in a donor bottle so that if necessary it can later be returned to the patient. If there is reliable evidence that the patient has not recently received *digitalis,* a rapid-acting digitalis preparation should be given. Lanatoside C, 1.6 mg, and digoxin, 1.5 mg—by vein—are equally effective. The management of tachycardia is dealt with elsewhere. *Ethacrynic acid* or *furosemide* produces a prompt diuresis after intravenous administration and either may be a useful adjunct. Infection should be treated with appropriate *antibiotics*. Pulmonary embolization is a frequent cause of acute pulmonary edema. The use of *anticoagulants* and indications for *surgery* are discussed elsewhere.

CARDIOVERSION

The term *cardioversion* was introduced to designate the restitution of sino-atrial rhythm after complete depolarization of the dysrhythmic heart by a transthoracic electrical impulse of high voltage and brief duration (Fig. 4-1). A direct-current capacitor discharge is

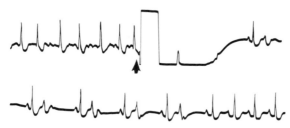

Fig. 4-1. Restoration of sinus rhythm following total cardiac depolarization in a patient with atrial fibrillation. The time of the condenser discharge is indicated by the arrow. Following a brief asystolic interval, a nodal beat appears, then probably a sinus beat distorted by the shifting base line, followed by a series of sinus beats with bigeminal ventricular premature beats, and finally a stable sinus rhythm. The morphology of P waves following cardioversion is initially often quite abnormal. Atrial function immediately after cardioversion has been shown to be hemodynamically ineffective. Hemodynamic improvement after cardioversion tends, therefore, to be delayed.

the preferred mode of delivering the electrical stimulus, since it can be precisely shaped and timed for greatest efficacy. Monophasic direct current is also less damaging to tissues than alternating current. Cardioversion carries a small but real risk of precipitating ventricular fibrillation. A synchronizing device to insure delivery of the electrical impulse outside the vulnerable period of cardiac depolarization minimizes the likelihood of this complication. High-energy electrical impulses traversing the chest wall excite a violent and painful clonic contraction of the chest muscles. Humane considerations, therefore, dictate the use of a brief general anesthesia just deep enough to assure amnesia.

The only absolute contraindication to cardioversion is digitalis intoxication. Electrical depolarization of the heart is the sole method of terminating ventricular fibrillation. Cardioversion is the treatment of choice when atrial tachycardia, atrial fibrillation, atrial flutter, nodal tachycardia, or ventricular tachycardia has precipitated life-threatening circulatory collapse. A good case for cardioversion can be made even when these rhythm disturbances are not catastrophic, since drug therapy is slower, less predictable, and probably not as safe.

Digitalis should be withheld for at least 24 hours and preferably longer before cardioversion. Quinidine or procaine amide are customarily given beforehand to the candidate for elective cardioversion on the chance that a therapeutic response might occur and on the assumption that the effectiveness of the depolarizing impulse is potentiated.

The details of cardioversion vary slightly with the type of instrument. Electrocardiographic leads will already have been attached. A precordial electrode may be attached for external pacing in the unlikely event that asystole persists after cardioversion. If the patient is conscious, anesthesia should be given by a skilled anesthesiologist. An intravenous drip is started. Thiopental, 200 to 400 mg, or some other short-acting barbiturate is injected rapidly into the tubing. Diazepam (Valium) has been recommended as an anesthetic agent but has no particular advantage over the barbiturates. Facilities for tracheal intubation should be at hand. One hundred percent oxygen is given by mask and bag. The synchronizer of the defibrillator is set, if necessary, to deliver the condenser discharge at the end of the QRS complex or at the beginning of the ST segment. Synchronization is, of course, unnecessary in ventricular fibrillation. Anterior and posterior electrodes provide a greater energy flux than electrodes placed anteriorly and laterally and hence permit the use of smaller condenser discharges. The skin over the upper left anterior chest and over the corresponding area posteriorly is briskly abraded with electrode paste. The weight of the patient holds the posterior electrode in place. The anterior electrode, well covered with electrode paste, is held firmly against the anterior chest wall. The cautious operator may wear an electrician's glove. The anesthetist and all others stand clear of the patient. An initial impulse of 100 to 150 joules (watt-seconds) is delivered and hyperoxygenation promptly restarted. After momentary asystole, normal sinus rhythm invariably appears if the heart can be depolarized. Several repetitions with increasing currents may be required to achieve cardiac depolarization. Oral maintenance therapy with quinidine or procaine amide may be initiated or continued, although it is virtually impossible to demon-strate that such prophylaxis is effective.

CARDIOPULMONARY RESUSCITATION

Energetic efforts should be made to restore life to any victim of circulatory arrest who is not clearly suffering from a terminal or hopelessly incapacitating disease. It is probably unwise to intervene more than 5 minutes after collapse or to continue resuscitative efforts if the pupils do not constrict promptly, lest a decerebrate vegetable be salvaged. Children and drowning victims are exceptions to this rule. Numerous excellent outlines of cardiopulmonary resuscitation are now available. Several points, nonetheless, merit particular emphasis.

1. Since cardiac arrest may befall anyone, anywhere, at any time, it is essential that all personnel who attend the sick be taught to take immediate and effective counteraction. A simple plan for cardiopul-monary resuscitation tailored to local needs should exist. All individ-uals involved must be frequently and conscientiously drilled in their respective roles. A team effort is required, but all efforts must be di-rected and coordinated by an acknowledged team leader. It must further be recognized that, particularly in small community hospi-tals, the crucial initial phases of cardiopulmonary resuscitation will have to be handled by specifically trained nursing personnel, since physicians will rarely be immediately available. There is an increas-ing impression, although as yet little documentation, that failure to institute resuscitative measures is more likely to invite the insinuation or formal accusation of malpractice than the unsuccessful applica-tion of such measures by nurses or nonprofessional personnel.

2. Unless a special resuscitation table or cart is used, it is best to place the patient on the floor to provide adequate support during sternal compression. Plywood panels inserted under the mattress are awkward and often ineffective.

3. Mouth-to-mouth insufflation is begun after clearing the airway and hyperextending the head. As soon as possible tracheal intubation should be done and ventilation with 100 percent oxygen maintained by bag.

4. If the heart does not start after a stiff blow to the precordium, sternal compression is begun and continued without interruption for *any* reason until an effective cardiac mechanism is restored.

5. An intravenous drip is started as soon as possible through a Rochester needle or a surgical cutdown. Sodium bicarbonate, 3.75 gm, is given immediately and every 5 minutes during resuscitation to combat acidosis.

6. Intracardiac epinephrine, 0.3 to 0.4 mg in a 1:1000 dilution is given early and repeatedly before electrical depolarization.

7. Ventricular fibrillation is treated by countershock, as described in the preceding section, using 400 joules. Persistent asystole usually indicates profound myocardial depression and rarely responds to transthoracic pacing stimuli.

8. The measures described are, in favorable circumstances, usually promptly effective. If all details of technique have been meticulously observed but circulatory arrest persists for more than 15 minutes, and if suitable facilities are available, consideration should be given to thoracotomy and direct cardiac compression to produce a larger stroke volume.

9. External cardiac compression is regularly attended by complications such as rib fracture and pneumothorax. Aspiration pneumonitis is common. Anoxic cerebral damage is a constant and unpredictable hazard. Acute renal tubular necrosis may occur if there has been a period of prolonged circulatory stagnation.

TACHYSYSTOLIC DYSRHYTHMIA

The mechanism of the cardiac rhythm can often be deduced from physical examination and is an unusually gratifying clinical exercise. An essential diagnostic maneuver is stimulation of the carotid sinuses. These baroreceptors are situated at the carotid bifurcations deep under the angles of the mandible. Firm massage, not occlusion, of the sinus against the transverse processes of the cervical vertebrae excites the sensory nerve endings in the sinus and evokes a powerful vagal reflex. The rate of discharge of the sino-atrial node and the speed of conduction through the atrioventricular nodal tissue are depressed. Indeed, in older subjects, in whom the reflex may be very sensitive, asystole long enough to cause cerebral ischemia and fainting may supervene. For this reason the patient should always be recumbent during stimulation of the carotid sinuses. Simultaneous stimulation of both carotid sinuses should never be done. Ectopic tachysystolic atrial foci may be transiently or permanently abolished by carotid sinus stimulation, which is, accordingly, diagnostic of and often curative in atrial tachycardia. Atrial fibrillation is not affected by carotid sinus stimulation, while characteristically in atrial flutter there may be an abrupt and momentary stepwise decrement in atrioventricular conduction. The carotid sinus reflex is usefully sensitized by morphine.

The electrocardiogram, of course, provides the definitive diagnosis of rhythm disturbances. The most satisfactory surface lead reflecting atrial activity is V_{3R} (Fig. 4-2). A continuous strip should be re-

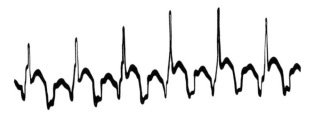

Fig. 4-2. Right atrial electrocardiogram. The large, narrow deflections are P waves, not apparent in surface leads which were typical of ventricular tachycardia.

corded before, during, and after massage of first the right, then the left, carotid sinus. A common diagnostic dilemma is the distinction between supraventricular tachycardia with fixed or functional bundle branch block and ventricular tachycardia. The response to carotid sinus stimulation may be both diagnostic and therapeutic, but the absence of a response has no significance. In such situations a bipolar esophageal lead is helpful. With this technique P waves are very large while QRS complexes are very small and diagnosis is usually easy. A newer and very safe technique, and one far more acceptable to queasy patients, is the passage into the right atrium of an electrode catheter either through a venous cutdown or through a large-bore needle. Since any low-resistance electrical connection between the heart and the exterior invites electrically induced ventricular fibrillation through inadvertent grounding, it is essential that the electrocardiograph used to record the intracavity electrocardiogram be adequately grounded; that the intracavity electrode be connected to the chest lead, *never* to the right leg lead; and that the patient not be connected to any other AC-powered device, whether or not it is operating.

SINUS TACHYCARDIA

In the adult, sinus tachycardia is defined as any heart rate over 100 per minute originating in the sinus node. Sinus tachycardia regularly occurs in response to emotion, to physical effort, and to catabolic states such as fever and thyrotoxicosis. Very rapid heart rates often raise the question of ectopic tachycardia. The electrocardiogram is, as a rule, diagnostic, the most useful features being small variations in rate in long lead strips and the bradycrotic response, no matter how slight, to carotid sinus stimulation. Treatment is directed toward the underlying cause. In some individuals sinus tachycardia and a hyperkinetic circulation appear to be due to overresponse to endogenous catecholamines. Reserpine (Serpacil), guanethidine (Ismelin), and propranolol (Inderal) may be useful in such situations since they tend to slow sinus tachycardia by catecholamine blockade or depletion.

PAROXYSMAL ATRIAL TACHYCARDIA

A common rhythm disturbance often occurring in healthy individuals, *paroxysmal atrial tachycardia,* is characterized by the abrupt onset of rapid, regular heart action of 150 to 200 beats per minute accompanied by varying degrees of apprehension, breathlessness, weakness, and ill-defined chest discomfort. If heart disease is present, complications such as angina pectoris, acute pulmonary edema, syncope, or congestive heart failure may be precipitated. Should the paroxysm last an hour or so, polyuria may ensue. Equally characteristically, the attack ceases abruptly after moments, hours, or, rarely, days. This feature is not apparent when the transition is to sinus tachycardia. Atrial tachycardia is a classic feature of the Wolff-Parkinson-White syndrome. The bizarre electrocardiogram may cause alarm if the underlying disorder is not known.

As a rule, paroxysmal atrial tachycardia occurs for no obvious reason. Often enough to require specific inquiry, however, attacks may be predictably induced by physical effort, fatigue, emotional stress, excessive smoking, alcoholic overindulgence, or infection. Attacks may occur frequently, may be separated by long intervals, or may come in clusters.

The diagnosis of paroxysmal atrial tachycardia can usually be inferred from the symptoms described. The differential diagnosis includes sinus tachycardia, atrioventricular nodal tachycardia, atrial fibrillation, atrial flutter, and ventricular tachycardia. A definitive diagnosis can be made only by electrocardiogram. Brief paroxysms may never be objectively diagnosed except by continuous electrocardiographic monitoring.

The victim of paroxysmal atrial tachycardia usually seeks medical attention only if the attack persists more than a few hours. Frequently he has learned from experience how to stop the rapid heart action by maneuvers such as breath-holding, swallowing, straining, or vomiting. A diagnostic and often curative procedure is carotid sinus stimulation. Carotid sinus massage should be done only with the utmost caution if at all in elderly subjects with extensive arteriosclerosis, since hemiplegia can be precipitated. Pressure on the eyeballs, a very effective method of eliciting vagal reflex activity, is to be condemned because of the hazard of retinal detachment.

Should carotid sinus stimulation prove ineffective, and should the electrocardiogram show the mechanism to be atrial tachycardia, the next move is to sensitize the vagal reflex mechanism. Morphine sulfate, 8 to 10 mg subcutaneously, is particularly effective and has the additional advantage of sedating the patient. Morphine should not, of course, be used when tachycardia recurs frequently, because of the danger of habituation. If this maneuver proves ineffective, a heavy dose of a short-acting barbiturate may be given. Ectopic tachycardia often subsides during the ensuing sleep.

If sedation does not work, if the patient is acutely uncomfortable, or if it appears that sustained rapid heart action threatens to aggravate underlying heart disease, a rapid-acting digitalis preparation should be administered. If it is certain that digitalis has not been previously taken, half an average digitalizing dose may be given, for instance, lanatoside C, 0.8 mg. Almost invariably there will be prompt reversion to sinus rhythm, due clearly to the extracardiac, vagotonic effects of the drug. In the occasional instance in which the dysrhythmia is judged to be life-threatening and these suggested modes of treatment are ineffective, recourse may be immediately had to electrical depolarization of the heart. This technique, described previously, carries virtually no hazard beyond that of the brief general anesthesia usually required.

The numerous unpleasant side effects caused by parasympathomimetic agents prohibit their use. The technique of breaking tachycardia by powerful baroreceptor stimulation with pressor amines is to be deprecated because of the hazard of uncontrolled hypertension or ventricular dysrhythmia.

It is desirable to impress upon the patient that, no matter how frightening, his rhythm disturbance is in itself benign. If simple measures suffice to break tachycardia, he should be shown how to apply these maneuvers.

A technique for breaking supraventricular tachycardia with which the writer has very limited experience is either to capture or to overdrive the atrium with a pacing catheter. This method is reported to be effective and at least as safe as cardioversion. It has the advantage over cardioversion in that it can be used in the digitalized patient.

Far less common is *paroxysmal nodal tachycardia,* clinically indistinguishable from atrial tachycardia and treated identically.

A special form of atrial tachycardia of entirely different significance and etiology is *atrial tachycardia with varying atrioventricular block,* a rhythm disturbance almost pathognomonic of digitalis intoxication (Fig. 4-3). As a primary disorder of the cardiac mecha-

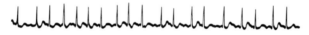

Fig. 4-3. Atrial tachycardia with varying atrioventricular block.

nism, it implies serious underlying heart disease. This form of atrial tachycardia should be suspected at the bedside when any digitalized patient known to have had a sinus mechanism is now found to have a rapid regular or an irregular rhythm; it may be diagnosed with considerable confidence when a patient with chronic atrial fibrillation is found inexplicably to have a regular rhythm.

Overdosage with digitalis is usually responsible for atrial tachycardia with varying atrioventricular block. Commonly, however, excessive potassium loss due to vigorous diuretic therapy or to acute gastroenteritis may be implicated.

Treatment consists of withdrawal of digitalis and the administration of potassium salts by mouth or parenterally, so long as kidney function is known to be adequate. Potassium chloride, 3.0 gm, may be given by mouth every 4 hours or 40 mEq per liter may be infused by vein. A good case can be made for the intravenous infusion of potassium, since the dose can be precisely adjusted while absorption from the gut may be erratic. Chelating agents have proved of little practical value. Sodium diphenylhydantoin (Dilantin) and the beta-adrenergic blocking agent propranolol are often effective in reversing the electrocardiographic manifestations of digitalis intoxication. The intravenous dose of the former is 100 to 300 mg and of the latter 2 to 5 mg. Since sodium diphenylhydantoin may improve atrioventricular conduction, it may be useful in the management of dysrhythmic or conduction disturbances induced by digitalis. Propranolol, on the other hand, should be reserved for ectopic rhythm disturbances including atrial paroxysmal tachycardia with varying block and should not be used in primary disturbances of atrioventricular conduction. Still entirely experimental is the technique of controlling the heart rate by paired electrical stimuli. Electrical depolarization of the heart to control atrial tachycardia caused by overdigitalization is unwarranted save in desperate situations, because of the hazard of precipitating uncontrollable ventricular dysrhythmia.

ATRIAL FLUTTER; ATRIAL FIBRILLATION

Atrial fibrillation frequently and *atrial flutter* almost invariably indicate serious heart disease. Pulmonary embolization as a precipitating factor should always be kept in mind. The subject typically presents himself because of uncomfortable, indeed alarming palpitations, breathlessness, and weakness. These complaints are due to a diminished stroke volume caused by the rapid ventricular rate, which shortens diastole so that adequate ventricular filling does not occur. When myocardial function is impaired by ischemic or hypertensive disease, or when mitral or aortic valve function is compromised, the rapid ventricular rate may precipitate acute left ventricular failure.

The diagnosis of atrial fibrillation can usually be made by auscultation. The distinction from the tumultuous rhythm caused by a rapidly *shifting atrial pacemaker* is, however, impossible to make except by electrocardiogram (Fig. 4-4). Atrial flutter or atrial tachycardia

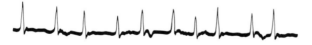

Fig. 4-4. Shifting atrial pacemaker. Clinical impression suggests that this is a pathological phenomenon often portending atrial fibrillation. By auscultation this mechanism is indistinguishable from atrial fibrillation.

with *varying atrioventricular block* also resembles atrial fibrillation (Figs. 4-5, 4-6). In theory, identification of rapid, regular f waves in

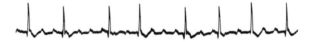

Fig. 4-5. Atrial flutter with varying atrioventricular block induced by digitalis. This is a notoriously unstable mechanism. The ventricular rate often rises to unacceptable levels on minimal exertion.

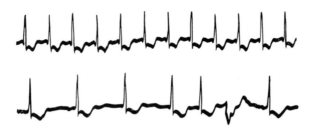

Fig. 4-6. Atrial fibrillation. The upper strip was recorded at the patient's first visit to the clinic after discharge from the hospital, the second after sedation and a night of rest. Clearly only the vagotonic effects of digitalis had been achieved.

the jugular vein at about 300 per minute verifies flutter. More practically, an abrupt halving of the rate to perhaps 75 per minute during carotid sinus stimulation confirms the diagnosis.

Atrial fibrillation and atrial flutter are usually well tolerated and rarely require emergency treatment. On the other hand, the patient with severe mitral stenosis or with a recent myocardial infarction may quickly be thrown into acute pulmonary edema. Rapid digitalization with lanatoside C, 1.6 mg, or digoxin, 1.5 mg, by vein, will, as a rule, promptly slow the ventricular response. Cardioversion should be seriously considered both as emergency and as definitive treatment, especially when the absence of serious heart disease indicates the likelihood that a sinus mechanism will be maintained.

VENTRICULAR TACHYCARDIA

Ventricular tachycardia is a rapid idioventricular tachysystolic mechanism averaging about 180 beats per minute (Fig. 4-7). The

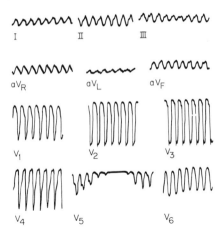

Fig. 4-7. Ventricular tachycardia. Absolute electrocardiographic confirmation requires demonstration of an independent atrial mechanism. See Figure 4-2.

electrocardiographic diagnosis depends on the demonstration of complete atrioventricular dissociation, which is usually difficult and requires the use of special leads. Ventricular tachycardia is often encountered in the early stage of acute myocardial infarction; it is a frequent complication of myocarditis of diverse etiologies; and it may be a manifestation of digitalis intoxication, particularly when there is serious underlying heart disease.

Ventricular tachycardia is especially feared because of its unpredictable tendency to disintegrate into ventricular fibrillation.

The patient with ventricular tachycardia may be little discommoded by rapid heart action, but like anyone with an excessively fast heart rate he is usually restless and uncomfortable. He may complain of chest pain, due either to pulmonary congestion, myocardial ischemia, or both. Acute left ventricular failure frequently supervenes. The bedside diagnosis of ventricular tachycardia can, in theory, be made by identifying cannon waves—that is, large atrial waves—in the jugular veins. These occur when the atrium contracts against the closed tricuspid valve. Practically, however, the diagnosis can be made only by electrocardiogram and even then with little confidence unless special techniques are used to identify atrial activity. Even then, unhappily, it may not be invariably possible to differentiate the rhythm from supraventricular tachycardia with aberration, since some patients with ventricular tachycardia have retrograde conduction to the atria.

From the therapeutic standpoint it is fortunate that the precise diagnosis of ventricular tachycardia is not of crucial importance, since both supraventricular tachycardia with bundle branch block and true ventricular tachycardia respond to the same management. The simplest, safest, and speediest treatment is now cardioversion. If a defibrillator is not available or it is elected not to employ cardioversion, lidocaine should be given by vein as a bolus of 50 to 100 mg and repeated several times as necessary. To protect against a recurrence of ventricular tachycardia, lidocaine, 1000 mg in 500 ml dextrose 5% in water, may be delivered intravenously at a rate sufficient to suppress ventricular ectopic activity, which may be as much as 2 ml per minute. Procaine amide or quinidine sulfate, 1000 mg in 500 ml of 5% dextrose and water, may also be given by vein. The electrocardiogram should be continuously monitored on an oscilloscope, or frequent electrocardiographic strips should be recorded. Further widening of the QRS complex or prolongation of the QT interval signifies serious myocardial depression and necessitates temporary discontinuance of any of these drugs. The arterial pressure should be measured frequently. Should the blood pressure fall with no deterioration of the electrocardiogram, the hypotension may be counteracted by administering a pressor amine while continuing the antifibrillatory agent. Lidocaine is the drug of choice, since it is less likely than procaine amide or quinidine to cause hypotension, and its duration of action is brief. Acute left ventricular failure associated with or precipitated by ventricular tachycardia requires rapid digitalization if digitalis has not previously been given. Since the continuous electrocardiographic monitoring of patients with acute myocardial infarction has become routine, a benign rhythm disturbance morphologically identical to ventricular tachycardia has been frequently encountered. The diagnostic difference is that the rate is slow. The mechanism is probably nodal with aberrant ventricular conduction. The disorder is paroxysmal, brief, self-limiting, and requires no treatment (Fig. 4-8).

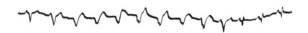

Fig. 4-8. So-called accelerated idioventricular rhythm with spontaneous reversion to normal sinus rhythm occurring in a patient with acute myocardial infarction. No hemodynamic deterioration is associated with this mechanism and no therapeutic intervention is indicated. Prognosis is apparently unimpaired, in contrast with most other rhythm disturbances complicating acute myocardial infarction.

VENTRICULAR FIBRILLATION

Ventricular fibrillation is totally disorganized, uncoordinated electrical activity of the ventricles (Fig. 4-9). The ventricles are non-

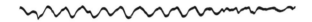

Fig. 4-9. Ventricular fibrillation. The electrocardiographic diagnosis of "dying heart" is no longer inevitable.

contractile and no stroke volume is generated. Irreversible cerebral anoxia takes place within a very few minutes. Profound metabolic acidosis develops rapidly, further depressing myocardial function. Ventricular fibrillation is a common lethal event in early acute myocardial infarction and is not closely correlated with the size of the infarct. Ventricular fibrillation may occur in the normal heart rendered anoxic from any cause or depressed by a variety of analgesic and anesthetic agents. Ventricular fibrillation regularly occurs in accidental electrocution.

The clinical features of ventricular fibrillation are those of death.

The treatment of ventricular fibrillation is covered in Cardiopulmonary Resuscitation, an earlier section of this chapter.

HEART-BLOCK

In an occasional individual, usually one with long-standing left ventricular hypertension whatever the cause, conduction through the atrioventricular node fails. This lapse of conduction is probably a common cause of sudden death. In some people, on the other hand, after a variable period of asystole, ventricular automatism asserts itself and an idioventricular rhythm is established. If the automatic focus is high, in the region of the atrioventricular node, the heart rate is between 50 and 70 beats per minute and the QRS complex resembles the normal. If, however, the idioventricular focus is low, the rate is slow and fixed, and there is marked aberrance of the QRS complex. The rate may be so slow that an adequate cardiac output is not generated. The patient is bedridden because of profound weakness, cerebral anoxia, and congestive heart failure. In still other individuals the idioventricular mechanism suddenly and unpredictably ceases. The clinical picture is that of cerebral anoxia, syncope, and convulsions, i.e., the Morgagni-Adams-Stokes syndrome. Congenital complete heart-block is usually, although not invariably, asymptomatic.

The diagnosis of heart-block is difficult when it occurs only transiently (Fig. 4-10). The history of fainting and convulsions quite

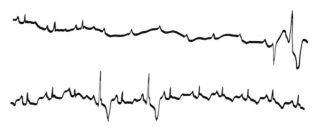

Fig. 4-10. Intermittent complete heart-block. Circulatory arrest of about 8 seconds is sufficient to cause loss of consciousness in young subjects; the interval is presumably shorter in the cerebrosclerotic patient.

naturally suggests primary neurological disease. Unless portable continuous-recording electrocardiographic equipment is available, documentation of the heart-block is virtually impossible until or unless it becomes fixed. The diagnosis of established complete heart-block is obvious but should be confirmed electrocardiographically.

Complete heart-block commonly presents as an emergency characterized by repeated episodes of asystole with syncope and anoxic convulsions. Isoproterenol (Isuprel), 5 mg in 1000 ml of 5% dextrose in water by vein, can usually be infused at a rate sufficient to maintain an adequate heart rate and prevent asystole. Continuous electrocardiographic monitoring is essential to adjust the rate of the infusion. Overdosage with isoproterenol is manifested by bizarre multifocal ventricular premature contractions. Isoproterenol may also be given sublingually. Because of tachyphylaxis, the drug is suitable only for emergency use.

Most patients with symptomatic heart-block require the implantation of a permanent cardiac pacemaker. Both in the urgent management of patients with complete heart-block and to prepare them for permanent pacemaker implantation, a transvenous intracardiac pacing catheter is indispensable. The insertion of the catheter is an easily learned technique that need not be confined to medical centers where cardiac catheterization is done routinely. The catheter is most easily and rapidly inserted via a median basilic vein. This route is not optimal because the catheter may be dislodged by even slight movement of the arm, which is difficult to immobilize without considerable discomfort to the patient. The right external jugular vein is, for the patient, a more comfortable site for the introduction of the pacing catheter. On occasion the femoral vein may be the best site for introduction of the pacing catheter. The pacing catheter is introduced through a nick in the vein and passed into the heart under fluoroscopic guidance. The catheter is then rotated medially, insinuated through the tricuspid valve into the right ventricle, and wedged firmly in the trabeculae of the right ventricular apex. Floating catheter techniques utilizing the antecubital or subclavian veins are effective in the hands of experienced operators but cannot be recommended for the occasional emergency situation in community hospitals. A battery-powered pacing unit is attached to the catheter and the heart rate set at 70 to 90 per minute. If available, a demand or standby type of pulse generator should be used in preference to a fixed-rate pacemaker to obviate the possibility of competition and of lethal stimulation of the ventricle during its excitable period. Under no circumstances, because of the hazard of ungrounded currents, should an externally powered pacemaker be used. The skin incision is closed and a loose loop of catheter sutured to the skin for fixation. The same technique is used for the permanent implantation of a transvenous pacemaker except, of course, that the proximal end of the catheter is attached to a sterile power pack buried in a subcutaneous pouch in the anterior chest wall. The simplicity and safety of this method commend it over the much more difficult and hazardous technique of transthoracic placement of epicardial leads. In life-threatening episodes of recurrent or persistent heart-block, a temporary endocardial pacing electrode may be introduced into either right or left ventricle by transthoracic puncture. A "permanent" pacemaker can later be installed at leisure, or the patient can be safely moved to a surgical center for this purpose.

Contrary to traditional notions, coronary heart disease is rarely a cause of permanent complete heart-block. Inferior wall infarctions are, however, rather typically complicated by transient atrioventricular dissociation. Although the ventricular rate is usually adequate and the conduction disturbance is short-lived, mortality is increased by the higher incidence of high-grade heart-block and of congestive failure. Prompt insertion of a transvenous pacemaker, even if only on a standby basis, is recommended if intravenous atropine sulfate, 1 to 3 mg, is ineffective. Complete heart-block following recurrent myocardial infarction in an individual with a prior anterior wall infarction is fortunately rare but is usually permanent, due to loss of both the direct and the collateral blood supplies of the atrioventricular node or to both bundle branches. Permanent pacing is indicated, although this decision cannot be made until after a trial of temporary pacing.

AIR EMBOLISM

Air embolism is fortunately a rare and almost invariably iatrogenic event likely, however, to occur more frequently as subclavian venous punctures and the insertion of central venous catheters become commonplace. The head-up position, and in particular hypovolemia, can create a negative pressure powerful enough to cause the rapid aspiration of large quantities of air into the superior vena cava and right atrium through even medium-sized tubing. In theory, under similar circumstances the aspiration of air through a short needle would be prevented by collapse of the walls of the vein downstream from the puncture site.

The mixture of blood and air forms a tenacious froth which produces an airlock of the right ventricular outflow tract and pulmonary capillaries. A precordial "millwheel" murmur is characteristically heard. Death occurs rapidly, since the heart is, in effect, tamponaded. Disaster may be averted, if the continued entrance of air into the right side of the heart can be stopped, by placing the victim in the left lateral decubitus position. In this posture the air rises as a bubble to the highest points in the venous system. If this level be above the tricuspid valve, the air is innocuous and is gradually resorbed. Needle aspiration of the right ventricle through a puncture adjacent to the lower left sternal border should be done if this simple gravitational maneuver is ineffective. In the rare event that a hyperbaric chamber were available, the rapid elevation of atmospheric pressure should compress the embolus to tolerable size.

HYPERKALEMIA

Serum potassium levels above 6.5 mEq per liter are potentially cardiotoxic (Fig. 4-11). Any seriously ill patient with diminished

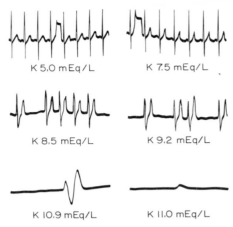

Fig. 4-11. Hyperkalemia (potassium poisoning) induced experimentally in a dog. The electrocardiograph is far more reliable than the flame photometer in detecting cardiotoxicity due to potassium.

renal function may develop a dangerously high serum potassium concentration. An elevated serum potassium level is easily recognized by sharply peaked T waves in the electrocardiogram. More advanced electrocardiographic evidences of potassium toxicity are prolongation of atrioventricular and intraventricular conduction, volleys of ventricular tachycardia, bradycardia, and ultimate disintegration of electrical activity. Pari passu there is progressive deterioration of the mechanical function of the heart.

Hyperkalemia must be aggressively treated as soon as recognized, since cardiac arrest may occur unpredictably. Raising the concentration of other serum cations blocks the toxic effects of potassium; this is most effectively achieved by the infusion of 5% sodium chloride in water. As a temporary measure, the excessive serum potassium may be sequestered intracellularly by the administration of 10% dextrose in water covered by crystalline insulin. If the situation is less threatening, the ion-exchange resin sodium polystyrene sulfonate (Kayexalate) may be given orally or rectally in a daily dosage of 15 gm. The preparation is extremely constipating, so that equal quantities of sorbitol and water should be given if the resin is administered orally, while the rectally administered resin must be recovered by copious lavage. Depending on the cause of renal insufficiency and the long-term prognosis, hemodialysis or peritoneal dialysis may be required.

Neurosurgical Emergencies 5

RICHARD A. LENDE

This review concerns primarily the evaluation of neurosurgical problems rather than treatment, which is necessarily limited in the emergency room. The indications but not the techniques are presented for x-ray contrast procedures which must be performed by trained specialists. A neurological examination should be performed if there is any question of impairment of the nervous system, but only selected aspects of that examination are touched upon here.

EVALUATION OF THE UNCONSCIOUS PATIENT

Airway

Impaired ventilation may be secondary to the neurological disability or may, in fact, be responsible for the unconsciousness. The airway should be evaluated initially before a full history is obtained. Whatever measures are necessary should be instituted to secure adequate ventilation: oxygen, suctioning, pharyngeal airway, endotracheal tube, or emergency tracheostomy.

Historical Considerations

The history may be absent or misleading. Impressions of the patient's previous condition should be obtained from observers before they leave the emergency room. It should be remembered that a patient may have fallen and struck his head or become involved in an automobile accident because he lost consciousness from an underlying cause such as an epileptic seizure, subarachnoid hemorrhage, or metabolic disorder. He may, of course, on admission be suffering from the primary disorder as well as the secondary head injury.

Vital Signs and Their Significance

Temperature, pulse, blood pressure, and respiration should be recorded as soon as practicable and followed intermittently to see if they indicate a trend. It is commonly taught that increasing intracranial pressure is accompanied by a rising systolic blood pressure, a widening pulse pressure, and a slowing pulse. Valuable as these signs often are, they are not to be relied upon to indicate the presence or absence of an intracranial mass that requires surgical attention. It is true that changes in vital signs accompany increasing intracranial pressure in the experimental animal. However, in complex head injuries the human patient may have progressive neurological deterioration to a point near death before a change in vital signs is remarkable. Generally patients with head injury alone do not show evidence of shock even though they may have lost blood from a scalp laceration. If the systolic pressure is low and the pulse rapid, a thorough search should be made for a cause such as a ruptured intra-abdominal viscus, a fractured femur, or a hemothorax. When one of these is present, priority is given to the treatment of shock and the condition responsible for it. The systolic pressure may be low in patients with head injuries who have also suffered paraplegia with loss of autonomic control below the level of a cord lesion.

Respiratory alterations are variable in head injuries. Commonly, with a severe brain injury or in a state of decerebrate rigidity, the patient exhibits a stertorous, labored respiration and secretions are not swallowed. Ventilation in such a case is helped by tracheostomy. However, if the patient is improving, a tracheostomy may be wisely forestalled for a period of observation, in the hope that adequate neurological control will be regained shortly. Cheyne-Stokes respirations may occur in more severe head injuries but do not reliably indicate prognosis or need for surgical intervention.

THE QUESTION OF ARTIFICIAL VENTILATION WHEN BREATHING STOPS. As death approaches, breathing ordinarily ceases before the heart stops in patients with neurological deterioration due to the effects of head injury, increased intracranial pressure, or stroke. Consequently, an opportunity is presented for institution of mechanical ventilation via an endotracheal tube or tracheostomy. Almost never does such a patient recover, regardless of what therapy is undertaken. However, life may be prolonged several days, during which time the patient is unresponsive to pain and has fixed dilated pupils. An ethical question is thus posed. It must be borne in mind that cases of unconsciousness due to metabolic, toxic, infectious, or other causes may need artificial respiration and may respond following adequate therapy. Seldom does the emergency-room physician question the institution of artificial ventilation, since he is preoccupied with the maintenance of life.

Patients dying from severe head injury are potential donors of organs for transplantation, and the ability to sustain the circulation of oxygenated blood to the organs to be transplanted is essential for their continued viability and function. When death from head injury seems imminent, the responsible relative should be contacted for permission to use the patient after death as a donor. Since there is constant need for cadaver organs it is important for all physicians involved in the care of patients with head injury to be alert to this possibility. Most hospitals have a committee of physicians who are not involved in the care of either donor or recipient to make the final decision, in such circumstances, that "brain death" has occurred.

Cervical Fracture in the Unconscious Patient

Injuries to the neck may accompany injuries to the head. In a state of unconsciousness the patient cannot volunteer information about this disability, and the physical examination may not demonstrate neck injury. Cervical spine x-rays should be taken if cervical spine injury is suspected. The point is mentioned because it is possible to convert an uncomplicated cervical fracture into one with a quadriplegia by inexpert flexion and positioning of the neck in the emergency room or on the radiological table.

Level of Consciousness

It is of the utmost practical importance to establish and record the patient's level of consciousness initially and periodically. A deepening level may indicate a progressive disorder which needs urgent remedy. A lightening level may indicate spontaneous recovery which needs only observation. The level of consciousness may be estimated by stimulating the patient and noting his response. Since the terms *confusion, stupor, semicoma,* and *coma* vary in meaning and usage among physicians, it is preferable to note in the chart the mode of stimulation and the manner of response.

In the deepest stages, near death, the patient may make no response to painful stimuli such as pinprick, rubbing the knuckle on the sternum with pressure, pressing the supraorbital nerve at its foramen, or pinching the tendons or finger webs. In this state the corneal reflex may be absent and the pupils fixed and dilated. At a less deep stage the patient may respond to pain by generalized or mass movement. In the condition of decerebrate rigidity a noxious stimulus may result in a tonic stiffening of the entire body. At a lighter stage the patient may withdraw the appropriate part of the body. In still lighter stages he may withdraw a part quickly and accurately on pinprick and may attempt to remove the noxious stimulus. Although unable to verbalize, he may respond on command to grasp the examiner's hand or to protrude his tongue. At a still lighter level he may give simple answers to simple questions and obey more complex commands. When able to talk he can be questioned concerning orientation in time and place. Direct questions must be asked, since it is possible for the patient to carry on a superficially clear conversation and be entirely disoriented in time. In recovery stages his only disability may be a slight but inappropriate confusion regarding recent events and current affairs. Amnesia for the events immediately preceding an injury is unfortunately often present, and the retrograde extent of amnesia has been used by some as an index of the severity of the injury.

Since a deepening unconsciousness is so significant, it is important not to obscure a trend in level of consciousness by administration of drugs which affect responsiveness. In particular, narcotics should not be given. Pupillary activity should likewise not be altered by administration of mydriatics when the level of consciousness is being followed with concern.

Differential Consideration of Unconsciousness

The following check list is provided because in many cases of unconsciousness the history is obscure:

1. Head injuries and their sequelae, including cerebral concussion and intracranial hematomas.

2. Cerebral anemia, including shock, cardiac arrhythmia and failure, general anemia, fainting, and moribund states.
3. Cerebral strokes, including embolism, hemorrhage, and thrombosis.
4. Poisoning, including narcotics and alcohol.
5. Psychogenic factors, including hysteria and psychosis.
6. Metabolic disorders, including acidosis, alkalosis, hypoglycemia, uremia, and hepatic failure.
7. Infections, including meningitis, encephalitis, and septic shock.
8. Epileptic seizures.
9. Intracranial tumor.
10. Subarachnoid hemorrhage.
11. Cerebral edema, including hypertensive encephalopathy.

HEAD INJURIES

The principle aim in treatment of head injuries is to prevent further damage. The patient with a head injury may be rendered worse by various sequelae, including the development of an intracranial hematoma which acts as a space-consuming lesion, the development of increased intracranial pressure without an associated clot, the development of infection which is provided ingress by the nature of the injury, or the development of epileptic seizures associated with cortical irritation. The preceding section, Evaluation of the Unconscious Patient, should be consulted in considering patients whose head injuries have resulted in unconsciousness.

Cerebral Concussion

There is no absolute definition of cerebral concussion. Concussion means simply a blow or a shaking. However, the term *cerebral concussion* is commonly used among neurosurgeons to indicate a state of unconsciousness caused by a blow to the head. The unconsciousness is ordinarily transient and is followed by more or less complete recovery. The term is sometimes modified by the adjective *severe* or *mild*. Concussion implies some interference with the function of the central core of the brain stem, which is concerned with consciousness —the reticular activating system. A frank cerebral contusion or laceration may be an accompaniment. Most head injuries which are brought to the emergency room are termed cerebral concussions, and usually a progressive spontaneous recovery occurs without specific treatment.

Any patient with a cerebral concussion should be admitted to the hospital for a period of observation, often for only overnight. It is not possible to foretell accurately on an initial evaluation which case will demand surgical attention. Less than 10 percent of patients with head injury involving cerebral concussion who are admitted to the emergency room will have an intracranial clot. Suspicion of such a lesion is raised in patients who are progressively deteriorating or who remain at an impaired state without recovery for a prolonged period. Consequently, the sequential recording of level of consciousness, neurological signs, and vital signs is of greatest importance in separating out those patients who may require evacuation of a clot.

Occasionally an incoherent patient exhibits an extreme exhausting restlessness such that he may injure himself. Tranquilizers or sedatives—paraldehyde, for example—may eventually be necessary but are always given with the awareness that responsiveness is thereby altered. Epileptic seizures occasionally occur and require treatment but they must be clearly differentiated from attacks of decerebrate rigidity (cerebellar fits), which are more common in severe head injuries and are not specifically treated in the emergency room.

Skull Fractures

In all cases of cerebral concussion skull roentgenograms are taken. These may indicate recent trauma by showing a linear skull fracture, which does not require specific treatment. Linear fractures per se do not reveal the extent of cerebral damage, which is our main concern, nor do they necessarily mark the location of an intracranial clot when one is present. An exception is the case of an extradural hematoma caused by bleeding from the middle meningeal artery, which may be torn by a fracture in the temporal region. A skull fracture is not a reliable guide to the severity of injury, since it may be absent in a case with very severe cerebral damage or present occasionally in a case without a history of loss of consciousness.

If a skull fracture is depressed into the substance of the brain, it should be surgically elevated in the operating room. If a scalp laceration overlies a depressed skull fracture, it must be considered a contaminated compound fracture and antibiotic coverage given. From such wounds brain substance or cerebrospinal fluid may exude.

These wounds should be covered simply with a sterile dressing in the emergency room. The patient is usually admitted directly to the operating room, where definitive care is given. A seemingly innocent scalp laceration sometimes overlies a significant depressed skull fracture. Such a fracture may be present in a perfectly alert patient who did not lose consciousness following an injury inflicted by a small, rapidly moving object—like a bullet or sharp hammer. Palpation is not reliable in the evaluation of depression of a fracture.

A leak of cerebrospinal fluid from the ear, the nose, or a wound is prima facie evidence of a skull fracture and dural tear. Most leaks will subside without surgical repair, but they should be given antibiotic coverage. Blood behind the ear drum may accompany a fracture of the base of the skull. The delayed appearance of subcutaneous blood over the mastoid or about the orbit suggests a nearby skull fracture. In all such cases hospital admission is necessary.

Intracranial Hematoma

An intracranial hematoma may develop following head injury and attain significant size. It is usually removed surgically when clinical evidence is supported by radiological evidence. In the unusual case in which a very rapid deterioration of level of consciousness is occurring in the emergency room or has occurred by reliable history, the patient is rushed to the operating room where a cranial opening may relieve a clot and save his life. It is seldom, however, that trephine or bur hole openings are done before cerebral angiography is performed to give radiological confirmation of a space-occupying lesion. Cerebral angiography is now a mainstay of diagnosis and is indicated in patients who show clinical evidence of neurological deterioration or who stay at an impaired level without improvement.

Extradural hematoma is much less common than subdural hematoma and may develop more rapidly, since it is usually of arterial origin. Acute subdural hematoma is likely to be associated with generalized brain damage; the prognosis is often poor even if the clot is successfully removed. In some cases the patient recovers consciousness following cerebral concussion only to lose consciousness again as a forming blood clot gains in size—the so-called lucid interval of extradural hematoma. Obviously, in the case of a longer period of unconsciousness, or a more rapidly developing clot, the lucid period would not manifest itself. An enlarging pupil is usually taken as evidence of distortion or stretching of the third nerve, and this may occur with development of a clot. The enlarged pupil is classically described as ipsilateral to the hematoma and associated with a contralateral hemiparesis. However, it is often observed in dealing with complex head injuries that the enlarged pupil and the hemiparesis do not reliably lateralize the clot. Plain skull roentgenograms may suggest a space-occupying lesion by a lateral shift of a calcified pineal gland. Cerebral angiograms dependably demonstrate the location and extent of most intracranial hematomas of surgical significance.

Subdural hematoma may present subacutely or chronically, simulating a brain tumor in all respects. Certain patients diagnosed as having a stroke may actually have a subdural hematoma. This is a particularly difficult clinical differentiation in the aged, where the history is clouded and a known chronic disease is present. No patient should be allowed to die in an undiagnosed coma without serious consideration of cerebral angiography.

Lumbar Puncture

Lumbar puncture is usually well tolerated by a patient but it must be remembered that in some cases of intracranial mass lesions the removal of spinal fluid will induce a shift of the intracranial contents with consequent increase of neurological disability or even death. In the case of a mass within the posterior fossa, lumbar puncture is more dangerous, since it may result in a downward shift with herniation of the medulla and cerebellar tonsils into the foramen magnum and consequent interference with medullary control of vital functions. In the emergency room the danger of lumbar puncture must be weighed against the value of the diagnostic information which is sought. In evaluating a head injury, lumbar puncture is rarely used and should not be done for the sake of completing a "neurological work-up." The information which may be obtained is of little diagnostic or prognostic value.

A lumbar puncture need not be performed in cases of head injury unless there are features which suggest another diagnosis. An intracranial clot is not suggested by blood in the cerebrospinal fluid; over half the cases of head injuries seen in the emergency room will have some blood in the cerebrospinal fluid. A hematoma is not necessarily suggested by a high cerebrospinal fluid pressure and may be present along with a normal pressure. There is likewise little purpose and considerable risk in performing a lumbar puncture in the emergency room when a brain tumor is seriously suspected; nonspecific information—that an elevated cerebrospinal fluid protein is present, for example—does not really add to the information obtained on history and examination which gave evidence of neurological disability. An elevated cerebrospinal fluid pressure may be found in any patient who is struggling or even holding his breath or holding himself tense.

A lumbar puncture is indicated and spinal fluid findings may be diagnostic in cases in which meningitis or spontaneous subarachnoid hemorrhage is clearly suggested. In both situations signs of meningeal irritation are usually present. If spontaneous subarachnoid hemorrhage from an intracranial aneurysm or angioma is suspected, it is of great importance to have a well-executed spinal tap, since the issue is confused in a traumatic tap where bleeding induced by the needle point has contaminated the spinal fluid specimen. The contamination may gradually clear as fluid is drained, or the centrifuged specimen may show a yellowish color indicating earlier bleeding. Lumbar puncture may also be done when it is desired to show the presence or absence of a spinal subarachnoid block by observing spinal fluid pressure changes on jugular compression (Queckenstedt's test). However, prudence must also be exercised in these cases, for there is a possibility of increasing neurological disability by the withdrawal of cerebrospinal fluid. (See Spinal Cord Compression, below.)

INCREASED INTRACRANIAL PRESSURE

Increased intracranial pressure is best evaluated during hospitalization. Unless the situation is very urgent, the work-up in the emergency room is usually limited to history, physical examination, and plain roentgenograms. In infants in whom the cranial sutures have not united, increased pressure may be clearly manifested by a tense fontanelle or, if prolonged, by an enlarged head. In children and adults it may be difficult to establish the presence of increased pressure in the emergency room. Few patients complaining of headache actually have increased pressure, and an increase of pressure may exist in a patient who does not complain of headache. Papilledema may not be seen in patients with increased pressure and may be present in patients without increased pressure.

Although it is possible to measure spinal fluid pressure on lumbar puncture, this procedure may be hazardous, as noted previously. There is little value in undertaking it in the emergency room when one encounters a progressive neurological disorder presumed to be due to a space-occupying lesion that will require extensive evaluation. If a suspicion of increased intracranial pressure is entertained on the basis of history and examination, skull roentgenograms should be made. Special x-ray procedures such as cerebral angiography or air contrast studies are usually done after hospital admission, but they may be indicated as emergency studies in the urgent case. A patient with increased intracranial pressure who is decompensating in the emergency room may be given urea or mannitol intravenously in an attempt to dehydrate the brain. A urinary catheter should be in place because of diuresis after administration. Reduction in pressure often ensues for a period of hours. Such attempts to reduce pressure osmotically are not indicated in the face of intracranial bleeding. Parenteral cortisone in high dosage may also be expected to reduce cerebral edema, although the effects are slower than with hypertonic agents, and such medication should not be begun unless there is a clear plan for continued management.

The most rapid method of reducing intracranial pressure in an emergency situation is by the introduction of a needle into the lateral ventricle or a pathological fluid-containing space. The needle is passed through a twist drill hole in the skull, and the procedure should be carried out by someone with neurosurgical knowledge. The subdural space in infants may be tapped by a sharp needle in the edge of the anterior fontanelle when subdural hematoma or effusion is suspected, but this procedure is ordinarily best delayed until after admission to the hospital ward.

SPINAL CORD COMPRESSION

Patients in whom spinal injury is suspected are ordinarily best transported in the supine position. Occasionally a patient who has a marked dorsal gibbus or who is in a fixed position of flexion because of trauma or kyphosis requires transportation on his side or even in the prone position. Moving from a stretcher without altering position significantly may be done by the combined efforts of a number of lifters, unless special facilities are available. In unconscious patients an unsuspected spinal injury may be aggravated by faulty positioning. It may be advantageous to take the history and do much of the examination while the patient is left on the stretcher in which he was carried into the emergency room.

If neurological examination shows a level of paralysis, a urinary catheter will be required. Associated injuries in the area of anesthesia should be excluded by examination. Lowered blood pressure may be encountered due to autonomic paralysis but this is usually not an indication for administration of blood. If an elevation of pressure is deemed desirable, a response may follow administration of plasma expander or other intravenous fluids. The patient may be placed on an orthopedic frame (such as the Foster or Stryker frame) in the emergency room when spinal immobilization at any level is desired. In all patients with areas of anesthesia, the danger of untoward pressures on skin surfaces should be considered from the outset.

Where examination suggests a cervical fracture, sandbags may be placed on either side of the head for immobilization. If a canvas head halter is available, it may be quickly applied and used to exert moderate traction on the head. Manual traction may also be used. Spine roentgenograms should be made as quickly as practicable with due precaution. Positioning should not be done by an unsupervised technician. If a significant cervical fracture is shown on a roentgenogram, skull tongs should be directly placed and tension applied— under local anesthesia in the emergency room if facilities permit.

If a subarachnoid block is suspected, Queckenstedt's test is sometimes applied to help determine the need for emergency surgical decompression, but only after the surgeon has been directly contacted and the desirability of the procedure discussed. It is easily performed by measuring the spinal fluid pressure below the level of the questioned block and noting the response to pressure on the jugular veins, which is induced by gradually inflating a sphygmomanometer cuff wrapped around the neck. A myelogram may be recommended by the surgeon to visualize the level of a possible spinal block. When spinal cord compression from a tumor is suspected, spinal roentgenograms are made, but a lumbar puncture in the emergency room is not recommended because of the danger of converting paresis into complete paralysis. The outlook for recovery after complete paraplegia from any cause is usually poor. Therefore, in cases of increasing paraparesis, a decision should be made quickly regarding the need for operation.

The Unconscious Patient 6

ALICE E. FRUEHAN

SPECIAL PROBLEMS

Before any attempt is made to establish a specific diagnosis in an unconscious patient, attention must be given to vital physiological functions, which may be primarily or secondarily deranged. Appropriate supportive therapy, when needed, is essential for patient survival no matter what the etiology of the coma.

1. Maintain airway, by intubation if necessary; suction to clear secretions; oxygen.
2. Treat shock, if present.
3. Position patient to avoid aspiration and injury.
4. Regulate temperature, if necessary.
5. Catheterize to relieve bladder distension.

DIFFERENTIAL DIAGNOSIS OF COMA

The unconscious patient offers to the clinical acumen of the physician a challenge perhaps unequaled by any other situation in the practice of medicine. A medical history is seldom available, unless family, friends, or past medical records can supply factual data. Patients with chronic illness may carry identifying cards or tags specifying their disease and drugs, and this information is invaluable. If no history is available, the physician is forced to proceed solely upon his recognition and interpretation of clinical signs and, helped by basic laboratory data, to arrive speedily at the correct diagnosis so that appropriate therapy may be started before too much time is lost. An organized approach and painstaking attention to detail are essential if the correct diagnosis is to be made. The differential diagnosis of coma outlined in Table 6-1 is offered as a comprehensive list of etiological factors, yet one which is simple enough to be used at the bedside. Each patient deserves complete consideration of both primary and secondary causes of coma, for multiple etiological factors are often involved and the less obvious may escape detection unless careful search is made.

EMERGENCY-ROOM CARE OF THE COMATOSE PATIENT

Work-Up

1. Obtain temperature, pulse, respiratory rate, and blood pressure.
2. Note color, cyanosis, skin turgor, and hydration; smell breath.
3. Do a neurological examination.
   a. Eyes: pupil size and reaction, eye deviation, extraocular movements; careful funduscopy
   b. Cranial nerves: especially facial asymmetry, integrity of gag reflex
   c. Neck: stiff or flaccid
   d. Extremities: position, muscle tone, reflexes, withdrawal response to pain
4. Complete physical examination, especially of:
   a. Heart
   b. Lungs
   c. Abdomen
   d. Pelvis and rectum
5. Catheterize.
6. Have laboratory tests done immediately.
   a. Complete blood count, serology, blood glucose, blood urea nitrogen, serum electrolytes including sodium, potassium, chloride, and carbon dioxide content

    b. Urinalysis

    c. Stool for occult blood

    d. Electrocardiogram in the elderly

    e. Chest roentgenogram

  7. Do special laboratory tests as outlined in Table 6-1.

Treatment

Therapy of the comatose patient begins in the emergency room. Once the diagnosis has been established, definitive treatment (see Table 6-1) can be initiated and continued during subsequent transfer to inpatient facilities.

Hospital Admission

All patients who are brought to the emergency room in coma should be admitted to the inpatient facilities after initial work-up is complete and appropriate treatment has been started. If partial or complete restoration of consciousness occurs in the emergency room, a short period of hospitalization is still advisable for observation. Transfer of the comatose patient should be made speedily and with care. Oxygen, suction, and other supportive apparatus should accompany him as needed; he should never be left unattended. Stretchers equipped with side rails should be used, and the patient should be tied securely in the prone position with the head tilted to one side to drain secretions.

Table 6-1. Emergency-Room Care of the Unconscious Patient

Differential Diagnosis	Comments	Special Tests	Emergency-Room Treatment
1. Intoxications			
a. Alcohol	History of ingestion. Odor of alcohol on breath. Must rule out head injury and all other causes of coma	Skull roentgenograms if head injury suspected. Stool for occult blood	If delirium tremens present, control with paraldehyde, 4 ml intramuscularly, or 5 to 10 ml of paraldehyde in oil by rectum. Start intravenous fluids slowly
b. Sedatives Barbiturates, various tranquilizers	History of available drugs from family, friends, druggist, physician. Police can assist in search for empty bottle or vial. Many tranquilizers have a bizarre clinical picture associated with overdosage which is difficult to recognize unless a specific history of ingestion can be obtained.	Blood barbiturate level. Analysis of gastric contents and urine. Consult poison-control center or handbook for specific drug ingested	Clear airway; assist respiration if needed. Gastric lavage if within 4 to 6 hours of ingestion. Start intravenous fluids. Consider hemodialysis if coma deepens. Consult poison-control center or handbook for specific drug ingested
c. Narcotic analgesics Morphine, meperidine, heroin, etc.	Pinpoint pupils. History of addiction. Puncture wounds along veins, thromboses, infection	—	Clear airway; assist respiration if needed. Give nalorphine hydrochloride, 5 to 10 mg, intravenously to combat respiratory depression (drug is contraindicated for barbiturates and other sedatives). Gastric lavage if within 4 to 6 hours of ingestion

2. Metabolic Disorders

	History	Laboratory	Treatment
a. Diabetic acidosis	History of diabetes. "Fruity" odor to breath, dehydration. Diabetic acidosis and hypoglycemia are sometimes difficult to distinguish clinically; diagnosis should always be confirmed by laboratory tests	Urine sugar and acetone Blood sugar Plasma acetone Serum electrolytes	Give regular insulin 50 to 100 units intramuscularly or intravenously, or initial insulin dosage required by plasma acetone dilution method. Start normal saline intravenously. If doubt exists between acidosis and hypoglycemia, treat first for hypoglycemia immediately after drawing blood sugar
b. Hypoglycemia	History of diabetes, or episodes of weakness, coma, or convulsions relieved by food	Blood sugar	Give 50 ml of 50% glucose intravenously, followed by infusion of 5% glucose
c. Uremia	History of renal disease, oliguria-anuria, etc. Uremic "frost," odor of breath	Urinalysis Blood urea nitrogen Serum creatinine Hematocrit Serum electrolytes	Assess status of fluid and electrolyte balance and start intravenous fluids accordingly
d. Addisonian crisis Primary or secondary to steroid withdrawal	History of adrenal insufficiency or chronic steroid therapy	Plasma cortisol Blood urea nitrogen Serum electrolytes	Give hydrocortisone, 100 mg intravenously. Start 5 or 10% glucose in normal saline
e. Hepatic coma	History and stigmata of liver disease. Coma often precipitated	Blood ammonia Serum bilirubin, SGOT,[a]	Start 5% glucose in water intravenously. If gastrointestinal

[a] Serum glutamic-oxalacetic transaminase.

Table 6-1 continued on pages 104-106

Table 6-1. (Continued)

Differential Diagnosis	Comments	Special Tests	Emergency-Room Treatment
		by gastrointestinal bleeding, infection, or high-protein diet	alkaline phosphatase, total protein and albumin: globulin ratio Blood sugar Stool for occult blood Culture suspected sites of infection	bleeding present, control blood loss, transfuse if necessary. If infection present, add appropriate antibiotics to intravenous infusion
f. Carbon dioxide narcosis	History and stigmata of chronic lung disease, usually with superimposed infection	Serum electrolytes Arterial pH, pCO_2, and pO_2 Culture sputum or endotracheal secretions and blood	Clear airway. Suction vigorously. Intubate, oxygenate. Assist ventilation with Ambu bag until clinical situation stabilizes, followed by respirator. Start intravenous fluids, with appropriate antibiotics added if infection present.
3. Severe systemic infection	Careful search for infection is indicated in any comatose patient. Fever and leukocytosis may be absent in elderly or debilitated patients	Lumbar puncture if there is no papilledema Cultures of blood, cerebrospinal fluid, and suspected foci of infection	Start intravenous fluids. Add appropriate antibiotics after cultures taken

4. Cardiovascular Disorders			
a. Shock and hypotension	Low blood pressure may accompany other causes of coma, but acute myocardial infarction and acute blood loss should always be excluded. Relative hypotension in the aged may be difficult to judge unless previous blood pressures are known	Electrocardiogram Hematocrit	Start intravenous fluids. Treat primary cause.
b. Arrhythmia	Complete heart-block, auricular or ventricular fibrillation, etc., may be transient, but if cerebral damage has occurred, coma may persist	Electrocardiogram	Pacemaker, defibrillator, digitalis, or procain amide may be necessary, depending upon specific arrhythmia present
c. Hypertensive encephalopathy	Extreme blood pressure elevation with grade III or IV retinopathy is an easy syndrome to recognize if other causes of coma can be excluded	Electrocardiogram	Start parenteral reserpine in initial doses not exceeding 0.5 to 1.0 mg or titrate blood pressure, under continuous supervision by physician, with trimethaphan, 0.1% intravenously, starting with about 60 drops (3 to 4 mg) per minute
5. Postconvulsive state	A flaccid postictal state may be difficult to diagnose if the history of epilepsy is not known. Focal neurological signs may not be present	Electroencephalogram if diagnosis is in doubt	Supportive care

Table 6-1. (*Continued*)

Differential Diagnosis	Comments	Special Tests	Emergency-Room Treatment
6. Alterations in body temperature			
a. Hyperthermia	Heatstroke should be easily recognized by the high temperature with complete absence of sweating		Cool with alcohol-water sponges and fan or cooling blanket
b. Hypothermia	Search for predisposing conditions such as alcoholism, metabolic disorders, stroke, myocardial infarction, infection, etc. Very low temperatures must be recorded by special rectal or esophageal thermometers	Electrocardiogram	Warm very slowly with blankets. Support respiration or use pacemaker if necessary
7. Meningitis	A stiff neck and blood or leukocytes in the cerebrospinal fluid are diagnostic of hemorrhage or infection in the meninges. Focal neurological signs may be absent	Lumbar puncture if there is no papilledema Complete examination of spinal fluid including smears and cultures If hemorrhage, consider cerebral angiography If infection, culture blood and suspected foci of infection Skull roentgenogram	Start intravenous fluids. Add appropriate antibiotics if infection present. Supportive care
8. Central nervous system lesions	Focal neurological signs with or without changes in the cerebrospinal fluid. Careful search for other causes of coma is essential; these may accentuate signs of previously existing central	Lumbar puncture if there is no papilledema Complete examination of spinal fluid including smears and cultures Skull roentgenogram	Start intravenous fluids. Supportive care

Vascular Emergencies 7

MAKIS J. TSAPOGAS

Vascular emergencies are occurring in significantly increasing numbers. This is clearly a result of the greater number of road and industrial accidents and the many more acts of violence. The complications of chronic vascular disease also contribute to this increase.

Rapid transportation, prompt diagnosis, and competent initial management, can considerably reduce the mortality and amputation rate, as early reconstruction of the injured vessels is the key to success. Progress in vascular surgery during the last 20 years has been impressive, and the results obtained today show a vast improvement over those previously obtained.

INITIAL ASSESSMENT AND IMMEDIATE MANAGEMENT

The plan of action in vascular emergencies depends on the presence and degree of shock and the seriousness of associated injuries. Rapid evaluation and resuscitation of the patient in shock must proceed simultaneously and without delay. Since speed is essential, teamwork is highly desirable. It is also important that a surgeon trained and experienced in vascular surgery be readily available for consultation in the emergency room.

Control of Hemorrhage

The control of bleeding is an essential feature of resuscitation. Digital pressure and elevation of the injured extremity, when feasible, are effective measures. Excellent results are obtained when the artery can be compressed against an underlying bone such as the femoral artery against the femur, the brachial artery against the humerus, and the aorta against the spine. A gaping wound can be packed with gauze which is kept in place by a tight bandage.

The pneumatic tourniquet or blood-pressure cuff is of only occasional use for control of bleeding from the extremities. It is mainly indicated in multiple injuries when it can be applied to one extremity while attention is given to other sites. The pressure in the tourniquet must be above the patient's systolic pressure. Lower pressure may aggravate bleeding by promoting venous congestion. The pneumatic tourniquet should be applied for the shortest possible time and maximally for no longer than an hour. If it has to be used for a longer period of time, it should be intermittently released. This may obviously be dangerous since torrential hemorrhage may suddenly occur and prove lethal to an already oligemic patient. Great caution is therefore required when releasing the tourniquet, and digital pressure should be applied during those intervals.

There is little justification today for the use of old-fashioned tourniquets. They may cause tissue and nerve damage when tightly applied, or if loose, they will act as venous tourniquets. They can only be used in life-threatening hemorrhage when no other means are effective or available.

Hemostatic clamps are not to be used on bleeding arteries in the emergency room, as they may increase damage to the vessel. As a result of this, grafting procedures may be necessary when simple suture of the injured vessel might have been adequate. Small atraumatic (bulldog) vascular clamps are useful only for bleeding arteries already exposed in the wound. Large-sized vascular atraumatic clamps should not be used, particularly on restless patients, as avulsion may occur. Surgical exploration of vascular injuries should be attempted only in the operating room.

Resuscitation

Control of hemorrhage is accompanied by general measures of resuscitation. Restoration of adequate circulating blood volume and satisfactory tissue perfusion are the primary aims. A wide-bore plastic cannula or catheter is inserted in a vein and blood is taken for typing and cross matching. Ringer's lactate is administered rapidly until compatible blood is available. A central venous catheter is also inserted and is a useful parameter for the regulation of the amount of fluids to be given. Overtransfusion of these patients should be avoided because of the risk of congestive heart failure and recurrence of bleeding. The patient is kept warm and the injured extremity is not exposed to intense heat or cold. Overheating increases metabolic requirements, and low temperature promotes vasoconstriction. Both conditions further embarrass the already compromised circulation in the extremity.

Temporary immobilization of unstable fractures by splinting is essential for the prevention of further vascular damage, particularly in restless patients.

Antibiotics are given in open injuries to control infection which would reduce the chance for successful reconstructive surgery. Tetanus immunization is also necessary.

Following resuscitative measures a rapid reevaluation of the patient's status is essential. When recovery from shock begins, the clinical signs may change. As the blood pressure rises, previously absent arterial pulses may return and a cool limb may become warm. Meticulous examination is necessary for correct evaluation and management. Comprehensive records of the patient's condition on arrival at the emergency room and following resuscitation are most important for appropriate assessment as well as for possible medicolegal action. The pulses of the injured extremity are checked and oscillometric recordings are also made. The skin temperature and the motor and sensory functions of the extremity are carefully tested.

TYPES OF VASCULAR EMERGENCIES

Vasospasm

Significant and symptomatic vasospasm usually follows vascular injuries or complications of chronic vascular disease, and may contribute in varying degree to the ischemia of the affected extremity. It is most often transient and may spontaneously regress within 4 to 6 hours. The emergency-room physician should not waste valuable time treating vasospasm. By thorough physical examination and arteriography, an underlying organic vascular lesion may be demonstrated.

Certain arteries, such as those of the upper extremity, are more susceptible to spasm than others. If vasospasm is considered a significant factor in ischemia and immediate surgical exploration is not anticipated, measures can be taken in the emergency room in an effort to release the increased vasomotor tone. Application of heat to the trunk and the unaffected extremities may cause reflex vasodilatation in the affected part. Intra-arterial injection of lidocaine and papaverine, along with peripheral nerve block, may be helpful. Sympathetic nerve blocks, when indicated, should not be carried out in the emergency room.

It should be emphasized that in most instances in which vasospasm is considered responsible for ischemia an underlying organic arterial lesion is the main cause.

Mechanical Injuries

The management of peripheral vascular injuries has significantly improved during the last 20 years as a result of the experience gained in wartime. In World War II, when ligation was the method of treating injured vessels, the amputation rate was 50 percent. In the Korean War immediate repair of the vessels was applied in 88 percent of arterial injuries and the amputation rate fell to 13 percent. Other factors have also contributed to the impressive improvement. Among these are: rapid transportation of the injured to the hospital, greater awareness of the likelihood of arterial injuries, abandonment of the use of tourniquets except on rare occasions, availability of blood and antibiotics, and the wider use of arteriography for prompt and accurate diagnosis.

PENETRATING WOUNDS. These wounds may vary from a puncture wound to an extensive gaping one because of laceration of the vessel or even its complete transection. This is usually followed by significant bleeding. It is worthy of note that complete vessel transection may cause less bleeding than partial laceration because the transected ends can retract effectively. Clot formation may sometimes control overt bleeding and therefore the vascular trauma may be overlooked.

BLUNT TRAUMA. This may result in contusion of the vessel, occlusion by intramural hematoma, or intimal tears which may be circumferential and become the nidus for thrombosis. Blunt vascular injury is usually more difficult to diagnose than is penetrating injury.

Complications may appear immediately or more often at a later stage when the damaged vessel becomes distended by constant intraluminal pressure.

Arterial injuries are often associated with trauma to the accompanying vein, nerves, or concomitant fractures or dislocations. Knowledge of the anatomy helps in suspecting such associated injuries. Reports from the Vietnam War indicate a 37.7 percent rate of concomitant venous injury, 28.5 percent of bone injury, and 42.4 percent of nerve injury. In axillary artery injuries the incidence of associated nerve injury is reported to be 90 percent.

TRAUMATIC ANEURYSM. If the injured artery communicates with a hematoma in a closed space, a traumatic aneurysm may form. This usually results from an injury caused by a blunt instrument. Bleeding or hematoma formation is particularly suspect if it is out of proportion to the otherwise innocuous appearance of a wound over the course of a major artery. A thrill and a systolic bruit can be heard on auscultation over the hematoma. When the traumatic aneurysm is located in a closed space such as the popliteal fossa, it eventually compresses major veins or nerves causing edema and/or paresthesia; thrombosis is a common complication.

ARTERIOVENOUS FISTULA. When an injured artery ruptures into the adjacent vein, an arteriovenous fistula forms. This may develop in any part of the body. The involved vessels dilate and a pulsatile mass forms. The vein drains a significant amount of blood from the artery. The clinical picture obviously depends on the location of the fistula as well as on its size. The most common physical sign is a machinery murmur over the lesion during both systole and diastole, its intensity depending on the size of the fistula. The pulse rate gradually increases and the diastolic pressure decreases. Application of pressure over the fistula causes bradycardia and raises the blood pressure (Branham's sign). This is of significant diagnostic importance. Locally the temperature is elevated and the veins are dilated and sometimes pulsatile. Large arteriovenous fistulas produce cardiac enlargement and increased cardiac output, which eventually will lead to heart failure. The O_2 content of the venous blood and the venous pressure are locally increased.

Early recognition of traumatic aneurysms and arteriovenous fistulas is usually difficult, as the full clinical picture does not develop until later. Auscultation of a bruit in the region of a recent wound will lead to the diagnosis. The characteristic findings in arteriovenous fistulas are decreased arterial circulation distal to the injury, with distended venous collaterals, and at later stages the signs and symptoms of high-output cardiac failure.

Careful early evaluation and prompt treatment are most important in minimizing complications. Surgical exploration is indicated when doubt exists.

Cuts of the Wrist and Throat

Cuts of the wrist and throat occur most commonly in attempted suicide. Caution is needed in dealing with these emergencies which at first sight may look like simple lacerations despite extensive injury to important structures. Exploration of the wound should be avoided and the extent of the injury should be assessed only in the operating room. Concomitant injuries of arteries, veins, nerves, and tendons should be anticipated in either type of wound. Control of arterial or venous bleeding in the emergency room is achieved by digital pressure or direct packing of the wound reinforced by a gentle compression dressing. Although it may be tempting to ligate or suture the bleeding vessel, this should never be considered, as it may leave the patient with serious residual circulatory insufficiency.

In lacerations of the throat it is most important to watch for respiratory obstruction by blood, foreign body, edema of the glottis, or compression bandage. Maintenance of an adequate airway is mandatory and tracheal intubation or tracheostomy should be performed if necessary. In deep wounds in the base of the neck the possibility of complicating pneumothorax should be kept in mind. Use of suction will clear mucus or blood obstructing the airway. Traumatic thrombosis of the internal carotid artery can result from penetrating as well as nonpenetrating injuries of the neck and will give the picture of cerebral ischemia. In such cases the diagnosis will be helped by angiography.

In vascular injury at the wrist, application of a resilient compression dressing and elevation of the hand above heart level usually control bleeding. Preoperative examination of the function of the hand is very important to detect motor or sensory loss in addition to circulatory embarrassment.

Vascular Injuries Associated with Fractures

Fractures of long bones may cause direct injury to adjacent arteries. The injury, if unrecognized and consequently not repaired, can lead to either immediate gangrene or delayed manifestations of arterial insufficiency. Injury to the radial and ulnar arteries usually results from fractures of the shaft of one or both forearm bones. The distal segments of these arteries, however, are more often occluded by compression from a hematoma or edema in the carpal tunnel. Fracture dislocation of the neck of the humerus may injure the axillary artery. The diagnosis of ischemia in the extremity should be made as soon as possible. The characteristic clinical features are pain, pallor, paralysis, and lack of pulse. Absence of the radial pulse is a significant early clinical finding. If flexion contracture is present, permanent damage is already established.

The immediate steps taken in the emergency room are directed toward improving the circulation in the extremity. The possibility of external pressure should be excluded by cutting through the entire length of any encircling bandage or plaster cast. If there is acute flexion of the injured elbow, this should be gently supported in a lesser degree of flexion. If gross deformity is present, early reduction is indicated, and if despite satisfactory reduction evidence of impaired arterial inflow persists, arteriography should be carried out to demonstrate the site and extent of the vascular injury. Necessary surgical measures to establish continuity of the vessel are carried out after reduction and immobilization of the fracture.

Fractures of the shaft of femur may injure the distal segment of the superficial femoral artery which is held in close contact with the bone by the fibrous arch of the adductor magnus muscle. Supracondylar fractures of the femur and oblique fractures of the upper third of the tibia and fibula are known to produce serious vascular injuries, which may result in gangrene of the foot unless promptly treated.

The application of an unpadded plaster cast to a fractured extremity soon after injury is dangerous. Pressure within the rigid cast may become so great that arterial flow may be obstructed and cause ischemic contracture or gangrene. It is therefore important in early treatment of displaced fractures to avoid unpadded plasters, and to leave the fingers and toes exposed in order to observe the circulation in the extremity carefully. Swelling can be minimized by elevation of the extremity. At the first sign of pallor or cyanosis of the toes or fingers, the plaster cast must be cut throughout its length.

Von Volkmann's ischemic contracture is a serious complication of fractures in which, as a result of partial interference to arterial inflow and venous outflow, there is progressive fibrosis of muscle groups, leading to functional loss and contracture. It most frequently attends fractures about the elbow, particularly supracondylar fractures of the humerus. These fractures tend to be unstable after reduction, and acute flexion of the elbow may be necessary to maintain the position of the fragments. Acute flexion at the elbow can cause compression of both arteries and veins, particularly those of the volar muscles of the forearm. The interference to blood flow is not sufficient to cause gangrene, but leads to increasing edema. The volar muscles are enveloped by the deep fascia, which, under the above conditions, leads to rising pressure in a closed space. A "claw hand" deformity is the eventual result.

Cold Injuries

IMMERSION OR TRENCH FOOT.   This condition results from prolonged exposure to cold or dampness at temperatures above freezing. It occurred extensively in the American armed forces in Europe during the winter of 1944–1945, when 45,000 cases of trench or immersion foot were reported. The typical history is that of prolonged immobility in damp or frankly wet footwear. The initial coldness and numbness are usually tolerated by the exposed individual until he returns to a warm environment. He then experiences severe burning pain with swelling and redness. In the initial period the extremity may be cold and pale, or blue, and the patient may complain of paresthesia. The peripheral pulses are usually difficult to palpate because of edema. Warming the leg produces hyperemia with return of the pulses unless there is underlying vascular pathology. Blisters filled with serous fluid form in the edematous skin. Ulceration with superimposed infection and gangrene may eventually occur. The burning sensation is persistent and most distressing for the patient. If improperly treated, the patient may be left with a permanently cold extremity which may be uncomfortable even in a warm environment. Hypersensitivity to cold is a frequent sequel. In the emergency room, it is imperative to prevent further damage to the affected extremity which is anesthetic and may be easily injured without the patient's being aware of it. It should be wrapped in cotton or wool and the weight of bed linen taken off by the use of a footboard. The leg is kept elevated to prevent edema. Even mild antiseptics and local heat are avoided, as these may further damage the skin. Intra-arterial injection of vasodilators may help but the effect is usually transient.

Similar changes occur in sailors immersed for nonlethal periods in cold seawater.

FROSTBITE.   In this condition actual freezing of tissues exposed to temperatures below 32°F occurs. The fingers, toes, ears, and nose are most commonly affected. Frostbite can be considered as analogous to burns in the grading of tissue damage. In the mild form, the affected part turns white or waxy and is numb. Rewarming produces a tingling feeling and no special therapy is required. A residual mild degree of susceptibility to refrosting may remain.

In a moderate degree of frostbite, blisters form and are followed by desquamation, as in severe sunburn. In the severe form, the skin and subcutaneous tissues are affected with loss of sensation and varying depths of necrosis.

Diagnosis in the emergency room is established from the history and the above-described manifestations. Rapid rewarming has been found to give the best results. The injured part is placed in warm water (about 99°F) and the temperature is kept steady. All wet and restricting clothes are removed. Caution should be taken to prevent additional injury to the anesthetic extremity. The patient is placed on chemotherapy to prevent infection of the frozen part. Intra-arterial injection of lidocaine and papaverine may be considered to release coexisting vasospasm in the initial management. Following rewarming, the extremity should be examined for the presence of pulses, the state of capillary filling, and for evidence of underlying arterial disease. When only one of the extremities is affected despite equal exposure to both limbs, this should be viewed with suspicion, as underlying atherosclerotic occlusive disease may be responsible. The patient with frostbite often has residual hypersensitivity to cold; therefore, he should be warned to protect himself from further exposure which may cause early tissue damage.

Radical débridement is contraindicated because the depth of injury is usually less than that estimated by the initial examiner.

COMPLICATIONS OF VASCULAR DISEASES

Acute Arterial Occlusion

The sudden cessation of blood flow in an artery, by embolism or by acute thrombosis, necessitates immediate recognition and management to prevent gangrene.

EMBOLISM. This is manifested by sudden pain followed by pallor and coldness in an extremity, usually in middle-aged or elderly patients with underlying heart disease. Atrial fibrillation, coronary thrombosis, and mitral stenosis are the most common predisposing processes leading to embolism. Sometimes, however, the source of the embolus is not found even after thorough examination. An arterial embolus travels in a continually narrowing stream until it becomes lodged usually at a bifurcation. Common sites are the femoral, the iliac, and the popliteal arteries. Anoxia is produced in tissues distal to the block, with immediate and severe pain, followed by motor and sensory deficits. Stagnation of blood distal to the block leads to thrombosis in the peripheral arterial channels. If the block persists long enough for the thrombosis to involve the small arteries diffusely, embolectomy will not restore flow and gangrene will follow. The need for early diagnosis and immediate operation is obvious. The optimum period for operation is within the first 5 to 6 hours after the occlusion has occurred. Surgical intervention during this period usually will give satisfactory results. Nevertheless embolectomy should still be done despite a longer time lag. On examination the involved extremity is pale and cold. Distal pulses and oscillometric deviations are absent, while those proximal to the block are present. This helps in locating the site of occlusion. With the passage of time the extremity will show gross ischemic changes. The skin becomes discolored and the presence of rigor in the muscles indicates irreversibility. Arteriography will accurately demonstrate the site of the block but it is not carried out if it will lead to undue delay of an imperative operation.

ACUTE ARTERIAL THROMBOSIS.   This often affects patients with a history of claudication or other ischemic symptoms. Thrombosis usually occurs in an arterial segment already narrowed by atherosclerosis. The presenting symptoms are similar to those seen in embolism although usually they are not as acute. This is attributed to the progressive nature of the atherosclerotic process which promotes the development of collateral circulation. However, relief of the obstruction is mandatory, as the prognosis is otherwise poor. Immediate thrombectomy is indicated and, if successful, consideration is given for a later elective reconstructive procedure.

INITIAL MANAGEMENT OF ACUTE ARTERIAL OCCLUSION.   The patient is kept in a warm environment and heat is applied to the trunk or the unaffected extremities to produce reflex vasodilatation in the ischemic limb. External trauma to the ischemic extremity should be prevented by wrapping it in a thick layer of cotton. When arterial spasm is considered a factor contributing to ischemia, lidocaine and papaverine injected intra-arterially may be helpful.

Ruptured Abdominal Aneurysm

Ruptured abdominal aortic aneurysm is one of the common emergencies caused by atherosclerosis. The usual history is that of an elderly male with previous low-grade back pain which suddenly increases in severity. The pain is persistent and not relieved by changing position or analgesics. Sometimes there may have been a preexisting pulsatile abdominal mass. The patient will usually present with a varying degree of shock owing to severe blood loss.

Aneurysms are most often of atherosclerotic origin and involve the lower abdominal aorta below the renal arteries. On examination a tender pulsatile mass is felt in the abdomen. The femoral pulses are usually present, and there is no evidence of ischemia in the lower extremities. Plain films of the abdomen in the anteroposterior, lateral, and oblique projections will, in the majority of cases, show a rim of calcification in the aortic region. Flank ecchymoses secondary to the retroperitoneal hemorrhage are sometimes present.

These patients need immediate operation in spite of their poor condition. An intravenous cannula or wide-bore catheter should be inserted and Ringer's lactate started until compatible blood is available. A catheter is inserted in the bladder to monitor urinary output. However, effective resuscitation is only achieved by the control of bleeding at operation. Valuable time should not be wasted in trying to restore the blood volume to normal levels by transfusion of fluids and blood, which are usually lost into the retroperitoneal space faster than they can be infused. Overenthusiastic resuscitation may result in exsanguination of the patient, since the rising blood pressure increases bleeding. Every effort should be made to expedite the transfer of the patient to the operating room.

Dissecting Aneurysm of the Aorta

In most instances this is the result of cystic medial necrosis and a tear in the overlying intima. The origin is most frequently found just beyond the aortic valve in the ascending aorta. Distally the extension is variable and therefore the clinical manifestations depend on the progress of the dissection. Paraplegia or hemiplegia are not uncommon, although abdominal symptoms predominate in other cases. A tearing agonizing pain in the back is initially experienced and shock may follow. Differentiation from acute myocardial infarction may be difficult. Early evaluation is important because the patient's condition may suddenly deteriorate. As the dissection progresses, the loosened intima may balloon into the lumen, thereby blocking the origin of the branches of the aorta, with symptoms dependent upon the specific vessels occluded. Murmurs may be produced by the turbulence through abnormal openings. The presence of an aortic diastolic murmur is of significant diagnostic value. A double aortic shadow, widening of the supracardiac space, and pleural effusion mainly on the left side are characteristic roentgenographic findings. The diagnosis is confirmed by aortography, which demonstrates the extent of the dissection. Since death may occur suddenly, the importance of speedy assessment and proper initial management cannot be overemphasized.

Venous Thrombosis and Pulmonary Embolism

Venous thrombosis may affect the superficial or deep veins most commonly in the lower extremity.

SUPERFICIAL VENOUS THROMBOSIS.   This results from trauma, injection of sclerosing agents, venous stasis, or infection. The intima is initially affected and thrombosis gradually follows. The thrombus is usually firmly attached to the wall of the vein and only rarely does it detach and cause pulmonary embolism.

On examination, the area over the thrombosed vein is warm and painful, and a tender cordlike vein is usually palpable. Swelling if present is slight. Venography is indicated only when concomitant deep vein thrombosis is suspected. The immediate management consists of rest and elevation of the leg. Active leg exercises are encouraged to prevent deep venous thrombosis. Antibiotics are given if infection is present. Anticoagulants are not indicated in superficial vein thrombosis, and thrombectomy is considered only when the thrombus extends into the femoral vein.

DEEP VENOUS THROMBOSIS.   Thrombi originate in the calf or the iliofemoral veins as a result of stasis, injury of the vein wall, or increased coagulability of the blood. Early recognition and treatment are important in preventing pulmonary embolism and chronic venous insufficiency of the extremity. Thrombosis of the calf veins is often difficult to diagnose owing to lack of early local signs. Unexplained mild pyrexia and tachycardia in a patient confined to bed should be suggestive of deep vein thrombosis. The patient may complain of aching pain and tenderness in the calf and ankle edema. Phlebography or the use of fibrinogen ^{125}I is indicated to detect the presence and extent of thrombosis. Early management includes elevation of the foot of the bed, active exercises of the leg, and administration of heparin or of thrombolytic enzymes under careful laboratory control.

ILIOFEMORAL VEIN THROMBOSIS. The thrombosis may start in the iliofemoral veins or extend from the calf veins. There is usually pain, tenderness, and marked swelling over the entire extremity, and the skin is tense and shiny. The thrombosis may be silent with pulmonary embolism as the first sign. Management is similar to that of calf vein thrombosis. In the early stages thrombectomy should be considered.

PHLEGMASIA CERULEA DOLENS. This is acute massive thrombosis of major venous trunks and their tributaries. It presents with severe pain, extensive edema, and discoloration of the extremity. A varying degree of shock is present, and the peripheral pulses may be diminished or absent because of swelling. The general management is similar to that described above. Thrombectomy is indicated, since gangrene may occur in some cases. Venous thrombosis less frequently occurs in the inferior vena cava, the superior vena cava, and the axillary vein.

PULMONARY EMBOLISM. This is the most serious complication of deep vein thrombosis. It is commonly seen in middle-aged and elderly patients confined to bed. The clinical picture depends on the size of the embolus, usually consisting of sudden severe pain in the chest, dyspnea, tachycardia, hemoptysis, and pyrexia. The presence of rales, decreased aeration, and a friction rub are the features of established pulmonary infarction. Massive embolism is followed by severe shock and cyanosis. Chest roentgenograms, the electrocardiogram, and blood gas determinations may help in the diagnosis which is established by lung scanning and pulmonary angiography. Immediate management consists of general measures to combat shock, such as intravenous fluids, oxygen administration, and analgesics. Anticoagulants or fibrinolytic enzymes are given under appropriate laboratory control. Embolectomy is considered in massive embolism not responding to medical treatment.

Rupture of Varicose Veins

Rupture of a varix in the leg is an uncommon occurrence and can be easily managed. The skin overlying the varix may be thin, owing to pressure, and may eventually erode. Hemorrhage can be significant, and attempts at reducing the flow in a standing or sitting position are ineffective. Elevation of the leg along with pressure over the bleeding site will rapidly control the hemorrhage. The patient who presents with this complication will require elective operation for varicose veins at a later date.

Acute Superior Mesenteric Occlusion

This may be due to embolism or thrombosis and affects the main stem of the artery or only one of its branches. With the passage of time, there is distal propagation of the thrombus. As embolism is a sudden phenomenon, there is no time for collateral circulation to develop and therefore the symptoms are very acute. Mesenteric artery thrombosis may present with a similar clinical picture. The onset, however, is usually gradual, as it occurs in a previously stenosed atherosclerotic vessel and there has been time for some collateral circulation to develop. On examination in the emergency room the patient complains of severe midabdominal pain which is at first colicky, but later becomes constant. There may be vomiting of bloody fluid and explosive bloody diarrhea. Later the bowel sounds disappear and the abdomen becomes diffusely tender with obvious muscle spasm. The temperature and pulse are raised and there are signs of increasing toxicity. Abdominal paracentesis may reveal blood-stained fluid with a characteristic odor. For resuscitation, intravenous fluids and blood are administered to replace blood lost in the bowel and peritoneal cavity. Antibiotics are given to control infection. Selective mesenteric arteriography is valuable in establishing the diagnosis.

Abdominal Emergencies   *8*

HAROLD F. WELCH

TRAUMA

Penetrating injuries of the abdomen are of two main types: (1) gunshot wounds and (2) stab wounds. Prognosis of all penetrating wounds is related to the degree of shock.

Penetrating Wounds

GUNSHOT WOUNDS. All gunshot wounds should be evaluated and managed with a view to immediate surgical intervention. The operating room should be alerted at once. Severe internal bleeding, which is the main cause of death in patients with gunshot wounds, can be controlled only by operation. Surgical exploration should be considered an integral part of resuscitation. The following measures should be taken:

1. Any bullet wound between nipples and midthigh must be regarded as possibly causing abdominal injury.
2. The patient should be moved as little as possible to minimize the possibility of resumption of bleeding. All clothes should be quickly cut away. Respiratory and cardiac status should be examined, the number of wounds tabulated, and the vital signs taken repeatedly. Cutdowns for infusion should be done if possible in upper ex-

tremities, as the inferior vena cava may be lacerated with abdominal penetrating wounds.

3. An intravenous infusion should be started, preferably by the insertion of a No. 17 or No. 18 French polyethylene catheter into an arm vein. The initial infusion should be 0.85% sodium chloride or Ringer's lactate solution.

4. A central venous pressure catheter should be inserted and serial measurements made in all patients in shock.

5. A Levin tube should be inserted for aspiration of the stomach and detection of possible gastric wounding.

6. The urinary bladder should be catheterized for detection of genitourinary injury and for following postoperative renal status.

7. Tetanus prophylaxis should be instituted.

8. No débridement or probing of the wound should be done in the emergency room.

9. X-ray examination will add little more than localization of missile and presence of bone injury. It is more important when there is no exit wound. The value of the roentgenograms must be weighed against condition of the patient and x-ray procedure should not interfere with the resuscitation.

10. Police officials, always in attendance on these cases, should be kept from treatment areas.

ACUTE STAB WOUNDS.   Since stab wounds may be treacherous, the wisest course, when there is a possibility of penetration of the abdominal wall, is to examine the parietal peritoneum. This can be done *only* in the operating room. If the parietal peritoneum is pierced, complete exploration is indicated. The following are essential to remember:

1. Probing the wound in the emergency room is useless and dangerous.

2. The stomach is aspirated; many patients will show recent alcohol ingestion. However, this ingestion should not be a deterrent to a needed operation.

3. Most deaths from stab wounds of the abdomen result from a large-vessel laceration, which in the majority of cases is rapidly fatal. However, if the patient is fortunate enough to reach the emergency room alive, immediate recognition of the problem and operative control of bleeding offer the only chance of survival.

4. Roentgenograms of the abdomen and chest may be taken if

exsanguinating hemorrhage is not judged to be the most immediate problem. They are more important where there is possibility of diaphragmatic laceration.

5. If the stab wound is over 3 hours old, vital signs are normal, and there is no evidence of peritoneal soiling or of hemorrhage, the patient may be admitted and observed for 24 to 48 hours.

6. A number of hospitals in large cities where abdominal stab wounds are frequent use the technique of injecting water-soluble contrast radiographic media into the tract of the stab wound to distinguish wounds which have penetrated the peritoneum from those which have not. Only patients whose wounds have penetrated the peritoneum are operated upon. The technique of injection is simple. A small catheter is introduced into the wound and a purse-string suture is placed about it to prevent reflux of the radiographic media. Injection is carried out using a hand syringe. The procedure has been safe and accurate in the hands of those reporting upon its use.

Nonpenetrating Wounds

Four out of five patients hospitalized for abdominal injury are suffering from blunt or nonpenetrating injury. Some 40 percent of these will have multiple injuries. Whereas diagnosis is not a problem in penetrating abdominal wounds because injury is always presumed, it is paramount in the nonpenetrating or blunt injury. The following are important:

1. A high degree of suspicion should be entertained. A knowledge of the anatomical configuration of the abdominal contents is necessary, as is a concern that this portion of the body is not overlooked in relation to other, more overt injuries.

2. The presence of shock should make one very suspicious of intra-abdominal injury. Certainly hypotension and tachycardia in the absence of other severe injuries should suggest hemoperitoneum.

3. Evidence of peritoneal irritation and/or of internal bleeding should be the object of the search when one sets out to investigate a possible abdominal injury.

4. Often what is considered trivial trauma will be enough to injure the spleen or liver. One must not be misled. A fall of 2 to 3 feet may be sufficient; falling from a bicycle is a common cause of ruptured spleen in children.

LIVER AND SPLEEN.   Both of these organs may be injured together when the trauma is severe. Injury of the liver or spleen is manifest by signs and symptoms of internal bleeding. If the hematocrit reading continues to fall in a suspected abdominal injury, it is safer to ascribe it to continued bleeding than to hemodilution. The following are important:

1. Pallor, low hematocrit, hypotension, tachycardia, elevated leukocyte count, fracture of the lower ribs, and abrasions and contusions of the lower chest margin and upper abdomen are clues which suggest splenic or hepatic injury. If there is associated tenderness with muscle spasm in the left or right upper quadrants, or pain on top of the shoulder, the evidence is nearly complete for a visceral injury.

2. Roentgenograms, particularly a plain abdominal film may show haziness suggesting hemoperitoneum or localized haziness with displacement of the stomach gas bubble. If there is any question of kidney injury, an intravenous pyelogram should be done before surgery.

3. Abdominal paracentesis should be done early in those cases where the indication for exploration is thought equivocal. A blunt 18 gauge needle can be used. However, a small plastic catheter introduced over a Rochester needle is safer and will give a more reliable result. The paracentesis should be done first in the left upper quadrant if a ruptured spleen is the prime concern. Ready aspiration of blood is confirmatory evidence for bleeding, and exploration is indicated. False negative results are more common, and the paracentesis may be repeated in another quadrant if believed necessary. It should be remembered that paracentesis supplements the clinical impression; it does not supplant a careful evaluation. Peritoneal lavage with 500 ml of 0.9% saline solution will increase diagnostic accuracy. In this test the finding of either gross blood or a leukocytosis exceeding 800 cells per ml^3 in the effluent is significant. The catheter is inserted in the midline through a short incision. Accurate hemostasis should be obtained to prevent false positive results.

Delayed rupture of the spleen secondary to a subcapsular hematoma should come to mind when a patient presents with signs of internal bleeding several days to a week after abdominal trauma.

PANCREAS.   Pancreatic injury is rarely diagnosed as such in the emergency room. It most commonly follows penetrating wounds of the gunshot variety where there is multiple organ damage. In blunt trauma, it is the complication of pseudocyst formation that gives the first belated notice of pancreatic injury, although acute transection of the pancreas with signs and symptoms of an acute surgical abdomen is being seen more often.

SMALL AND LARGE INTESTINE.   Blunt trauma rarely injures the mobile portion of the bowel, as is often noted with a penetrating injury. Occasionally, actual disruption or perforation of the first portion of the jejunum will occur and the patient will rapidly develop signs of peritonitis. Usually in blunt trauma, the force of sudden deceleration is directed at the moorings of the bowel and tears of the mesentery are the most commonly seen injury. These may lead to bleeding or to devitalization of the bowel, the signs and symptoms of which are those of strangulation.

In certain compression injuries of the upper abdomen, the retroperitoneal duodenum may be compressed against the vertebrae and be lacerated or devitalized. The history of the injury is often quite important in making the diagnosis, although generally it is made only on exploration usually a few days after admission when persistent vomiting, upper abdominal tenderness, and gastrointestinal bleeding are noted.

SAFETY (SEAT) BELT INJURIES.   It must be emphasized that hundreds of lives have been saved by wearing a safety belt for each injury attributed to their use.

Both the lap-type safety belt and the shoulder-strap type have been associated with injuries to the soft parts and skeletal system. Abdominal injury is more frequent with the lap type than with the shoulder strap. When properly applied the lap-type snugly engages the bony pelvis just below the anterior-superior iliac spines. Under these circumstances there is little likelihood of intraperitoneal visceral injury (with the exception of the gravid uterus at term) upon impact at sublethal speed.

When the lap belt is loosely worn, however, shearing injury to the abdominal wall, as well as injury to almost all intra-abdominal viscera and the vertebral column, have all been reported. The mark of the belt may actually be left on the skin, or a hematoma may form, either of which suggest that the belt may have contributed to the injury of other structures.

The shoulder strap has also been the cause of a variety of abdominal, as well as thoracic injuries. Most spectacular are the decapitating injuries which have occurred when upon impact a door springs open and the driver (or occupant) is ejected while wearing a shoulder strap.

Maximum safety is provided by a combination of the lap belt and shoulder harness.

RECTAL INJURIES. Occasionally children will suffer trauma to the rectum or perianal area from falling and impaling themselves on sharp fences or tree branches. Since it may be difficult in the emergency room to estimate the seriousness of the injury, these children should be admitted where they can be observed and have sigmoidoscopic examination if necessary.

Patients with compressed-air injuries of the rectum, usually the result of a sadistic joke, should be considered as having a rupture of the bowel if there is any lower abdominal tenderness; they should be prepared for immediate surgery.

ABDOMINAL WALL AND RETROPERITONEAL INJURIES. Injuries confined to these areas well may simulate injuries to the abdominal organs; it may be difficult to differentiate between the tenderness and muscle spasm resulting from muscular injury and that of true peritoneal irritation. Retroperitoneal bleeding and contusion often produce adynamic ileus. Fractures of the transverse process of the lumbar spine, obliteration of the psoas muscle shadow on x-ray, and a negative paracentesis may help to solve the problem, although it is not usually resolved without repeated observation of the patient over a period of time.

THE ACUTE ABDOMEN

Patients with abdominal complaints should be placed in a private cubicle and should not be neglected in the press of other emergencies. They should be evaluated soon after their admission to the emergency room and a rapid estimate made of the seriousness of their problem.

The patient should be prepared by the nurse; his pulse, blood pressure, and temperature should be taken; and he should be completely undressed. It is a dangerous compromise to try to examine a patient through an aperture in his clothing. The basic evaluation of a person with an abdominal complaint is directed at determining whether the condition calls for surgery or not. If so, is an immediate operation necessary or can the patient be safely observed? In order to come to a conclusion regarding his disposition, a presumptive diagnosis must be made. Three basic questions should first be answered: Has the patient perforated a hollow viscus? Is he bleeding? Is he obstructed? In essence, how advanced is the inflammatory process, how severe the hemorrhage, how complete the obstruction? The history and complete physical examination, with the aid of a few laboratory examinations and x-ray, should enable the examiner to come to a rapid decision as to disposition and further treatment.

The history as taken in the emergency room should be aimed at securing a quick estimate of the problem. It is not a narrative but a purposeful cross-examination. Obviously, the more experienced the interrogator, the more pertinent the answers. The patient should be observed carefully during the history to see whether he exhibits restlessness, flaring of the alare nasi, or other overt manifestations of illness. It should be remembered that pain cannot be measured but only evaluated. Pain of more than four hours' duration is usually significant, while pain of lesser duration, i.e., one to two hours, without signs and symptoms of strangulation or peritonitis can often be safely observed. In women, the relation of the onset of pain should be correlated with the phase of the patient's menstrual cycle. Patients who have been chronically ill often have a lower threshold of pain.

Onset of Pain

Sudden abrupt pain often indicates a sudden occlusive process or a perforation of a viscus. Such entities as a ruptured ectopic pregnancy, perforated ulcer, mesenteric vascular occlusion, splenic or renal infarct, and ruptured corpus luteum should all be considered if the onset of pain is abrupt and severe. Pain which begins suddenly but reaches a maximum more slowly should suggest pancreatitis, ureteral stones, or cholecystitis. Appendicitis always must be kept in mind; this is the most common pathological process seen in patients complaining of abdominal pain in the emergency room.

Character of Pain

The colicky, episodic, paroxysmal pain of an obstructed hollow tube such as the ureter, intestine, or bile ducts is often diagnostic. The rhythmic periodicity of pain or waves of pain is characteristic of intestinal obstruction. In large-bowel obstruction this crampy pain is confined to the lower abdomen and is not as severe as that of small-bowel obstruction, in which it is characteristically periumbilical. The patient should be questioned carefully as to the presence of obstipation, or other changes in bowel habits if there is evidence of obstruction. The femoral and inguinal areas should be searched for presence of a hernia.

Radiation of Pain

Certain disorders will have typical patterns of pain radiation, which may be diagnostic. Ureteral pain is often referred to the groin and testicle; pain in the area of the scapula and/or right upper quadrant may be diagnostic of cholecystitis; collections of blood or pus under the diaphragm often will cause aching pain in the top of the shoulder. Ruptured or leaking aneurysms will give pain in the lumbosacral area and occasionally in the upper thighs. Other symptoms associated with the pain should be elucidated. Vomiting, anorexia, difficulty in urination, and obstipation should all be investigated and related to the onset of disease. The order of development of symptoms is important, especially in acute appendicitis, where the periumbilical or epigastric pain precedes the nausea and vomiting by a few hours.

Previous Hospitalization and Abdominal Operations

It is particularly important to know whether there has been hospitalization or abdominal surgery in the past. Many patients with pancreatitis, pelvic inflammatory disease, kidney stones, or peptic ulcer may have had previous admissions for these recurring problems. Knowledge of past surgery may be essential to correct interpretation of the new complaints. A telephone call to the record room of the previous admitting hospital often proves enlightening. Also, relatives or friends accompanying the patient to the emergency room should be questioned; they may well add to the validity of the history, especially in the very young or elderly. One must not be beguiled into minimizing the complaints of patients known for their hypochondriacal tendencies. Drug addicts may be extremely clever in their portrayal of a patient with abdominal pain. The severe symptoms they relate, however, are not in accord with the physical findings. Careful physical examination may also reveal evidence of their addiction, such as scarring of the arms with thrombosis of the superficial veins. These patients are usually wary of admission to the hospital.

Physical Examination

Palpation of the abdomen is the most important facet of the physical examination. It should be done gently, avoiding the area designated by the patient as the most tender until last. It is helpful to distract the patient, especially if he is a child, while palpating the abdomen. Observing facial expressions of the patient during the examination often gives a clue to the seriousness of the problem. During the examination the left side is compared to the right, the degree of spasm is noted, the amounts of pressure needed to elicit tenderness are compared, and masses are searched for. Rebound tenderness is elicited last. Obviously one tries to reduce the voluntary responses and looks for involuntary reflexes secondary to peritoneal irritation. If a pulsating mass is felt and the patient is complaining of sudden abdominal pain radiating to the flanks or upper thighs, the possibility of a leaking abdominal aneurysm is most likely and the patient's subsequent work-up should be managed with this as the most likely diagnosis.

AUSCULTATION. The absence of bowel sounds in a patient with abdominal complaints is an extremely serious sign, for it indicates paralysis of the bowel, often secondary to generalized peritonitis. A reflex ileus is seen in some retroperitoneal injuries; however, usually this is not the ominous silence of generalized peritonitis. The abdomen should be listened to for three minutes in either of the two lower quadrants. Sounds of intestinal obstruction are usually characteristic, with crescendo waves reaching a maximum coincident with crampy pain. High-pitched tinkling sounds may be heard between the intervals of the pain. These sounds, together with the distended, tympanitic abdomen and the x-ray observations, should lead one to an early presumptive diagnosis of intestinal obstruction.

PERCUSSION. Percussion has a limited value in the physical examination in the emergency room. Fluid waves and shifting dullness may be difficult to detect and more difficult to interpret. However, the detection of tympany aids in the diagnosis of intestinal obstruction or gastric dilatation. Distension of the cecum as revealed by percussion should lead the examiner to suspect appendicitis or sigmoid obstruction.

RECTAL EXAMINATION. The rectal examination in adults and children should be an integral part of the physical examination and should not be omitted on the assumption that others will do it eventually after the patient is admitted. Although the pain may be confined to the upper abdomen and not patently associated with bowel complaints, the examiner should still check the rectum noting whether the ampulla is empty, whether masses can be palpated, and whether tenderness is present. In general, the findings on rectal examination in infants and small children under the age of 7 or 8 are hard to interpret. Patients complaining of rectal pain should have anoscopic examination. To be worthwhile, this should be done with good lighting. Occasionally the condition is too painful and the patient will have to be admitted to be examined under anesthesia. To persist in trying to examine patients with severe rectal pain without anesthesia is often frustrating and usually unrewarding.

Patients with knifelike pain in the anal region on defecation will usually demonstrate an anal fissure in the posterior midline. Those with fever and inability to sit, presenting with induration in the perianal region, will usually have ischiorectal abscess. Fluctuance is a late manifestation and is not necessary for the diagnosis of ischiorectal abscess. Admission to the hospital for early incision and drainage is indicated.

VAGINAL EXAMINATION. The vaginal examination is essential in women complaining of lower abdominal discomfort. Anyone so examined in the emergency room should be prepared by the nurse and put in stirrups to make the examination complete. A vaginal smear should first be obtained for bacteriological evaluation. Milking the urethra for pus is important if gonorrhea is present, for associated urethritis is a common accompaniment. Bimanual palpation and combined rectal and vaginal examination are essential. Examination of patients in whom the problem of rape has been implicated should be extremely thorough and if possible done by a competent gynecologist, inasmuch as litigation will be involved. See Chapter 10.

External Hernias

Indirect inguinal, femoral, and umbilical hernias present as acute emergencies when they suddenly become irreducible. This event may or may not be attended by local pain and tenderness. Regardless of the presence or absence of symptoms and signs suggesting strangulation, an acutely incarcerated hernia must be considered strangulated until proved otherwise. An attempt at reduction by gentle taxis is justified in acutely incarcerated hernias without significant local pain or tenderness. Small doses of morphine and barbiturates may increase the likelihood of success of reduction by promoting muscular relaxation. When successful reduction has been accomplished, operative repair need not be done on an emergency basis, but operation should not be unduly delayed, for the likelihood of recurrent incarceration is great.

Patients presenting with clinical evidence of acute intestinal obstruction as well as patients with local pain, tenderness, edema, or redness of the skin are surgical emergencies. Operation should be performed as soon as fluid and electrolyte replacement therapy has progressed sufficiently to assure an adequate urinary output.

Place of Roentgenograms in the Diagnosis of Acute Abdomen

Roentgenograms may be invaluable in confirming certain diagnoses. However, the physician should be able to estimate the seriousness of the problem without them. It must be recognized that the value of the roentgenogram lies in accurate interpretation. One of the dangers of ordering roentgenograms is that the gravely ill patient may be stranded in the radiology department waiting for confirmatory films when he should be receiving treatment in preparation for operation.

In ordering roentgenograms, the physician should specify exactly what he wants, not leaving the choice of films to the technician. It is important to include the diaphragm when one is looking for free air as well as a lower abdominal film when one is interested in establishing the presence or absence of kidney or ureteral stones. A film of the chest should always be included when abdominal films are ordered. More importantly, the physician ordering the studies should review them himself, as he is the most familiar with the clinical findings and can relate them to the roentgenograms.

Laboratory Aids in the Diagnosis of Acute Abdomen

The number of laboratory tests that can be made is limited essentially by the time of the day and the imagination of the physician.

Practically speaking, the diagnostic studies, apart from the examination of the urine, a complete blood count, and a few other relevant tests such as those for amylase and blood urea nitrogen, should be accomplished after admission.

1. A clean catch specimen of urine from a male or a catheterized specimen from a female should be examined for leukocytes and erythrocytes. The urine should also be tested for sugar and albumin.

2. A complete blood count should be made with a differential count of the leukocytes.

3. A serum amylase test should also be made in patients with abdominal pain when diagnosis is obscure.

4. If a patient has a history of any internal or gastrointestinal bleeding, he should be typed and cross matched upon admission or entrance to the emergency room without waiting for the hemoglobin determination and hematocrit if the physical examination indicates that he is in shock or appears to be severely anemic.

5. Diagnostic paracentesis will rarely be necessary, but occasionally, when a patient's condition is critical and the need for further information is imperative, it is required. The aspiration of bile, exudate, or bloody transudate may clinch the diagnosis. Paracentesis should be avoided, however, if the patient is distended or if there are numerous abdominal surgical scars.

Treatment of the Acute Abdomen in the
Emergency Room

The treatment of the acute abdomen in the emergency room should be supportive only. At the time blood for laboratory examinations is drawn, intravenous therapy should be started, preferably with a large-gauge needle. Dehydrated patients with a history of vomiting should be given a balanced salt solution before admission to the floor. Patients with a history and evidence of gastrointestinal bleeding should be assessed as to the extent of hemorrhage and have their blood typed and cross matched in preparation for transfusion. The amount of blood requested to be typed and cross matched is dependent upon the condition and the patient. Generally, a patient appearing with hypotension, a rapid pulse, and a history of gastrointestinal bleeding should have a minimum of three units of blood cross matched. Patients admitted in shock from bleeding should not be moved from the emergency room until resuscitated unless there is evidence that bleeding is massive and the resuscitation ineffectual without immediate surgical intervention. Those in whom immediate operation is indicated, as for a perforated ulcer, are best prepared for operation while in the emergency room. A Levin tube should be inserted and also a retention catheter, especially in older men.

Observation

Certain patients should be placed in the observation unit until the diagnosis becomes clear. In general, it is wiser to admit the patient to the hospital than to send him home if the examining physician is unsure of the problem. Not uncommonly, the diagnosis becomes apparent only after repeated examination. Surgical consultation should be obtained before admission or shortly after, so that the sequential examinations can be made by the person who will be responsible for operative management if it becomes necessary. In the majority of cases the problem will be reasonably resolved within 24 hours and the patient discharged or admitted to the general hospital. The lessening of abdominal pain, the return of appetite, and the presence of normal vital signs are encouraging, while the persistence of tenderness, anorexia, and leukocytosis is disquieting. During an initial period of indecision, the patient should be hydrated with intravenous fluids, given nothing by mouth, and observed frequently. The natural history of appendicitis may go from vague symptoms to obvious perforation in four to six hours, and only by frequent examinations can such a catastrophe be avoided. Narcotics should not be given during the period of observation unless a surgeon has come to a decision concerning the diagnosis and believes they will not confuse his further examination.

Urological Emergencies 9

HAROLD E. MARDEN, JR.

Genitourinary injuries usually occur in association with damage to other areas of the body and may therefore be overlooked with disastrous consequences unless an effort is made to discover their presence and extent as soon as possible. A urine specimen should be obtained, by catheterization if necessary, and examined in all patients with a history of major trauma. The abdomen, flanks, genitalia, and rectum should be checked. If the urine is clear microscopically and these areas are normal to physical examination, major urological injury is very unlikely. If there is hematuria, obstruction to passage of a soft rubber catheter, or tenderness or mass in any of the above areas, further studies must be carried out. These should be done as soon as possible, preferably before the patient leaves the emergency room. They are usually carried out as soon as an airway has been established, external bleeding controlled, and treatment of shock begun. Trying to evaluate the upper urinary tracts with a patient in deepening shock or with the abdomen open on the operating table is highly undesirable and can be avoided by early diagnostic studies.

INJURIES

Kidney

Blows to the flank, lumbar area, or lower lateral rib cage can cause kidney injuries. On the left the spleen is often injured as well,

and on the right the liver. There is hematuria except very occasionally when the renal vascular pedicle has been completely severed. If
there is significant bleeding into the perirenal space, tenderness,
abdominal muscle spasm, and a flank mass will be observed. These
signs should be checked for repeatedly to see if they are present or
are increasing. The patient's hematocrit and urine should also be
followed as indications of the continuing degree of hemorrhage.
An intravenous pyelogram without bowel preparation or dehydration should be done immediately. A double or larger dose of contrast material is often useful if there is poor concentration and
visualization with the usual dose. The injured side should be examined for extravasation, loss of psoas shadow, and normal renal
outline (psoas shadow normally not visible in 20 percent) and function. It should also be noted whether the uninjured kidney appears
normal in case the damaged one needs to be removed. Unless there
is evidence of extravasation by x-ray or clinical signs of massive
continuing hemorrhage, most renal injuries can be treated by rest
and observation and only about 5 percent will require operation.
Renal angiography and retrograde pyelography are of use occasionally. Abnormal kidneys, especially if they are enlarged, are more
easily injured than normal ones. When hematuria results from
minor injury, preexisting renal disease should be suspected.

Bladder

Bladder injuries result from blows to the abdomen when the
bladder is full or nearly so, since it is very difficult to injure an
empty bladder. Therefore, there is widespread infiltration of large
amounts of urine around and/or into the peritoneal cavity, depending on the site of rupture. Signs of peritoneal irritation will develop
although it may be several hours before they appear. Shifting dullness can sometimes be elicited. The diagnosis should be suspected if
there is hematuria or the patient cannot void and if there is only a
small amount of bloody urine in the bladder on catheterization. The
diagnosis may be established by doing a cystogram or cystourethrogram with 50 to 100 ml of contrast material. It will be hard to irrigate
the catheter. If injected fluid cannot be aspirated out again, large
amounts of irrigating fluid should not be introduced.

Delay in the recognition of bladder rupture increases the risk of
peritonitis or retroperitoneal infection due to the presence of urine
and of an opening into the urinary tract. Early drainage of the

areas of extravasation and of the bladder is required as well as closure of the bladder laceration.

Urethra

Urethral injuries usually occur from indirect trauma with fractures of the bony pelvis. The urethra is partially or completely torn across between the apex of the prostate and the urogenital diaphragm. If the tear is complete, the ends will be separated by several centimeters and will also be out of line so that a catheter cannot be inserted into the bladder. Damage to the anterior urethra can occur from lacerations, from sharp instruments, or from straddle injuries. Fractures of the pelvis or lacerations or subcutaneous hematomas in the vicinity of the anterior urethra require examination of the urine and further investigation if erythrocytes are found. If a soft rubber catheter cannot be passed easily, a cystourethrogram should be carried out by injecting contrast material through the external urethral meatus. If the urethra is injured above the urogenital diaphragm, there will be dissection of blood and urine retroperitoneally around the bony pelvis as well as extravasation of the contrast material by roentgenogram. Bleeding is usually considerable because of the extensive venous plexus around the prostate and bladder neck. Early evacuation of the blood and urine and drainage of the pelvis and bladder are necessary. There is some debate as to the best time to repair the urethra but that is beyond the scope of this chapter.

Partial tears can be treated by indwelling catheters alone, if a catheter can be inserted. Forceful repeated attempts at instrumentation should not be made. Injuries to the urethra from instrumentation are common and may be treated by indwelling catheters, if insertion is possible, and antibiotics. If catheterization cannot be accomplished easily, a suprapubic trochar cystostomy may be done, in the emergency room if necessary.

GENITOURINARY INFECTIONS

Urethritis

Gonorrhea is caused by *Neisseria gonorrhoeae*. After an incubation period of 2 to 7 days, severe dysuria with urinary frequency and urethral discharge appear. Previous infection does not give immunity. Gram stain of the urethral discharge is 98 percent accurate in the male so that culture is not usually necessary. The organism can be grown on chocolate or ascitic fluid agar under CO_2. Fluorescent antibody techniques can be useful, especially in women. The usual therapy is 300,000 to 500,000 units penicillin daily for 3 days or about 1,000,000 units of one of the prolonged-action forms of penicillin. The resistance of the *Gonococcus* is gradually increasing throughout the world so that larger and larger doses of penicillin are being required. Chloramphenicol or tetracyclines can be used as an alternative, usually 500 mg four times a day for 5 days. The patient should be reexamined after treatment to be sure of cure. Serological tests for syphilis should be done after 1 and 4 months.

Nonspecific urethritis or prostatitis presents with similar but usually milder symptoms. Most of the common organisms of urinary infections can be found on smear or culture, as well as fungi, trichomonads, L organisms, *Candida albicans, Schistosoma, Mimea,* and *Neisseria catarrhalis.* Which if any of these are the true causative agents is questionable. Response will usually occur to sulfa drugs, nitrofurantoin, or broad-spectrum antibiotics, but cultures with drug-sensitivity determinations should be done in order to select the appropriate drug and dosage better.

Ulcerated Lesions of the Genitalia

In *syphilis* the primary lesion, the chancre, may range from a small inconspicuous papule to a large, sharply punched out, non-tender ulcer appearing 2 to 8 weeks after exposure. Moist papules from secondary lues may also appear. Diagnosis is by dark-field examination of fresh fluid from the lesion. The primary lesion may be present for 1 or more weeks before the serology becomes positive. Treatment consists of 2,400,000 units benzathine penicillin or 4,800,-000 units procaine penicillin in oil and aluminum monostearate in divided doses of 1,200,000 each. Thirty grams tetracycline over 20 to 25 days may also be used. The lesions are noninfectious within 24 hours of the beginning of therapy.

Chancroid is caused by *Haemophilus ducreyi* and is usually characterized by a rapidly growing, destructive, painful, eroding ulcer. Incubation period is 3 to 5 days. Diagnosis is by smear or culture of the ulcer or enlarged inguinal nodes. The organism is a small gram-negative rod which grows best on blood agar. Response will usually occur to chloramphenicol.

Granuloma inguinale appears as an elevated soft papule or serpiginous ulcer. The causative agent is *Donovania granulomatis* and the incubation period is 8 days to 12 weeks. Donovan bodies are seen in phagocytes and are small, deeply staining, round or rodlike bodies, best demonstrated by Wright's stain. Diagnosis is made by smear of the lesion after the removal of crusts.

Nonspecific balanoposthitis may be confused with any of the above and must be differentiated by smear and culture. Treatment is by saline soaks, broad-spectrum antibiotics, and dorsal slit if needed.

Neoplasms must also be considered in all penile lesions, especially in the uncircumcised.

Urinary Infections

Urinary infections may be mild to very severe. There is usually dysuria and urinary frequency but there also may be severe suprapubic and/or flank pain, fever, nausea, and vomiting. The extent of treatment depends upon the severity of the acute process. If the patient is able to retain oral fluids in large amounts and does not have an excessively high fever or evidence of shock, hospitalization is not usually necessary. A gram stain of the urinary sediment is the most useful procedure when the patient is first seen, but cultures with drug-sensitivity determinations should also be started.

The most common organisms in descending order of frequency are *Escherichia coli, Aerobacter aerogenes, Proteus* organisms, *Pseudomonas aeruginosa,* staphylococci, and streptococci. Acute infections will usually respond to sulfa drugs, nitrofurantoin, or broad-spectrum antibiotics. The most important aspect of care is to be sure that the patient is followed closely thereafter and treated long enough to give the best chance of permanent cure of the infection; 3 weeks is the minimum time desirable for drug therapy of an acute infection.

Septicemia

Urinary tract infection, especially after instrumentation, may be accompanied by septicemia with endotoxic shock. Early recognition greatly influences the mortality rate which is distressingly high at best. The most common etiologic agents are *E. coli, A. aerogenes, Proteus* organisms, *Pseudomonas aeruginosa,* staphylococci, and streptococci. Any patient who suddenly develops a high fever, tachycardia, hypotension, or oliguria, along with other symptoms of urinary infection, especially after urinary tract instrumentation, should be suspected of having septicemia. Urine and blood cultures must be made, but treatment should be started immediately without waiting for results. The following are the general principles of treatment, but the details will need to be varied according to the circumstances:

1. Drain any urinary tract obstruction or other accumulation of pus.

2. Monitor the central venous pressure and the pH, pCO_2 and pO_2 of arterial blood if possible.

3. Give large doses of antibiotics parenterally to cover all the likely organisms, such as penicillin, 5 to 10 million units intravenously, kanamycin sulfate, 15 mg per kilogram per day intramuscularly in divided doses 6 to 8 hours apart.

4. Parenteral fluids regulated according to the central venous pressure and urine output plus perhaps intravenous mannitol.

5. Give isoproterenol hydrochloride intravenously at rate of 0.5 to 30 μg/minute using solution of 1 mg in 500 ml 5% glucose in water. Adjust rate on basis of pulse rate, central venous pressure, blood pressure, and urine output.

6. Intubation and respiratory assistance may be needed, depending upon the blood gas findings.

URETERAL COLIC

Ureteral colic is seen very commonly in an emergency room, and there is often a previous history of urinary tract disease to help. Severe colicky flank pain, radiating into the scrotum or vulva on the affected side, and microscopic hematuria will usually make the diagnosis, but there can be confusion with appendicitis, gastroenteritis, vasitis, and pyelonephritis. The responsible physician should examine a fresh urine specimen microscopically himself. The few blood cells present will often hemolyze if the urine is allowed to stand around. It is often advisable to have someone watch the patient void because of the frequency with which addicts will use pretended colic in an attempt to obtain drugs. I have never seen a patient with active ureteral colic who did not have microscopic hematuria if the urine was examined promptly. One should therefore be suspicious when none is found.

If the differential diagnosis is at all doubtful, an emergency intravenous pyelogram can be made without preparation. The patients are usually dehydrated anyway from anorexia and vomiting, and laxatives or enemas will only make their paralytic ileus worse.

ACUTE URINARY RETENTION

There are a number of different reasons for urinary retention, and, unless the patient has had previous similar episodes, the differential diagnosis must be made rather hurriedly in a patient who is in severe distress. Injudicious instrumentation can lead to grave or even fatal complications, or, by the production of a false passage, cause continuing difficulties in instrumentation throughout the patient's life. A small, soft rubber catheter, preferably with a coudé tip, and much lubrication should be tried first. If it cannot be passed, Phillips filiforms and followers are the safest and most useful instruments and should be available in all emergency rooms. If used properly these are entirely safe. Metal sounds and catheter stylets should never be used except in very experienced hands; even then they are hazardous. Urethral strictures and prostatic enlargements are the most common causes of obstruction. Strictures can be dilated with filiforms and followers to No. 18 or No. 20 French and referred for further dilatation at intervals. Prostatic urethral obstructions are usually best treated by an indwelling catheter and hospitalization.

Instrumentation should be avoided as much as possible in the presence of infection.

Urinary retention due to meatal stricture is not uncommon, especially in children who have been circumcised. It can be treated by urethral meatotomy under local anesthesia.

Urinary retention may be the presenting symptom of neurological disease, particularly multiple sclerosis, poliomyelitis, or herniated intervertebral disk. These should be borne in mind whenever no apparent reason can be found for urinary retention. Acute spinal cord injuries require early insertion of an indwelling catheter. Permanent damage to the bladder can result from overdistension and is easily avoided if thought of.

ACUTE SCROTAL PAIN AND SWELLING

A number of pathological conditions which must be differentiated promptly for proper treatment are manifested in scrotal pain and swelling.

Torsion of the spermatic cord is an acute surgical emergency requiring immediate operation and detorsion if the testis is to be saved. Since this occurs usually in the teens and twenties, salvage is obviously important, and unless correction is carried out within several hours gangrene of the testis will occur. Torsion is characterized by sudden onset with severe pain, shock, nausea, and vomiting. On examination the testis is high in the scrotum and extremely tender. Elevation of the testis increases the pain (Plehn's sign). The urine is normal. (There may be a history of previous similar episodes with spontaneous remission.)

Torsion of the appendix testis (hydatid of Morgagni) has similar but milder symptoms with less local and systemic reaction.

Acute epididymitis comes on more gradually with milder systemic complaints. If there is not too much swelling, the enlarged epididymis can be distinguished from the testis, which is normal. Elevation of the testis reduces the pain. There will often be pyuria and prostatic enlargement and tenderness. If the differential diagnosis between this and torsion is in doubt, the scrotum should be explored, since no harm will result if epididymitis is present and an ischemic testis may be saved.

Incarcerated or strangulated hernia can be confused if careful physical examination is not done. Presence of bowel sounds or an impulse on coughing or straining are of help in differentiation.

An acute hydrocele may occur with any inflammatory process in the scrotum and make examination difficult. If necessary this can be evacuated with a syringe and needle in order better to palpate the testes and appendages. One must, of course, be sure he is not dealing with a hernia before using this procedure.

HEMATURIA

A common presenting complaint with a number of acute urological problems is hematuria. Injuries, calculi, neoplasms, and urinary infections are often associated with bleeding. Whenever possible, except in injuries, an emergency cystoscopy should be done, since the source of bleeding can be identified much more easily and certainly while it is going on. If the opportunity is lost, the bleeding may cease, adding greatly to the extent, cost, discomfort, and inaccuracy of investigation.

PHIMOSIS AND PARAPHIMOSIS

Phimosis, or the inability to retract the foreskin, causes problems by promoting infection from poor drainage under the foreskin or occasionally by interfering with urination. If the infection is severe or there is sufficient narrowing to cause urinary retention, a dorsal slit is necessary. This can be done under local anesthesia by infiltrating the dorsal prepuce and then making a longitudinal incision down to about 0.5 cm from the coronal sulcus through both layers. Bleeders are ligated, and the skin and mucosa approximated along the edges. It is not advisable to do a circumcision under these conditions.

Paraphimosis, or entrapment of a tight foreskin behind the glans penis, can usually be reduced by maintaining steady traction on the foreskin with pressure on the glans to reduce edema. This maneuver may need to be kept up for several minutes. If it fails, a dorsal slit is necessary.

Obstetrical and Gynecological Emergencies

10

MANUEL J. PEARL

Obstetrical and gynecological emergency problems the physician may be called upon to handle in the hospital emergency room may vary from acute discomforts of minor consequence (vaginitis, dysmenorrhea) to life-threatening situations requiring prompt diagnosis and management. The most acute life-threatening situations are generally associated with vaginal hemorrhage and shock. However, fulminating toxemia of pregnancy and acute pelvic peritonitis also constitute serious emergencies.

VAGINAL HEMORRHAGE

A comprehensive consideration of all causes of vaginal bleeding would necessitate a complete treatise on obstetrical and gynecological pathology. In terms of emergency treatment, it is sufficient to indicate certain broad categories which require special attention. In the nonpregnant state only unusually heavy bleeding warrants emergency care. It should be emphasized, however, that any amount of vaginal bleeding associated with a known or suspected pregnancy should be regarded as an emergency until the condition is adequately evaluated and at least a tentative diagnosis established. Bleeding associated with gestational disorders may become profuse with alarming suddenness. It is helpful to remember the few general causes of massive or profuse bleeding, so-called gushing or flooding. These are (1) pregnancy complications, (2) genital cancer, (3) submucous myoma, and (4) dysfunctional uterine bleeding.

Pregnancy

ANTEPARTUM—LESS THAN 20 WEEKS' GESTATION

ABORTION. The diagnosis of abortion is made on the basis of a history of amenorrhea or a missed period, cramping, vaginal bleeding, and the findings on pelvic examination. The patient may or may not describe the passage of "tissue" or an actual embryo or fetus. All tissue passed spontaneously should be carefully inspected and preserved in fixative for histological study and identification in the pathology laboratory.

If, on pelvic examination, the uterus is enlarged, the cervix is closed, and the bleeding is minimal, a diagnosis of "threatened abortion" is made and the patient is managed by observation, bed rest, and inderdiction of coitus. Progesterone therapy, e.g., hydroxy-progesterone caproate (Delalutin), 500 mg intramuscularly, or medroxyprogesterone acetate (Provera) tablets, 10 mg twice a day, may be prescribed. Some patients may warrant hospitalization for further observation; the majority are allowed to return home on the above-mentioned regimen.

If the pelvic findings are equivocal and the diagnosis of pregnancy is uncertain, a pregnancy test may be rapidly performed in the emergency room to help clarify the diagnosis. An immunological test system, utilizing latex particles coated with human chorionic gonadotropin and an antihuman chorionic gonadotropic serum, provides a commercially available slide test which can be performed and read in 3 minutes. In such a system, inhibition of agglutination indicates a positive test for pregnancy. These tests are accurate, rapid, and easy to perform. The earliest time that the test may be considered to be reliably positive is approximately 2 weeks after the first missed period. Negative results of the test do not exclude pregnancy.

If the cervix is open, the abortion is inevitable, and if the membranes are ruptured, it is imminent. If tissue has been passed or if placental tissue is visible or palpable in the cervical os, the abortion is incomplete. Under these circumstances the patient should be admitted to the hospital. No measures are necessary in the emergency room unless profuse bleeding is present. If the patient is bleeding profusely and if the gestation sac (chorionic vesicle) or placental tissue is lying free in the cervical canal, it may be gently removed with ovum forceps. An intravenous infusion of 5% dextrose in water containing 10 units of oxytocin should be started. Removal of products of conception may rapidly control the bleeding. However, on no account should the uterine cavity be sounded or explored in the emergency room, as this procedure may result in aggravation of the bleeding, perforation, or infection. All cases of inevitable and incomplete abortion should be scheduled for dilatation and curettage in the operating room at the earliest suitable time following immediate routine blood work, urinalysis, and cross match. Cases presenting in hypovolemic shock require prompt blood replacement and measures to combat shock while arrangements are made with the operating room for immediate evacuation and curettage of the uterus.

The possibility of "induced" abortion should always be considered in emergency-room cases. A fever of 100.4°F or more warrants the designation "septic abortion" and strongly suggests a prior attempt to interrupt the pregnancy. A positive history is usually difficult to obtain under these circumstances, but if such an abortion is suspected, a detailed description of the course of events helps the emergency physician to assess the case properly. Specific inquiry should be directed to the use of mechanical devices or chemical douches. Detection of crepitus on pelvic examination suggests clostridial infection. Abdominal x-rays are indicated to exclude the presence of a foreign body and "free air" secondary to uterine perforation. Induced abortions may lead to hemorrhagic shock, septic shock, hemolysis, jaundice, disseminated intravascular coagulation with hypofibrinogenemia, septic pulmonary embolization, and acute renal failure. It is important to realize that unless the physician is oriented to the possibility of septic abortion, symptoms referable to the cardiovascular, respiratory, or gastrointestinal systems along with signs of general toxicity may serve to divert attention from the pelvis. Mild vaginal bleeding often seems insignificant in the presence of tachycardia, hypotension, dyspnea, chest pain, vomiting, abdominal distension, dehydration, and electrolyte imbalance. Under these circumstances, *the primary diagnosis of "septic abortion" is often needlessly delayed*. It is, therefore, of great importance to have a competent pelvic examination performed as part of the initial survey of the patient. Once the diagnosis is established, the patient should immediately be admitted to the hospital and appropriate studies (cervical smears and culture, blood and urine cultures, electrolytes, central venous pressure, etc.) should be promptly initiated. The emergency-room physician may make an important contribution to the management of the patient by being able to establish a prompt diagnosis.

Occasionally, potassium permanganate tablets are inserted in the vagina as an abortifacient. They cause characteristic chemical ulceration of the vaginal walls at areas of contact ("kissing ulcers") which may bleed profusely. Any visible remaining potassium permanganate should be removed with forceps and the vagina irrigated with copious amounts of saline. If the bleeding persists, a tight vaginal pack is inserted. The patient is then transferred to the operating room where suture ligature is employed to arrest the bleeding.

ECTOPIC PREGNANCY. Only rarely is ectopic pregnancy associated with heavy vaginal bleeding. The bleeding is characteristically mild, intermittent, and often dark brown in color. The association of vaginal bleeding with abdominal pain in any female patient of reproductive age should bring to mind the possibility of ectopic pregnancy. Nausea, diarrhea, and frequency of micturition are not infrequent. A history of missed period, faintness or dizziness, and shoulder pain corroborates the diagnosis. Pallor, tachycardia, hypotension, abdominal tenderness, palpation of a tender boggy fullness in the cul-de-sac, and pain on motion of the cervix strongly suggest the diagnosis of ruptured ectopic pregnancy. The patient should be promptly cross matched and scheduled for emergency laparotomy without delay.

When the diagnosis is equivocal or uncertain, a careful history and pelvic examination will usually lead to the correct diagnosis. Lateralizing pain or tenderness on motion of the cervix and the presence or suggestion of a mass or fullness in either adnexal area should arouse a strong suspicion of ectopic pregnancy. Differential diagnosis will include threatened abortion, pelvic inflammatory disease, endometriosis, corpus luteum cyst, or other ovarian cyst. Not infrequently, cases of unruptured ectopic pregnancy are erroneously diagnosed in the emergency room as mild pelvic inflammatory disease, treated with penicillin, and sent home. To avoid this error, it is important always to have a high index of suspicion for ectopic pregnancy. Symptoms and signs which are predominantly unilateral, normal temperature, normal leukocyte count, and normal sedimentation rate do *not* support a diagnosis of pelvic inflammatory disease but are entirely consistent with ectopic pregnancy. Reasonable suspicion of ectopic pregnancy warrants immediate hospitalization for continued observation and further studies. Culdocentesis should not be performed in the emergency room, since the procedure is not infallible and could be misleading if relied upon to the exclusion of other measures. If there is sufficient suspicion to warrant performance of culdocentesis, it should be performed in the operating room in conjunction with an examination under anesthesia and any other diagnostic procedure that may seem indicated (dilatation and curettage, culdoscopy, culdotomy, laparotomy).

HYDATIDIFORM MOLE. A history of prolonged and persistent bleeding during the first trimester of pregnancy in the face of a growing uterus or one that seems larger than anticipated by menstrual data should suggest the possibility of hydatidiform mole. The passage of vesicles that can be recognized by the physician as mole tissue establishes the diagnosis. A history of persistent or intermittent bleeding following a recent term pregnancy, abortion, or mole should likewise bring to mind the possibility of trophoblastic disease. A pregnancy test should be performed. Pelvic examination will reveal an enlarged, soft, and boggy uterus. Vaginal bleeding may be profuse. Emergency-room management is limited to intravenous infusion therapy and cross matching for blood transfusion as arrangements are made for hospital admission.

ANTEPARTUM—MORE THAN 20 WEEKS' GESTATION. Patients who present with vaginal bleeding in the third trimester or late second trimester are better handled in the maternity unit than in the emergency room. Apart from local lesions of the lower genital tract, bleeding at this stage of pregnancy generally indicates one of three things: (1) *labor*—the bleeding representing a heavy "show" signaling the onset of labor; (2) *abruptio placentae*—bleeding generally associated with abdominal pain; or (3) *placenta praevia*—generally painless bleeding.

In all instances of third-trimester bleeding, rectal or vaginal examination should not be performed for fear of precipitating an exsanguinating hemorrhage in consequence of a placenta praevia. Vital signs should be monitored. Abdominal examination will document the presence or absence of uterine contractions as well as fetal presentation and heart tones. Blood should be obtained for clotting studies and an intravenous infusion should be started immediately with a large-gauge needle or intravenous catheter and cross match performed. More complete evaluation in the emergency room under such circumstances may only lose valuable time and delay definitive diagnosis and management. Patients arriving in the emergency room are best directed straight to the labor-delivery room for evaluation.

INTRAPARTUM.   Intrapartum hemorrhage may be due to premature separation of the placenta, placenta praevia, cervical lacerations, rupture of the uterus, or rupture of vasa praevia.

If a patient arrives in the emergency room in labor, with vaginal bleeding, she should not be evaluated but immediately redirected to the labor-delivery room. The only exception would be an unregistered patient who arrives in the emergency room rather than on the maternity floor with the baby in the process of delivery, i.e., with the presenting part crowning. Under these circumstances an episiotomy should be made and the baby delivered as atraumatically as possible. The cord should be divided between clamps, and the placenta should be delivered if it has been spontaneously expressed into the lower birth canal. The patient should then be transferred to the delivery room immediately for proper inspection and evaluation of the entire birth canal and further management. Blood should be cross matched at once and an intravenous infusion started.

POSTPARTUM

IMMEDIATE.   Immediate postpartum hemorrhage occurs within the first 24 hours of delivery. It may be due to retained placenta or placental fragments; uterine atony; cervical, vaginal, or perineal lacerations; uterine rupture; or possible coagulation defect.

A patient may appear in the emergency room with immediate postpartum hemorrhage, having delivered at home or en route to the hospital. She should be evaluated for vital signs and have blood drawn for blood counts and cross matching. An intravenous infusion should be started. Pelvic examination should be deferred to the operating room, as the entire birth canal needs to be meticulously evaluated.

DELAYED.   Excessive uterine bleeding after the first 24 hours and up to a month following delivery may be due to retained secundine or subinvolution of the placental site. Profuse bleeding may occur. Measures to combat shock and to replace blood should be promptly instituted. Intravenous ergonovine, 0.2 mg or oxytocin, 10 units in 1000 cc 5% dextrose in water, should be administered. The patient should be admitted to the hospital. If the bleeding is significant, dilatation and curettage should not be delayed. There is no reason to pack the uterus prior to dilatation and curettage.

THE SYNDROME OF HYPOFIBRINOGENEMIA AND INCOAGULABLE BLOOD IN OBSTETRICS. Failure of the blood to clot may constitute a grave obstetrical emergency. This condition may complicate a variety of obstetrical situations but ordinarily occurs in association with abruptio placentae, amniotic fluid embolus, prolonged retention of a dead fetus in utero, and septic abortion. There are two main mechanisms responsible for the development of the coagulation defect. The more common mechanism involves the liberation of large amounts of tissue thromboplastin from the placenta, decidua, or amniotic fluid into the retroplacental site or general maternal circulation. This gives rise to excessive fibrin deposition, effectively defibrinating the circulating blood. Less often, there is excess activation of the fibrinolytic system resulting in pathological fibrinolysis and enzymatic degradation of the fibrinogen molecule. In either event fibrinogen is low or absent in the plasma, and the blood fails to clot. The physician should be alerted to this diagnosis by the recognition of the primary diagnosis (e.g., abruptio placentae) and the observation that there are no clots in the vagina. A clinical diagnosis of coagulation defect is confirmed by drawing 5 ml of blood in a test tube and observing it for clot formation. Failure of the blood to clot by 15 minutes or formation of a poor clot that fragments or lyses within one hour establishes the diagnosis. Any patient suspected of having this disorder should be immediately cross matched and transferred to the delivery-room unit.

Genital Cancer

Profuse vaginal bleeding may result from carcinoma of the cervix. It is usually possible to identify the source of hemorrhage, by inspection and palpation, as an irregular, fungating, necrotic lesion of the cervix. A few yards of gauze tightly packed against the bleeding cervix and filling the vagina may serve as a useful expedient to effect prompt hemostasis. The leading end of the gauze may be saturated in formalin or negatol to produce a local protein coagulant effect on the bleeding surfaces. When the bleeding is coming from within the uterine cavity (cancer of the endometrium), packing is of no avail and the patient should be prepared for immediate dilatation and curettage.

Submucous Myoma

Profuse vaginal bleeding associated with palpation of an irregularly enlarged uterus suggests the diagnosis of submucous myoma. Occasionally a submucous myoma is small and solitary in a uterus of approximately normal size and configuration. The patient should be scheduled for immediate dilatation and curettage. Prompt hysterectomy is sometimes necessary.

Dysfunctional Uterine Bleeding

Abnormal uterine bleeding occurring in the absence of discernible pelvic pathology and not due to pregnancy, systemic disease, blood dyscrasia, or specific major endocrinopathy is termed dysfunctional bleeding. It is due to an intrinsic endocrine defect in the hypothalamic-pituitary-ovarian axis that regulates normal menstrual function. The bleeding is most often of an anovular nature. If the bleeding is profuse, immediate dilatation and curettage is the treatment of choice in most adult patients. This serves to exclude organic endometrial pathology, to allow histological assessment of the hormonal status of the endometrium, and to effect prompt hemostasis. In menarchial and adolescent girls, rapid hemostasis may be achieved by suitable hormone therapy. For this purpose, a large dose of rapid-acting estrogen and progesterone should be administered parenterally. Premarin, 20 mg intravenously, and progesterone in oil, 100 mg intramuscularly, may be used to initiate therapy. The dose may be repeated in several hours. Simultaneously, one of the potent synthetic oral progestins should be started, e.g., norethindrone (Norlutin), 10 mg by mouth three or four times per day for 10 to 20 days. A close follow-up of these patients is mandatory.

Patients taking oral contraceptive tablets occasionally experience breakthrough bleeding, but this is seldom severe. When profuse bleeding occurs, it may be due to "skipping pills" or to an occult endometrial pathological condition. Prompt dilatation and curettage are usually indicated. Transient hemostasis may be frequently achieved by immediate ingestion of two or three tablets of the contraceptive formulation, repeated every 6 to 8 hours until the bleeding has been controlled or dilatation and curettage have been performed.

Patients utilizing an intra-uterine device for contraception will occasionally present in the emergency room because of excessive bleeding with a period or between periods. Under such circumstances it is usually best to remove the device. This is easily accomplished by simply identifying the attached suture protruding from the cervix, grasping it with forceps and gently pulling the device from the uterus. If the bleeding is profuse, the patient is best admitted to the hospital for dilatation and curettage.

ECTOPIC PREGNANCY. Ruptured ectopic pregnancy with hemoperitoneum may occur in the absence of overt vaginal bleeding. A history suggestive of ectopic pregnancy has been previously detailed. Pallor, tachycardia, restlessness, abdominal tenderness, and a tender bulge or fullness in the cul-de-sac strongly suggest the diagnosis. In addition to tubal pregnancy, ovarian and abdominal pregnancy may likewise cause massive intraperitoneal hemorrhage.

PERFORATED UTERUS. Perforated uterus is usually sustained as a result of an attempted criminal abortion or a bullet or stab wound of a pregnant abdomen. Prompt abdominal exploration is indicated.

RUPTURED UTERUS. Rupture of the uterus occurs most often in labor and is usually due to dehiscence of a uterine scar (cesarean section, myomectomy) or neglected obstructed labor. Other common causes of uterine rupture (oxytocin stimulation, version extraction, forceps) preclude its occurrence outside the hospital. Not infrequently a cesarean section scar ruptures spontaneously prior to the onset of labor, sometimes (though rarely) as early as 16 weeks' gestation. Immediate abdominal exploration is indicated.

CONCEALED ABRUPTIO PLACENTAE. In approximately 10 percent of cases of abruptio placentae the hemorrhage is concealed, being confined by the remaining placental attachment and dissecting into the muscular wall of the uterus. These cases almost invariably represent the more severe forms of abruptio that readily lead to profound shock, hypofibrinogenemia, and acute renal shutdown. Diagnosis is based on the history of sudden acute abdominal pain and the findings of uterine tenderness, increased uterine tone or rigidity, and evidence of fetal distress or fetal demise. An intravenous infusion should be started immediately, blood should be cross matched, and the patient should be immediately transferred to the delivery room for vaginal examination and definitive treatment.

ENDOTOXIC SHOCK

Septic shock always represents a very serious emergency that is associated with a high mortality. Only prompt recognition and early vigorous treatment improve the salvage rate. Delay in diagnosis or treatment may spell the difference between life and death.

The condition occurs predominantly in association with septic abortion. It may also occur as a complication of chorioamnionitis in consequence of prolonged premature rupture of the membranes at or near term, and as a complication of puerperal sepsis. Acute pyelonephritis and acute pelvic inflammatory disease with tubo-ovarian abscess may also be complicated by septic shock. The condition is due to endotoxemia. Any patient suspected of harboring a gram-negative infection in whom the clinical picture of pyrexia, tachycardia, hypotension, and oliguria is present should be regarded as manifesting endotoxic shock. At different stages in the evolution of the clinical picture the temperature may be subnormal, the pulse may be bounding and normal in rate, and the skin may be flushed and dry. Cervical, urine, and blood cultures should be obtained and prompt, vigorous treatment with antibiotics and corticosteroids initiated. When endotoxic shock is associated with intra-uterine infection, the uterus should be evacuated under antibiotic coverage. Hysterectomy may be necessary.

AMNIOTIC FLUID EMBOLUS

If a patient is brought to the emergency room in a state of vascular collapse with a history of having delivered her baby at home a short time before, following a rapid tumultuous labor, the diagnosis of amniotic fluid embolus should be entertained. A history of vascular collapse, dyspnea, and cyanosis occurring very suddenly during or immediately after labor or delivery is characteristic. If the patient survives the first few hours, hypofibrinogenemic hemorrhage may ensue as well as acute tubular necrosis.

Emergency treatment for acute cor pulmonale and pulmonary edema should be instituted including positive-pressure oxygen, intravenous aminophylline, and digitalization. Atropine and vasopressor agents may also be indicated, as may blood and fibrinogen replacement. After initial emergency evaluation and treatment the patient should be transferred to the delivery room, where the uterine cavity should be manually explored to exclude retained placental fragments and rupture of the uterus. This accident is hyperacute in onset and is generally fatal.

PUERPERAL INVERSION OF THE UTERUS

A rare obstetrical complication sometimes associated with profound shock—puerperal inversion of the uterus—generally occurs during or immediately following the third stage of labor. Most often it is due to ill-advised traction on the cord or improper expression of the placenta, but it may take place spontaneously in consequence of sudden increases in intra-abdominal pressure (e.g., bearing down, coughing) in the presence of a markedly atonic uterine fundus. The corpus drops into the vagina. If the placenta is still adherent, profuse hemorrhage may occur but does not do so invariably. If a patient has delivered outside the hospital and is brought into the emergency room in shock, this condition if present becomes apparent on direct examination. Mortality rises as recognition is delayed. Shock should be promptly treated with intravenous infusions and blood replacement. The patient is admitted for prompt reduction of the inverted uterus.

PREECLAMPSIA AND ECLAMPSIA

Preeclampsia and eclampsia constitute serious obstetrical complications that significantly increase both maternal and perinatal mortality. Severe preeclampsia constitutes a true obstetric emergency as eclampsia may be imminent. A gravida beyond 24 weeks' gestation who complains of severe headache, blurring of vision, or epigastric pain, whose blood pressure is higher than 160/110 mm Hg, and whose urine shows 3+ to 4+ proteinuria should be considered a severe preeclampsia case. Oliguria and heart failure are other signs of grave preeclampsia. A hematocrit reading and urinalysis should be performed immediately (serial determination of these parameters is used to follow the patient's course over the subsequent 24 hours). Magnesium sulfate, 4 gm, should be given slowly, intravenously, over a period of 5 to 15 minutes, and an intravenous infusion of

1000 ml 5% dextrose in water containing 10 mg of magnesium sulfate started. This is infused at a rate sufficient to deliver magnesium sulfate 1 mg per hour. The patient is hospitalized for continued observation and definitive management. *It cannot be overemphasized that there is no ambulatory treatment for severe toxemia. Once the diagnosis is made, the patient must be hospitalized.*

Eclampsia is the clinical end stage of the toxemic process. Approximately 25 percent of cases of eclampsia occur in the immediate postpartum period. Should a patient arrive in the emergency room following or during an eclamptic seizure, the following steps must be taken: The patient is placed in a bed or stretcher with padded side rails, and an indwelling urethral catheter is inserted. A tongue blade covered with cotton and gauze is put between the teeth to prevent the tongue from being bitten. Suction is employed to prevent the aspiration of vomitus, saliva, and nasopharyngeal secretion. An oropharyngeal airway is inserted and oxygen administered by mask or nasal catheter if there is any evidence of cyanosis. The patient is suitably restrained during a seizure. Magnesium sulfate, 4 to 6 mg, in a 50% solution, is slowly administered intravenously followed by 10 mg in 1000 ml 5% dextrose and water infused at the rate of 1 gm per hour. Sodium amobarbital (Amytal), 250 to 500 mg, may also be slowly administered intravenously. An ampule of 10 ml 10% calcium gluconate should be kept immediately available to counteract a rare overdosage of magnesium sulfate. Hypertonic glucose (20%) may be effectively used, if administered rapidly, to produce an osmotic diuresis. Pulse rate, blood pressure, respiratory rate, knee jerks, temperature, and urine volume are carefully monitored. The occasional postictal or comatose patient will benefit from prompt tracheostomy to insure adequate respiratory exchange and tracheal toilet. As soon as the patient's condition is temporarily stabilized, she should be transferred to the maternity unit for further management.

As with septic abortion, so with toxemia of pregnancy, the emergency-room physician who is not oriented to consider specific complications of pregnancy will sometimes fail to make a correct diagnosis on initial survey of the patient. Headache, loss of visual acuity, nausea, vomiting and abdominal pain sometimes lead the physician to consider a primary neurovascular diagnosis (e.g., essential hypertension) or gastrointestinal diagnosis (e.g., peptic ulcer or gastroenteritis) rather than the true obstetrical diagnosis. Such errors should not occur. Hypertension and proteinuria in a pregnant woman, regardless of other symptoms, means toxemia of pregnancy. It is of great importance to establish a prompt diagnosis and to initiate magnesium sulfate therapy.

ACUTE ABDOMEN

Surgical

RUPTURED OVARIAN CYST. Nonneoplastic ovarian cysts are more prone to rupture than are neoplastic cysts. The most common types of ovarian cyst that may rupture are follicle cysts, corpus luteum cysts, theca-lutein cysts, and endometrial ("chocolate") cysts. If there is no significant intraperitoneal bleeding associated with the rupture, the clinical picture is often not impressive. The patient complains of abdominal pain. Objective findings may be minimal. Tenderness to direct palpation of the lower abdomen is usually elicited, as is pelvic tenderness on vaginal palpation of the adnexal areas. Bleeding is usually slight from endometrial cysts, but pain and tenderness are often marked. Hemorrhage into an ovarian cyst may give rise to distressing pain and sudden enlargement of the cyst. Significant intra-abdominal bleeding due to rupture of vessels in the cyst wall is unlikely, but when it occurs it may produce shock and a clinical picture identical with that of ruptured ectopic pregnancy.

Of the neoplastic cysts, the dermoid cyst is the most common and also the most prone to rupture. The sebaceous contents of dermoid cysts may be very irritating to the peritoneum and produce a marked peritoneal reaction. Malignant cysts may also undergo spontaneous perforation or rupture.

The diagnosis of ruptured ovarian cysts requires immediate hospitalization. In most instances laparotomy is indicated.

TORSION OF OVARIAN CYST. Pedunculated ovarian tumors (as well as pedunculated subserous myomas) sometimes undergo torsion causing unilateral abdominal and pelvic pain that may be referred to the flanks. When circulatory impairment results in infarction and hemorrhage into the mass, signs of adjacent peritoneal irritation become manifest, namely, tenderness and guarding. The abdomen is frequently distended. Nausea and vomiting are often associated symptoms, and low-grade fever and leukocytosis frequently coexist. It may be possible to elicit a history of one or more milder episodes of pain, in the recent past, of a transient and self-limiting nature.

Pelvic examination reveals an exquisitely tender, poorly movable adnexal mass.

Rarely a normal adnexa undergoes torsion leading to infarction of the ovary. This is more likely to occur in children but its occurrence in adults is documented.

In all these cases abdominal exploration is indicated.

RUPTURE OF TUBO-OVARIAN ABSCESS.   A high mortality attends the rupture of a tubo-ovarian abscess. The preoperative clinical diagnosis is often difficult to make. If an outpatient, under treatment for acute exacerbation of pelvic inflammatory disease, has palpable adnexal inflammatory masses and shows sudden clinical deterioration, this diagnosis should be strongly suspected. High fever, chills, toxic facies, tachycardia, hypotension, and generalized peritonitis bespeak the gravity of the condition. Surgery offers a better prognosis than conservative management in this desperately ill patient.

ECTOPIC PREGNANCY.   The differential diagnosis of the acute abdomen in any female patient of reproductive age must include consideration of ectopic pregnancy even in the absence of overt vaginal bleeding or evidence of hemoperitoneum. A careful history, pelvic examination by an experienced examiner, and a high index of suspicion are required to make the diagnosis in these cases.

Medical

ACUTE SALPINGITIS.   It is generally believed that gonorrhea remains the principal type of acute purulent salpingitis encountered in clinical practice; however, the coliform organisms are frequently found either as primary agents or as secondary invaders. The patient usually presents with acute generalized lower abdominal pain, anorexia, nausea and vomiting, fever, and often chills. There is likely to be marked lower abdominal tenderness as well as rebound tenderness and guarding. Pelvic examination reveals tenderness on manipulating the cervix to either side as well as on direct palpation of the adnexal areas. Leukocytosis is the rule. Smears and cultures should be obtained from the cervix, and urethra and penicillin or broad-spectrum antibiotic therapy should be initiated. Mild cases may be managed on an outpatient basis with careful follow-up. Any suggestion of pelvic peritonitis is an indication for prompt hospitalization.

UNRUPTURED TUBO-OVARIAN ABSCESS. Acute salpingitis may progress to pyosalpinx, tubo-ovarian abscess, or pelvic abscess. Pain and fever may persist or recur, and nausea, vomiting, and abdominal distension due to ileus may supervene. Sometimes it is possible to outline a firm adnexal mass in an acutely tender pelvis. Leukocytosis and elevated sedimentation rate are almost invariable. Cervical and blood cultures should be obtained. The patient should be hospitalized for nasogastric suction, parenteral fluid therapy, intravenous antibiotic therapy, and careful observation for resolution of the peritoneal signs. Acute progression of a tubo-ovarian abscess during medical therapy indicates surgical removal prior to rupture, if possible.

Evidence of a fluctuant mass in the cul-de-sac requires prompt surgical drainage by posterior culdotomy in the operating room.

POSTABORTAL AND PUERPERAL SEPSIS. Acute endometritis may become manifest within a few days following abortion or delivery. The usual spread is directly to the pelvic supporting tissues, causing parametritis, pelvic cellulitis, and, at times, a suppurative pelvic thrombophlebitis. Fever and chills are prominent symptoms, but pain is often only mild or moderate. The uterus is characteristically tender to palpation. In milder cases only fever may be present with no localizing signs or symptoms. Uterine and blood cultures should be obtained. Treatment involves vigorous antibiotic therapy after appropriate cultures have been obtained. Recurrent chills and a swinging temperature course suggest septic embolization secondary to a suppurative pelvic thrombophlebitis.

This condition carries a high mortality and often requires ligation of the inferior vena cava and ovarian veins to avert a fatal outcome.

DEGENERATION OF A MYOMA. Acute degeneration may result in sudden symptoms in preexisting uterine myomas. Infection, carneous degeneration, and necrosis may cause localized pain, low-grade fever, leukocytosis, and an accelerated sedimentation rate. "Red degeneration" of a myoma in pregnancy is associated with extravasation of blood into the tumor. This condition can usually be adequately managed with analgesics, bed rest, and antibiotics to prevent or control associated infection. In most instances operation is eventually indicated on an elective basis.

PELVIC PAIN

Dysmenorrhea

Menstrual pain is frequent during adolescence and is occasionally severe and incapacitating. It is usually sharp and colicky and is typically located in the hypogastrium. It most often develops concommitantly with the menstrual flow, but may precede the flow by hours or 1 or 2 days. It may be accompanied by nausea, vomiting, and faintness. Severe dysmenorrhea may occasion an emergency-room visit. A history of previous episodes can usually be elicited. The patient will often appear pale and in obvious distress. She will complain of agonizing pain not controlled by the usual proprietary household analgesics. General and pelvic examination and associated laboratory studies (c.b.c., E.S.R., and urinalysis) are normal. The patient should be given 100 mg meperidine (Demerol) intramuscularly, reassured, and observed for a short period of time. A prescription may be given for codeine tablets, as necessary.

Mittelschmerz

Ovulatory or midcycle pain is relatively common in older teen-agers and is associated with rupture of the graafian follicle and extrusion of the ovum. The discomfort is usually mild and fleeting, but may, on occasion, be continuous and severe and last several hours or days. The pain is usually located in one or other lower quadrant of the abdomen and may be associated with nausea and vomiting. There is usually a history of similar prior episodes. Gross vaginal bleeding is rare but midcycle staining may accompany the pain. On examination, there is no fever and no palpable mass. There may be mild tenderness in one or other lower quadrant of the abdomen and corresponding mild unilateral adnexal tenderness. Diagnosis is made on the basis of a typical history, absence of peritoneal signs, and the characteristic time in the cycle. Simple analgesia and reassurance are all that are needed.

On occasion, there may be guarding and even rigidity in the lower abdomen, suggesting the possibility of appendicitis, pelvic inflammatory disease, or accidents to an ovarian cyst. Syncope and abdominal distension may suggest hemoperitoneum secondary to ectopic pregnancy. Such cases are rare and are due to significant intraperitoneal bleeding. Hospitalization is required for more definitive diagnostic measures. These include: observation with serial laboratory studies, examination under anesthesia, culdoscopy, laparoscopy, or laparotomy.

Intra-uterine Device

Wearers of an intra-uterine device will occasionally present with severe pelvic pain, crampy or continuous, for which they seek immediate relief. Such pain is usually not associated with a perforation of the uterus but is due to excessive uterine irritabilty secondary to the presence of an intracavitary foreign body. Pelvic and laboratory findings are normal. The device should be removed and a simple analgesic prescribed.

GENITAL INJURIES

Nonspecific Trauma

VULVAR AND VAGINAL LACERATIONS. Direct trauma to the genital area may produce lacerations of the vulva which can extend into the vagina. Such injuries are sometimes sustained by children during play. Significant bleeding may ensue, although it is usually self-limiting. The external genitalia must be carefully examined in good light in order to assess the extent of the injury. The entire vagina must likewise be visualized so as not to overlook an associated separate vaginal injury. The clitoris and urethra should be carefully examined. Voided urine should be screened for hematuria. There should be no hesitancy in passing a catheter if any doubt exists as to the integrity of the urethra. The area should be cleansed with surgical soap and water, and antiseptic solution applied prior to suture repair under local anesthesia.

It may be impossible adequately to examine or treat a frightened child in the emergency room. Under such circumstances it is prudent to admit the patient to the hospital overnight in order to carry out the examination and repair in the operating room under general anesthesia. More extensive injuries in adults are likewise better handled in the operating room. With proper local cleansing and aseptic technique, it is not necessary to use prophylactic antibiotics for minor injuries. Protection against tetanus is generally indicated.

VULVAR AND VAGINAL VARICES. Rupture of a vaginal varix is a rare event. Vulvar varices occur more commonly and are found predominantly in association with pregnancy in women of very high parity. Occasionally such a varix ruptures spontaneously or secondary to mild local trauma. Bleeding can be profuse. Emergency treatment consists of digital compression with a sponge or gauze. The offending vessel should then be ligated or a segment excised.

VULVAR AND PERINEAL HEMATOMAS. Apart from postepisiotomy hematomas, most vulvar hematomas occur secondary to direct blows or penetrating wounds involving the vulva and perineum. Straddle falls are a frequent variety of trauma. Owing to the loose texture of the vulvar tissues, hematomas form readily and spread rapidly. A swelling may be seen to expand under direct observation and may achieve very large proportions. The swelling spreads posteriorly to the perianal region and anteriorly to the mons pubis. The swelling is bounded medially by the median perineal raphe and may involve the ischiorectal fossa, being limited by the infralevator fascia. The subperitoneal type of hemorrhage may dissect along the paravaginal tissues and into the pelvic extraperitoneal space so as to balloon out the broad ligament and even ascend toward the kidney. Most hematomas are self-limiting in extent and require only careful observation, serial hematocrit determinations, ice packs, analgesics, and usually prophylactic antibiotics. If a hematoma is seen to be enlarging, the patient should be promptly prepared for the operating room for incision, evacuation, and attempt to suture the bleeding vessel.

Sexual Trauma

Coital trauma sufficient to cause introital lacerations occurs infrequently. Bleeding ranges from scant to severe. Predisposing factors include the gravid and puerperal state associated with increased vascularity and friability of tissues, gross anatomical abnormality, genital infantilism, and brutal phallic intromission (e.g., in an alcoholic state). Such injuries should be fully assessed and repaired as outlined for nonspecific genital injuries.

DEFLORATION. Penile penetration of a virginal introitus usually involves dilatation and sometimes minor laceration of the hymeneal ring. Slight bleeding is common but is self-limited and usually does not come to medical attention. Rarely, a girl is brought to the emergency room with brisk genital bleeding following the first intromission. Following evaluation of the injury, hemostasis can usually be readily achieved with a few fine chromic catgut sutures. If adequate evaluation and repair are difficult to achieve because of the patient's embarrassment and trepidation, she should be hospitalized for hemostatic repair and hymenotomy in the operating room.

RAPE. The physician is often called upon to examine a patient in the emergency room in order to supply medical evidence bearing on the allegation of rape. Rape is sexual intercourse with a woman against her will. It may be accomplished by abuse of a helpless or disabled female, by physical force, and by intimidation. False accusations of rape are frequent. There appear to be many pretended cases. False accusations may be made erroneously or willfully from ulterior motives. The question for the physician to decide is not whether the patient has been raped but whether the findings of his examination reveal that the patient was or was not a party to sexual intercourse (or attempted intercourse) within the approximate time indicated. This is the only opinion he should render.

Medical evaluation of an alleged case of rape should proceed along the following lines:

1. Obtain a general history with particular emphasis on the patient's own account of the incident.

2. Note the patient's appearance, behavior, and state of mind.

3. Examine the clothing (particularly underclothing) for tears, stains, etc.

4. Look for abrasions, contusions, ecchymoses, and other marks of force or violence.

5. Examine the perineum, thighs, and external genitalia for evidence of trauma and suggestion of semen about the vulva or in matted pubic hair.

6. Perform a speculum examination of the vagina for evidence of seminal fluid. Obtain both vaginal and cervical smears for microscopic examination. The presence or absence of motile or nonmotile sperm should be noted for each specimen examined.

7. Examine cervical and urethral smears for gonococci and obtain cultures.

8. Perform bimanual pelvic examination.

9. Record all findings in writing, in full, immediately following these examinations.

LOWER GENITAL TRACT INFECTIONS

Vulvovaginal infections are not usually sufficiently acute or distressing to require emergency treatment. Nevertheless, occasionally a patient seeks emergency care for relief of intolerable pruritus vulvae. Copious vaginal discharge, itching, and burning are classic symptoms of acute vaginitis. Many times there is associated acute vulvitis.

Trichomoniasis

Vaginal infestation with *Trichomonas vaginalis* is extremely common and probably represents the most frequent form of vaginitis encountered. The patient may be asymptomatic or exceedingly uncomfortable. Frequently, the characteristic creamy discharge is seen at the introitus spilling out of the vagina. Speculum examination reveals more of this same discharge that is typically bubbly or frothy. Petechiae on the cervix or vagina are likewise characteristic.

The diagnosis is made by microscopic demonstration of the trichomonads in a wet mount of the vaginal discharge. A drop of the discharge is mixed with a drop of normal saline solution on a slide and the preparation is examined, preferably without a coverslip, for evidence of motile, oval flagellates. The vagina may be cleansed with aqueous benzalkonium chloride (Zephiran) or thimerosal (Merthiolate) solution in order to remove the irritating discharges immediately. Metronidazole (Flagyl), 250 mg by mouth three times a day for 10 days, provides the most prompt and effective relief and is curative in a high percentage of cases. Sitz baths may be prescribed.

Candidiasis (Moniliasis)

Candidial vulvovaginitis is often characterized by intense itching, and the vulva may show evidence of excoriation. The typical gross appearance is that of a curdy, white vaginal discharge, and thrushlike patches may be seen on the vaginal or cervical mucous membrane and about the introitus. The diagnosis is confirmed by positive microscopic identification of mycelia or hyphae on a direct smear of the exudate. A swab of the discharge may also be plated out on a Nickerson's slant for culture. The culture tube is read in 24 to 48 hours.

The treatment that affords the most prompt relief from exasperating pruritus consists of liberal painting of the entire vagina and vulva with a 1% aqueous solution of gentian violet. The patient will be perfectly content to accept the messiness of the treatment in exchange for the gratifying relief from the severe pruritus. Nystatin (Mycostatin) vaginal suppositories may then be prescribed, to be inserted twice a day. Treatment should be continued for 2 to 4 weeks.

Nonspecific Vaginitis

A symptomatic vaginal discharge with evidence of vaginal exudate, irritation, and inflammation may represent a nonspecific vaginitis if *Trichomonas* and *Candida* are excluded by both direct smear and culture. Some cases are due to *Haemophilus vaginalis,* others to a mixture of organisms including normal flora plus various strains of *Streptococcus, Staphylococcus,* and colon bacillus. It is helpful to cleanse the vagina with surgical soap and water and to prescribe a triple sulfa vaginal cream.

A very malodorous vaginal discharge suggests the possibility of a forgotten foreign body. This is usually a menstrual tampon. Removal affords prompt relief.

Bacterial Infection

Acute suppurative vaginitis due to pyogenic organisms is not commonly seen but may occur secondary to gross contamination particularly in debilitated or chronically ill patients. A direct smear of the exudate should be gram-stained and examined and appropriate bacterial cultures obtained. The vagina should be scrubbed with surgical soap and water and proper hygiene and perineal care prescribed. Nitrofurazone (Furacin) vaginal suppositories, to be inserted twice a day, should also be prescribed.

Gonorrheal vulvovaginitis is rare in the adult patient but occasionally occurs in children. There may be an associated profuse vaginal discharge and local irritation. Gram stain of a direct smear reveals gram-negative intracellular diplococci. A swab should be rapidly plated in an attempt to obtain a positive culture. Specific therapy consists of penicillin starting intramuscularly, followed by a 5-day course of oral penicillin.

In the adult, gonorrhea of the lower genital tract is often manifest as an acute bartholinitis. However, other organisms may be responsible for acute inflammation of this accessory sex gland. Treatment consists of rest, sitz baths, analgesics, and penicillin. When abscess formation is evident, incision and drainage should be performed as soon as fluctuation is present. The abscess may be incised in the emergency room under ethyl chloride spray but is usually best handled in the operating room, where adequate incision, drainage, and packing can be insured. Following incision and drainage there is immediate relief of pain, and healing is usually rapid thereafter.

FETAL EMERGENCIES

Occasionally a pregnant patient is brought to the emergency room presenting a fetal rather than a maternal emergency. The following situations may occur.

Prolapsed Cord

The umbilical cord may be seen prolapsed through the introitus and lying outside the vulva. The patient may or may not be in labor. Sterile gloves should be donned and the cord should be palpated for the presence or absence of pulsations. If no pulsations are felt, the fetus is assumed to have died and the emergency is thereby terminated. The patient should not be further examined in the emergency room but transferred immediately to the delivery room.

If pulsations are palpable, the patient should be placed at once in the Trendelenburg or knee-chest position and the hand should be inserted along the cord into the vagina and to the cervix. The degree of cervical dilatation and nature and station of the presenting part will thus be ascertained. The presenting part should be gently dislodged digitally so as to obviate compression of the cord between the presenting part and the bony pelvis. With the hand maintained in the vagina in order to keep pressure off the cord, the patient is quickly transferred to the operating room, where an immediate decision is made whether to proceed with cesarean section or to effect prompt vaginal delivery if obstetrically feasible.

Prolapsed Arm

A prolapsed arm is sometimes seen with a shoulder presentation when the membranes are ruptured. This accident generally occurs only in neglected labors or in unregistered patients who have had no medical care. The fetal heart tones should be auscultated but no vaginal manipulations or examinations undertaken in the emergency room. The patient should be directed to the operating room in anticipation of immediate cesarean section. Vaginal examination in the operating room will determine the definitive management; with rare exception, it will consist of prompt cesarean section.

Prolapsed Foot

The appearance of one foot or both feet outside the vulva need not occasion great alarm; it occurs not infrequently with footling breech presentations long before actual delivery. The fetal heart tones should be auscultated. Vaginal examination should not be performed. The patient should be immediately transferred to the delivery room for definitive examination.

If, however, the breech is already delivered as far as the umbilicus or farther, the remainder of the delivery should be completed as atraumatically as possible. The fetal back must be kept anterior. It may be necessary to assist with delivery of the arms. This is done by gently rotating the body so as to bring one shoulder anterior under the symphysis, thus facilitating delivery of the anterior arm, then rotating in the opposite direction to bring the posterior shoulder anterior. Delivery of the head, which in this case comes afterward, is accomplished by passing one hand along the posterior vaginal wall in order to flex the fetal head by exerting pressure with two fingers over the malar eminences while two fingers of the other hand exert gentle traction on the shoulders. Premature traction on the breech must be avoided. It is always proper to make a liberal episiotomy for a breech delivery. Following any delivery in the emergency room, the patient should be transferred to the delivery room for complete and thorough examination of the entire birth canal.

PEDIATRIC EMERGENCIES

Pediatric emergencies of a gynecological nature are uncommon; nevertheless, they do occur and hence deserve appropriate consideration. The conditions encountered fall into the following categories.

Bleeding

Vaginal bleeding in a child invariably alarms the mother, who may promptly bring the child for medical examination. The bleeding is practically never of serious proportions. A detailed history should be obtained including specific inquiry as to whether the child had inadvertently ingested any sex steroid medication such as oral contraceptive formulations. The breasts and external genitalia should be examined for evidence of precocious sexual development. A gentle rectal examination should be performed in order to determine the possible presence of a foreign body in the vagina and to detect a possible pelvic mass or palpable ovarian enlargement. If the physical examination serves to exclude gross organic disease and the bleeding is presumed to be of a functional nature, the patient should be referred to a suitable consultant for appropriate investigations. If a foreign body in the vagina is detected on rectal palpation, an attempt may be made to remove it by means of a Kelly clamp or a long, thin, nasal forceps. If this is not possible, the child should be hospitalized for vaginoscopy and removal of the foreign body under general anesthesia.

Trauma

Genital trauma to a child is generally sustained by way of straddle falls, injury while climbing a fence, a kick in the perineum, and so forth. The resultant injury usually takes the form of single or multiple lacerations, ecchymoses, and vulvar hematomas. These are assessed and managed in accordance with principles outlined under Genital Injuries, Nonspecific Trauma, earlier in this chapter. Any child with a vaginal wound should be examined under anesthesia.

Infection

Gonococcal vulvovaginitis in premenarchal children is generally acquired through cross infection from other girls or from an infected attendant or parent. It is relatively uncommon. Trichomonad and candidial vulvovaginitis are also uncommon in the child, although the latter may be seen more frequently as a sequel to broad-spectrum antibiotic therapy. Streptococci, staphylococci, pneumococci, and colon bacilli may cause occasional infections. Nonspecific vaginitis occurs most commonly in the child. It may, on occasion, be associated with pinworms which should be searched for by conventional means. The vaginal discharge should be examined for ova. Also, a foreign body in the vagina should always be excluded by rectal palpation and vaginoscopy where possible. Pencils, crayons, pins, beads, bits of cloth or paper, etc., may find their way into the vagina. A foreign body generally gives rise to a serosanguineous or purulosanguineous discharge. Treatment is predicated on specific diagnosis.

Congenital Anomalies

The congenital anomaly most likely to occasion an emergency visit is an imperforate hymen. This is largely an inconsequential anomaly and is often not discovered till the menarche. With the first menses, which may occur at age 10 or 11, symptoms arise due to the development of a hematocolpos. Not infrequently several menstrual cycles occur before the patient is brought to medical attention with symptoms of cyclic lower abdominal pain, awareness of a suprapubic mass, and occasionally urinary retention. Examination of the introitus will reveal a bulging cystic mass. The patient should be hospitalized for hymenectomy in order to release the accumulated menstrual blood. Occasionally, hematometra and hematosalpinx further complicate the problem. Antibiotics are indicated, for the accumulated bloody discharge serves as a good nidus for potential infection.

General Principles in the Management of Wounds

11

CHARLES ECKERT

Most wounds seen in the emergency room are small, superficial, and not associated with significant derangement of vital functions. In such "minor wounds" definitive treatment should be given in the emergency room and follow-up care provided on an ambulatory basis. Persons with extensive wounds, neglected or infected wounds, and wounds involving nerves, musculotendinous structures, major blood vessels, or body cavities should all be admitted to the hospital for definitive care in the operating room.

The objectives of wound management are the same regardless of severity, mechanism, or anatomical site: (1) healing, preferably by primary intention, should take place as rapidly as possible; (2) function is to be maintained or restored; and (3) scarring and deformity are to be minimized.

PRELIMINARY PROCEDURES

Evaluation of the Patient

A rapid assessment of the condition of the patient should precede the taking of a detailed history or inspection of wounds. Adequacy of the airway, the presence of shock, the level of consciousness, and the presence of associated major injuries, particularly those necessitating immediate splinting, all take precedence over management of the wound. The presence of continued bleeding of major proportions requires rapid measures for control, since this is the most important initial step in the management of shock.

Hemorrhage is usually best controlled by the application of direct pressure using aseptic precautions. When this is impossible, direct transfer to the operating room is probably best. Seldom is it advisable or possible to apply hemostatic forceps and ligatures to major vessels in the emergency room. Pneumatic tourniquets can be used safely and expeditiously in some cases, but most tourniquets used for first aid are ineffective and hazardous. Tourniquets which have been applied before the patient was transported to the emergency room should be removed and the interval between their application and removal noted.

History

While evaluation of the patient is in process and thereafter, the history should be obtained from the patient or a credible witness, if one is available. The history should include the mechanism of injury, the approximate time of occurrence, local care previously given, the condition of the patient at the time of injury, and the extent of contamination.

A history of *tetanus immunization* with toxoid, including the dates of primary immunization and of booster injections, is to be obtained in all wounded patients. In nonimmunized patients it is necessary to determine whether tetanus antitoxin has previously been given, and, if so, whether any allergic reaction has been experienced. A history of the presence of *allergic reactions* in general should also be sought, but specifically one must inquire into reactions to local anesthetic agents and to antimicrobials. In *animal bites,* of particular concern are the species involved, the condition of the animal, with emphasis on clinical manifestations of rabies, and the availability of the animal for observation.

Physical Examination

A complete physical examination is to be done on all patients seen in the emergency room. In the wounded patient this will have been accomplished in the initial evaluation of the patient, but special attention must be given the wounded part, directed toward determining the presence of concomitant injuries to sensory or motor nerves, tendons, or underlying bone. Special reference to specific aspects of examination of the hand and cranium will be found in Chapters 5 and 13.

Inspection of the Wound

Dressings should be removed by preference in those areas of the emergency room devoted to the definitive care of lacerations. The immediate availability of sterile dressings, irrigating and cleansing solutions, and a suture tray should be assured. Figure 11-1 shows a typical tray used for suture of lacerations at the Albany Medical Center Hospital.

The wound is examined to determine its extent, the presence of foreign material, damage to surrounding epithelium, and evidence of devitalization. If the dressing prior to removal interfered with complete functional evaluation of the part, the examination should be completed.

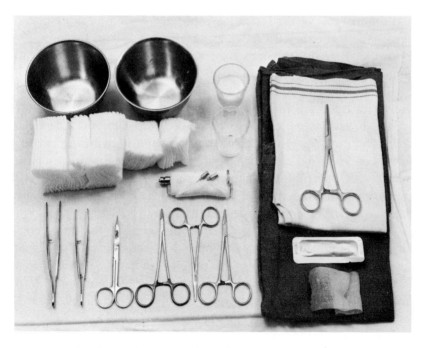

Fig. 11-1. Sterile tray for suture of lacerations.

TYPES OF WOUNDS

Lacerations

Based on the time elapsed since the injury, the degree of contamination, and the anatomical site involved, a decision can now be made regarding the advisability of managing the wound by primary closure as opposed to delayed primary closure. The so-called golden period during which primary closure can be carried out with impunity is usually considered to be 6 hours. However, when contamination is minimal and the area involved has a good blood supply (hand, scalp, face, anterior neck), this period can be extended to 12 hours with reasonable safety.

The skin surrounding the laceration is shaved (exception: eyebrows), then cleansed with an antiseptic detergent (pHisoHex) or a liquid soap containing 3% hexachlorophene, and sterile 0.85% saline solution for 10 minutes. The wound itself should not be included in this step, but following scrubbing of the skin the wound is copiously irrigated with saline solution. Sterile drapes are applied and the margins of the laceration infiltrated with a local anesthetic agent. We use either 0.5% lidocaine (Xylocaine) or 1% procaine (Novocain). Débridement is then carried out by excision of dead and devitalized tissue. Irregular and beveled skin edges are trimmed, but no attempt is made to "excise the wound." Foreign material, if present, is removed. Bleeding vessels are clamped with "mosquito" arterial hemostats and ligated with 5-0 chromic catgut. The deep fascia or galea aponeurotica, if involved, is sutured with interrupted sutures of 3-0 or 4-0 chromic catgut. The skin margins are approximated with interrupted subcuticular sutures of the same material; and to prevent overriding of the skin, skin sutures of 5-0 silk are taken at $\frac{1}{16}$ inch from the edges of the wound.

An alternative method of closure of the skin is the so-called nonsuture technique, in which already prepared commercially available "butterflies" are used. When the skin is accurately approximated in this way, excellent cosmetic results are possible. However, dead space must be obliterated and overriding absolutely avoided, regardless of the method used for closure of the skin.

When the wound is thought to be particularly prone to infection either because of delay, contamination of the skin at the time of wounding, contamination of the object inflicting the wound, or contamination subsequent to wounding, treatment by *delayed primary closure* should be elected. In this case the wound is handled identically with that which is to be closed primarily, up to the point of closure itself. After débridement is complete and hemostasis obtained, a small tampon of fine-mesh gauze is inserted in the wound and an occlusive dressing applied. In the absence of excessive drainage, odor, pain, or fever, the dressing is not disturbed for 4 days. At this time the wound is inspected, the fine-mesh gauze tampon being moistened with saline solution to assist in its removal. If the wound is grossly clean, it can be closed by either suture or nonsuture technique at this time. The optimum period for closure of wounds handled in this manner is 4 to 8 days. Beyond this time closure is impractical because healing will have progressed sufficiently to limit mobilization of the wound margins, and healing will proceed by secondary intention. Except in the case of human bites or comparable contamination of the wound, we seldom resort to delayed primary closure of lacerations of the face or hands.

The routine adjuvant use of antimicrobial agents is not recommended in the treatment of patients with lacerations except when the likelihood of infection is great. In such cases 1,200,000 units of phenoxymethyl penicillin is given daily in divided doses, unless a history of penicillin sensitivity has been elicited. Under these circumstances tetracycline is substituted, using 1 gm per day in four divided doses.

Tetanus prophylaxis is a necessary consideration in all wounds, including lacerations, since *Clostridium tetani* is so widespread in nature. However, lacerations sustained from household utensils when the skin is clean present little risk.

Follow-up at regular intervals, particularly in the first 72 hours after injury, is most important if infections occurring in the wound are not to be neglected. This by preference should be done by the same physician responsible for primary treatment, but if "on-call" schedules make it impractical, the patient should be seen by an alternate physician. The first visit should be at a minimum of 24 hours after initial treatment. The appearance of pain, fever, or drainage at any time is pathognomonic of infection. In all cases, however, the wound should be inspected and, if clean, simply redressed. If infection is suspected, one or two adjacent sutures should be removed after the wound has been painted with an antiseptic, such as vinylpyrrolidone-iodine complex (Betadine). A sterile probe should then be inserted. If pus is present, a culture should be obtained and adequate drainage then provided by the removal of additional sutures. The opened wound should be irrigated with saline solution and loosely packed with fine-mesh gauze. When evidence of invasive infections, such as extensive cellulitis, lymphangitis, lymphadenitis, fever, and leukocytosis, is present, the patient should be admitted to the hospital for further treatment. If systemic manifestations of infection are absent, continued ambulatory care is feasible. Pending the results of culture and the determination of antimicrobial sensitivities, it is best to start treatment with penicillin, using either phenoxymethyl penicillin orally or procaine penicillin intramuscularly.

The patient should be advised to rest, but more specifically the involved part is placed at rest, either by splinting or by means of bulky dressings. Use of wet dressings and local heat is probably unnecessary under the above circumstances. Subsequent wound cleansing and redressing on a daily basis are indicated. In some extensive lacerations which become infected following primary closure, the time requisite for healing can be shortened by secondary closure after the wound margins are covered by healthy granulation tissue.

Removal of sutures in cleanly healed lacerations varies with the anatomical site involved. On the face or scalp, skin sutures should be removed within 24–48 hours of closure; on the back they should be left in place for 8–10 days; on the palm of the hand they should not be removed for a full 2 weeks.

Abrasions

Characteristically, abrasions are associated with considerable local pain. In most instances they are managed by simple cleansing with an antiseptic detergent without anesthesia followed by the application of a nonadhering layer of sterile fine-mesh material and an occlusive dressing. Complete healing usually requires from 10 to 14 days. In some abrasions particulate matter is ground into the dermis and if not removed may leave unsightly tattoo-like marks. When such foreign particles are present, they must be removed as completely as possible by scrubbing with a sterile brush and antiseptic detergent solution. Anesthesia will be required. For small lesions, field block with a local anesthetic will suffice; for large lesions, general anesthesia is necessary.

Puncture Wounds

Puncture wounds are most commonly incurred by stepping on boards with projecting nails, accidental (or intentional) stabbing with ice picks, knives, and so forth. When both the skin and the offending object are known to be clean, the skin is thoroughly cleaned and a sterile dressing applied. In most instances, however, these circumstances do not hold, and more aggressive treatment is indicated. After the skin has been cleansed, the area is anesthetized by local infiltration, the skin margins, if irregular and devitalized, are excised, and the wound is opened. Foreign material is removed, hemostasis is obtained, and after thorough irrigation with 0.85% saline solution the wound is packed with fine-mesh gauze and a sterile dressing applied. In most cases the pack is removed in 24 hours and the edges are allowed to fall together. When the edges are separated, they can be handled by delayed primary closure.

Animal Bites

Animal bites are essentially puncture wounds in which both contamination and tissue injury are likely to be greater than in puncture wounds produced by inanimate objects. Generally the mouths of carnivorous animals harbor a greater number and variety of pathogenic microorganisms than do those of herbivorous animals, but none exceed man in the likelihood and severity of infected wounds resulting from contact with the teeth. In this country dog bites are by far the most common animal bites treated in emergency rooms.

Aside from the question of rabies, treatment of animal bites is essentially the same as that for other puncture wounds. Many surgeons routinely close dog bites after cleansing and débridement. We believe, however, that it is safest to treat them by delayed primary closure with the exception of those on the face and hands. The latter are carefully closed for cosmetic reasons, and because of the excellent blood supply they seldom become infected. The use of fuming nitric acid and other comparable agents recommended in former years has been abandoned as more harmful than helpful.

Human bites deserve special mention because of the severe necrotizing infections which commonly result from the anaerobic and microaerophilic organisms present in the human mouth. *These wounds should never be closed,* and antimicrobial prophylaxis should be instituted in all but the most trivial human bite wounds. The hand is the most common site of injury, as it is often the result of a blow on the mouth with the closed fist. The wound is located over the metacarpal heads and frequently involves the metacarpophalangeal joint. Infection in these cases is very likely to produce serious disability. After thorough cleansing and débridement, the wound is packed open and the hand immobilized in the position of function. Except in the case of a small superficial wound, the patient with a human-bite wound should be admitted to the hospital for wound care as described above.

Frostbite

Prolonged exposure to temperatures below freezing results in progressive necrosis. This is secondary to ice crystal formation within cells and decreased oxygenation from progressive vascular thrombosis. Frostbite affects primarily exposed and peripheral portions of the body, thus the nose, ears, toes and feet, and fingers and hands are most frequently affected. The involved part is cold and pale; as rewarming progresses it becomes red to cyanotic, swollen, and finally blisters form.

Treatment in the emergency room consists of rewarming by immersion in water at temperatures ranging from 100 to 110° F. The part should be protected from injury and infection. Débridement should be minimal, for the extent of tissue damage is always less than that suggested by the early appearance of the part.

MANAGEMENT

Dressing the Wound

In its simplest form the wound dressing attempts to maintain the aseptic environment in which wound management is begun. Further, the dressing may be used to minimize edema or actual bleeding into the wound area by the application of pressure. Splinting also is useful, up to a point, in aiding in the healing of wounds. It must be recognized, however, that within a matter of hours the cleanly incised, sutured wound will be sealed from the environment and can be left exposed with no greater risk of infection than in the wound covered by layers of sterile gauze. In the same few hours bacteria on the skin surface grow beneath the sterile gauze and constitute as great or a greater source of contamination than ambient organisms in a clean environment. In the application of pressure dressings, a narrow path is trod between inadequate pressure on the one side and dangerous excess on the other. While movement at the wound margins is undesirable, prolonged splinting leads to joint changes and atrophy. Pressure dressings are not a substitute for adequate hemostasis at the time of wound management.

From this brief discussion of the pros and cons of dressings, it is apparent that common sense and judgment influence the type of dressing applied to wounds to a greater extent than do scientific certitudes which can be formulated into rules. In the ambulatory care of patients with wounds, follow-up at short intervals is impossible; accordingly, in the use of dressings it is better to err on the side of safety than to risk pressure necrosis or devitalization due to circulatory embarrassment. Dressings should be kept simple, with a layer of nonadhering material placed adjacent to the wound and sufficient sterile gauze applied to absorb anticipated drainage of bloody ooze from the wound. If a circular bandage is applied, it should not be excessively tight but should be anchored securely to the skin above and below with adhesive tape to prevent slipping. Splints, when used, should be well padded. The patient should certainly be told to return if a dressing is inadvertently loosened, is contaminated, or for any reason proves inadequate, as well as when pain, anesthesia, paresthesia, change in color, or marked swelling is noted.

Tetanus Prophylaxis

The procedure recommended conforms in general to the recommendations of the Committee on Trauma of the American College of Surgeons. In all wounds in which the possibility of contamination by dirt or soil exists there is need for tetanus prophylaxis. Thoughtful consideration of this statement will lead to the conclusion that few wounds will not be included.

1. Of greatest importance in tetanus prophylaxis is proper *meticulous care of the wound,* including irrigation, débridement of dead and devitalized tissue, and removal of foreign bodies.

2. Every patient should receive tetanus toxoid at the time of in-

jury, as a booster for those previously immunized or as the initial immunizing dose, unless he has received a booster or completed his immunization within the past 12 months.

3. Patients not previously immunized should receive 250 units of human tetanus-immune globulin.

In wounds of slight to moderate severity which have been promptly and properly treated, antibiotic prophylaxis should be instituted. In patients not sensitive to penicillin, 1,200,000 units of benzathine penicillin G (Bicillin), administered in a deep intramuscular injection, are recommended. Penicillin-sensitive patients should be given tetracycline 0.5 gm four times a day by mouth for 3 weeks.

4. Every wounded patient should receive a written record of immunization procedures and be instructed to carry it with him. If necessary, arrangements should be made for him to complete active immunization.

5. Basic immunization with alum-precipitated toxoid requires three injections spaced at 4 to 6 weeks between the first two injections and 6 to 12 months between the second and third. If fluid toxoid is used, four injections are preferable, allowing 4 to 6 weeks between the first three injections and 6 to 12 months between the third and fourth injections.

Gas Gangrene

Adequate wound toilet and the exercise of good judgment in the selection of wounds for primary closure as opposed to delayed primary closure are the best prophylaxis against gas gangrene. Use of mixed gas bacillus antitoxin on a prophylactic basis is *not* recommended, and penicillin prophylaxis is not a substitute for the adequate removal of foreign material and excision of dead and devitalized tissue.

Rabies Prophylaxis

Prophylaxis against rabies must be considered in all individuals who sustain animal bites and those who are in contact with bat excreta, since the bat population in this country is highly infected. The latter situation arises commonly among cave explorers. When patients who have been bitten by dogs are seen in the emergency room, the police should be notified, so they may take proper precautions to assure that the dog will be observed for the minimal 10-day period.

In former years, when vaccine was prepared from brain tissue, serious reactions were so common that its use was omitted in many patients who were actually at risk. With the development of the duck-embryo vaccine, this situation no longer applies, and the following recommendations of the World Health Organization's expert committee on rabies should be observed.

1. If contact with the rabid animal has been indirect or if there has been only a lick on unabraded skin, no exposure is considered to have occurred and vaccine is not recommended.

2. If the exposure was mild, i.e., a lick on unabraded skin or on mucosal surfaces, or for single bites *not* on the head, neck, face, or arm: (a) if the animal is healthy at the time of exposure, withhold vaccine, but observe the animal for 10 days; (b) if during the 10-day observation period the animal is proved to have rabies or becomes clinically suspect, start vaccine immediately; (c) if the animal has signs indicating possible rabies at the time of exposure, start vaccine immediately, but stop injections if the animal is normal on the fifth day of exposure; (d) if the animal is rabid, if it escapes or is killed, or if its condition is unknown, give complete course of vaccine, and if the biting animal is wild, also give rabies antiserum.

3. If exposure was severe (multiple bites or single bites on the head, neck, face, or arm), the indications for giving vaccine are the same as in mild exposure (see 2 above). In addition, in every category, the administration of rabies antiserum is recommended.

Serum administered concurrently with vaccine interferes with the development of active immunity. If serum is used, supplementary doses of vaccine 10 and 20 days after the last usual dose are recommended.

Side-effects of Duck Embryo Vaccine

Severe reactions to duck embryo vaccine are very infrequent. Local reactions consist of tenderness at the site of injection, erythema and induration, and regional lymphadenopathy. Systemic sensitivity may be encountered, including urticaria and dyspnea. Three cases of anaphylactic shock have been reported. Therefore, in patients with a history of allergy, skin testing is advisable before the vaccine is given.

Two patients have been reported with symptoms suggesting encephalitis and two with transverse myelitis; all four patients recovered completely. It is recommended by the manufacturer that "if symptoms appear that indicate central-nervous-system involvement, vaccine injections should be discontinued."

Orthopedic Injuries 12

DONALD B. KETTELKAMP

The purpose of this chapter is to present a guide to the emergency-room care of patients with musculoskeletal injuries. The physical and roentgenographic examinations and the procedures performed in the emergency room will be discussed and, for the definitive care of patients with injuries which require hospital care, the reader is referred to the standard fracture texts.

PHYSICAL EXAMINATION

The patient's hospital record constitutes part of the emergency-room care. The portion of the record pertaining to orthopedic injuries should be completed as soon as the patient's injuries permit. An accurate description of the injuries and a statement of the status of peripheral innervation and vascular supply should be included in the report. The examiner should also record the date and time of the examination. All extremity injuries require continued observation of the neurovascular status and only with an accurate examination, including the time of that examination, can changes be determined.

Spine

The patient's neck and back should be gently palpated for areas of tenderness before he is moved. This can be done easily by depressing the mattress with one hand and sliding the other hand under the patient. Head halter traction, sandbags on each side of the head, or a firm collar support should be applied if a cervical fracture is suspected. Portable lateral roentgenograms should be taken *before* the patient is moved. If a fracture is not present and if the roentgenograms are normal, the range of active motion to the point of pain should be noted. Reflexes should be checked on all unfractured extremities and sensation to pinprick, including the perineal area, noted. Finger and toe motion is also noted. A more detailed examination can then be made if there are no obvious fractures and if movement will not adversely affect associated injuries.

Extremities

Dislocations and angulated fractures should be obvious at inspection and the part moved carefully and only sufficiently to improve alignment and obtain roentgenograms. The extremities should be carefully palpated for areas of tenderness.

Sensation to pinprick and peripheral pulses are examined in each extremity and with particular care distally to the site of fracture. The examiner must know the cutaneous and motor innervation of the major peripheral nerves.

If the patient is conscious, he should be asked to move each extremity in turn within the limits of pain. If he is unconscious, each extremity should be examined, palpated, and, if it is not obviously injured, passively moved through a range of motion.

Examination as outlined is usually sufficient for the upper extremity with the exception of the hand (see Chapter 13). In the lower extremity the knee, foot, and ankle require special comment.

KNEE.   The majority of knee injuries involve the ligaments and meniscus rather than bone. The collateral ligaments, joint line, tibial plateau, and femoral condyles must be carefully palpated to determine the site of injury. If the tibial plateau or femoral condyles are tender, roentgenograms to rule out fracture must be taken prior to further examination. In the absence of fractures the examiner must determine if the knee can fully extend and if there is ligamentous injury. A massive effusion or hemarthrosis can limit extension. The examiner may need to aspirate the knee under aseptic conditions to determine if the knee can fully extend. The collateral ligaments are examined with the knee in 20 degrees of flexion. The examiner abducts the tibia to test the lateral collateral ligament. The anterior cruciate ligament is examined by flexing the knee to 90 degrees, fixing the foot, and pulling the proximal tibia forward. The posterior cruciate is examined with the knee in the same position as for the anterior cruciate but by pushing the tibia posteriorly. Further, with a posterior cruciate and capsular tear the knee may be hyperextended. The methods of examining the menisci are usually not possible after an acute injury.

FOOT AND ANKLE.   Both ligament injuries and fractures are common. Areas of swelling and tenderness should be carefully noted and appropriate roentgenograms always obtained.

Rupture of the Achilles tendon should be suspected if the patient has heel and calf pain. A palpable defect is present, but after swelling has occurred the defect may no longer be felt. Plantar flexion is weak. The foot does not plantar-flex well when the calf muscles are squeezed and the patient has a flatfoot gait. Rupture of the plantaris tendon may occasionally be confused with rupture of the Achilles tendon. With rupture of the plantaris tendon there is no palpable defect, the patient can contract the gastrosoleus muscles, and plantar flexion of the foot does occur when the examiner squeezes the patient's calf.

ROENTGENOGRAPHIC EXAMINATION

Roentgenographic examination is a mandatory part of the orthopedic examination both medically and legally. Sufficient and appropriate roentgenograms to establish a diagnosis must be obtained on any suspected fracture. On the other hand, improper and unnecessary roentgenograms are to be discouraged because of the excessive exposure and the delay in treatment which results. Roentgenograms should also be taken after reduction or after the application of skeletal traction.

It is the attending surgeon's responsibility—and it cannot be delegated to an x-ray technician—to be certain that no further injury is sustained by the patient during the roentgenographic examination. This requires that he control the injured part during placement and removal of the cassettes.

Extremities

The minimum number of roentgenograms required for examination of an extremity are two: the anteroposterior (AP) and the lateral views. Additional views depend on the part examined and the suspected injury. The minimum views for the most frequently examined areas are as follows:

Hand: AP, lateral, and oblique.

Wrist: AP and lateral. The navicular view is necessary when there is tenderness in the anatomical snuffbox.

Elbow: AP and lateral are standard. However, oblique views are frequently necessary, particularly for suspected radial head fractures.

Shoulders: AP views in neutral, internal, and external rotation, axillary, and transthoracic views are used individually or in combination, depending on the type of injury.

Sternoclavicular joint: This joint is difficult to visualize adequately and requires an oblique view which eliminates the factor of superimposition over the vertebral column. Tomograms may be helpful.

Knee: Patellar, notch, and oblique views of the tibial plateau in addition to the AP and lateral may be necessary.

Ankle: An AP view which shows the mortise well and a lateral are minimum. An oblique view will frequently show a fracture of the lateral malleolus which is not otherwise visible. AP and lateral views of the entire fibula in addition to the ankle views are indicated when only the medial malleolus is fractured or when diastasis of the distal tibiofibular joint is suspected.

Foot: AP, lateral, and oblique views are minimum.

Comparison views of the uninjured extremity are frequently of value in establishing the diagnosis, particularly in children.

Spine

Roentgenograms are indicated in all cases of injury to the back or neck. Films of the cervical spine should also be obtained in all cases of head injury. Although roentgenograms of better quality can usually be obtained on the x-ray table, the patient should not be moved until unstable injuries have been ruled out. A portable lateral roentgenogram of the injured area should be taken and read. If an unstable fracture or fracture dislocation of the cervical spine is visualized, skeletal traction using tongs should be applied to stabilize the spine prior to further roentgenographic examination. If the lateral view is normal, the AP and odontoid views are obtained by sliding the cassette under the patient. Oblique views can be obtained with the cassette in the same position by angling the x-ray tube about 45 to 50 degrees.

MULTIPLE INJURIES AND MULTIPLE FRACTURES

The patient who has sustained multiple injuries including fractures presents many problems in diagnosis and treatment. Because fractures are often more obvious than injuries to intrathoracic or abdominal viscera or the brain, it is appropriate to emphasize again the importance of early recognition and treatment of these life-endangering injuries. The emergency-room treatment of the orthopedic injuries will frequently depend on whether or not anesthesia can or will be given, since all of these patients will be admitted. When anesthesia is necessary because of other severe injuries, the necessary orthopedic procedures which will not further jeopardize the patient should be carried out at the same time. If the patient's condition prohibits anesthesia, the fractures should be aligned and immobilized with a cast or traction in the emergency room.

Priority of Care of Orthopedic Injuries

There is also priority of care in handling multiple orthopedic injuries. This can be determined by answering the following questions.

1. What injuries endanger life or limb?
   Some fractures and fracture-dislocations of the spine and some of the very severe open fractures are examples.
2. What injuries are particularly prone to produce shock?
   Fractures of the pelvis and of the shaft of the femur are examples.
3. What injuries have a poor prognosis when treatment is delayed?
   Fracture-dislocations of the hip or talus and open fractures are examples.

4. What injuries are suitable for immediate immobilization or traction with definitive treatment at a later time?

Fractures of the hip and unstable fractures of the shafts of the radius and ulna are examples.

5. What injuries can be treated in a definitive manner without harm to a severely injured patient?

Distal forearm fractures, most fractures of the humerus, and skeletal traction for fractures of the femoral shaft are examples.

OPEN FRACTURES

Open fractures are always emergencies. The time between the injury and débridement in the operating room must be kept to the minimum if infection is to be avoided. The emergency-room care consists of examination of the patient, splinting the extremity and applying a sterile dressing to the wound, drawing blood for typing and cross matching, and starting intravenous fluids. An intravenous antibiotic, usually penicillin, is added to the intravenous fluids. Prophylactic measures against tetanus and gas gangrene should be taken and are discussed elsewhere in this text.

Occasionally the surgeon is confronted with an open fracture in a patient to whom anesthesia is a greater threat to life than the fracture. In this situation débridement should be done in the operating room using local infiltration with 1% lidocaine (Xylocaine) or procaine. The wound is cleaned with saline irrigation, and devitalized tissue and foreign material are removed. If the débridement has been less than optimum because of the limitations of anesthesia, the wound should not be sutured but a simple sterile gauze dressing should be applied with a layer of nonadhering petroleum jelly gauze next to the wound. Subsequently the part is immobilized in traction or a plaster cast. A second débridement may be performed as soon as the patient's condition permits, or, if the wound is satisfactory, secondary closure may be done.

SPLINTING FOR TRANSPORTATION

A fracture should be handled as little as possible consistent with obtaining reduction and immobilization. The surgeon must keep this in mind when determining whether to splint a fracture in the emergency room when definitive treatment will be administered soon. Splinting should not be used to enable untrained personnel to handle the fracture for roentgenographic or other examinations.

Intrahospital Splinting

The injured part should be placed in a comfortable, stable position. The upper extremity can be placed against the side of the chest and abdomen or on a pillow, whichever requires the least motion at the fracture site. If the patient is ambulatory, a sling or sling and swathe may be used. Occasionally the pneumatic splint can be used to advantage on a forearm fracture. Definitive care should be given as soon as possible. The lower extremity should be aligned and supported on a pillow or in a pillow splint. The cardboard or air splint will also provide good temporary immobilization for ankle and tibial injuries. Splints must be adequately padded to avoid producing pressure necrosis.

Interhospital Splinting

An injured patient should not be transferred from one hospital to another during the immediate postinjury period unless emergency procedures are required which cannot be performed at the first hospital.

The best splint for most ankle, tibia, wrist, forearm, and elbow injuries is a plaster cast. This is applied after alignment or reduction of the fracture has been obtained. The danger with a cast results from pressure and circulatory embarrassment due to swelling. It can be decreased by splitting the cast prior to transport so that it can be spread during transit if necessary. The second-best method is to bivalve the cast and leave the extremity in the posterior half. Well-padded metal, air, and cardboard splints may also be used. Fractures of the humerus are best treated with a coaptation splint, sling, and swathe as previously described. A sling and swathe are usually adequate for shoulder injuries. Fractures of the femur can be splinted on a well-padded and carefully applied full-ring Thomas splint. Care must be taken to avoid pressure necrosis from the ring and from the strapping about the foot and ankle. Patients with fractures of the pelvis and spine are best moved on a padded inflexible flat surface. Basket stretchers should not be used because it is difficult to move the patient in and out of them without flexing the spine.

TRACTION

Traction may be used to obtain reduction, to maintain reduction, and to immobilize the injured extremity. It may be used as definitive treatment or as a temporary method of immobilization prior to other procedures. The two basic types, skin traction and skeletal traction, will be discussed separately.

Skin Traction

Skin traction is suitable when not over 10 and preferably 5 pounds of traction will be required. It is thus limited to the treatment of fractures in small children and temporary immobilization for comfort in adults. It can easily be applied in the emergency room.

METHOD.   The basic method of application is used for any type of skin traction. Variations will be noted under specific types.

The skin is painted with tincture of benzoin or Ace adherent. Shaving the part first is not necessary but makes removal of the skin tapes more comfortable. The malleoli and heel, condyles of the humerus, or distal radius and ulna are padded with several layers of sheet wadding. Two strips of moleskin are cut as wide as can be placed about the part and long enough to be attached to a foot piece or block of wood. The moleskin is then placed on the skin, and care must be taken to apply it smoothly because blisters will occur under wrinkles. An elastic bandage is then wrapped under the moleskin from the toes to the ankle and over the moleskin above the malleoli. When skin traction is applied to the forearm, an elastic bandage is not required distally to the wrist, but a crosspiece should be applied for the hand to grasp and there must be room for a full range of finger motion. Traction is applied by hanging the weights from the rope attached to the foot piece or wooden block.

TYPES AND USES OF SKIN TRACTION

1. *Bryant's traction* (Fig. 12-1) is used to treat femoral shaft fractures in infants. The patient must be under 40 pounds in weight and under 4 years of age, and *not* have tight hamstrings. The hamstring tightness is checked by extending the knee and flexing the hip on the uninjured side. The leg must go to 90 degrees of flexion without resistance.

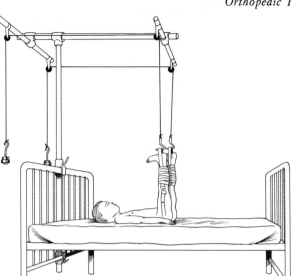

Fig. 12-1. Bryant's traction. Skin traction is applied to both lower extremities, and sufficient weight is used so that the buttocks just clear the bed. (Figs. 12-1–12-5, 12-7, and 12-8 from G. Schmeisser, Jr. [7]. *A Clinical Manual of Orthopedic Traction Techniques.* Philadelphia: Saunders, 1963. Reproduced by courtesy of the author and the publisher.)

Skin traction is applied to both legs distal to the fracture site. Both legs are then suspended with sufficient weight to have the buttocks just clear the bed.

Complications—ischemic necrosis of muscle resembling Volkmann's contracture in the forearm, and ulcerations of the skin beneath the moleskin—may occur on either side, and close observation is necessary if Bryant's traction is used.

2. *Russell's traction* (Fig. 12-2) is used for femoral shaft fractures, particularly in children under 8 years of age. The pad under the distal femur and knee can be made by placing a large piece of felt inside some tubular stockinette. Pressure on the peroneal nerve and fibular head must be carefully avoided.

3. *Buck's traction* (Fig. 12-3) may be used for temporary immobilization of hip fractures prior to operative fixation and for immobilizing or straightening a knee.

4. *Dunlop's traction* (Fig. 12-4) is used for supracondylar fractures of the humerus in children. It can also be used to control the forearm when applying skeletal traction through the olecranon.

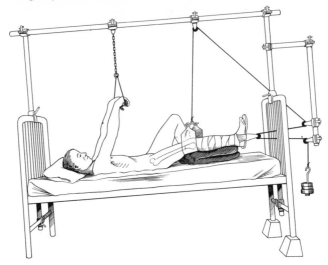

Fig. 12-2.   Russell's traction. (From Schmeisser [7].)

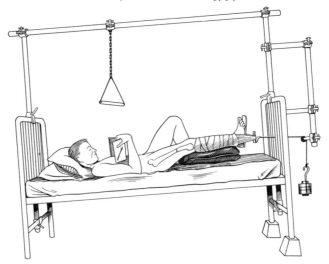

Fig. 12-3.   Buck's traction. The leg must be supported so that the heel just clears the bed to avoid pressure necrosis of the heel. (From Schmeisser [7].)

Skeletal Traction

Skeletal traction is a definitive method of treating some long bone fractures. It is preferable to skin traction where more than 10 pounds of weight must be used and when traction will be necessary for a long period. Because skeletal traction can usually be applied

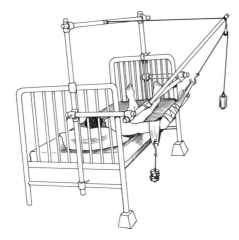

Fig. 12-4. Dunlop's traction. (From Schmeisser [7].)

in the emergency room it is particularly useful when the patient's other injuries preclude general anesthesia.

GENERAL METHODS. The insertion of a Steinmann pin or Kirschner wire through a bone requires strict adherence to aseptic technique to minimize the risk of infection. The area of insertion should be shaved. A sufficient area of skin to avoid contamination of the site is then prepared. Gloves, mask, and sterile instruments should be used. The skin is prepared by cleansing it with ether, alcohol, and Betadine, or other suitable methods of skin preparation. The prepared area is then draped with sterile towels.

The skin, subcutaneous tissue, and periosteum along the tract of the pin are infiltrated with 1% lidocaine or procaine. A small incision in the direction of pull of the traction is made in the skin at the site of insertion. The pin or wire is then inserted with a hand drill perpendicular to the anticipated line of traction—usually perpendicular, that is, to the longitudinal axis of the bone. When the pin tents the skin on the opposite side, the skin is incised. After the pin is through the bone sufficiently for application of the traction bow, the drill is removed and gauze sponges are placed over the skin incisions. The sponges are soaked with an antiseptic solution or collodion. The traction bow is then applied and excess pin cut off. Corks or tape are placed over the cut wire ends. Rope and weights are attached to the traction bow and the extremity is suspended in the appropriate manner for the fracture being treated.

The general rule in choosing the transfixation wire is to choose the smallest diameter which will withstand the amount of traction needed. A small *Kirschner wire* injures a minimal amount of bone and carries a minimal risk of pin tract infection but is more likely to break or cut through the bone. A large *Steinmann pin* damages more bone and has an increased risk of pin tract infection but will tolerate heavy traction with little risk of cutting through the bone. The ideal size is usually between these extremes.

Steinmann pins and Kirschner wires may be either smooth or threaded. The smooth wires are stronger for a given diameter and are easier to remove but tend to slide in the bone, increasing the risk of infection and pressure necrosis from the traction bow. The threaded wires require a drill for removal but do not slide. In general we prefer threaded wires.

SPECIFIC METHODS

CALCANEUS. The major disadvantage to calcaneal traction is the risk of an infection which is difficult to treat. The preferred site for insertion is 1 inch distal and 1 inch posterior to the lateral malleolus and 1½ inches distal and 1½ inches posterior to the medial malleolus. The pin is inserted from the lateral side. Care must be taken to avoid the posterior tibial vessels and nerves and the tendons on the medial side. Os calcis traction may be used in calcaneal fractures with loss of tuber-joint angle and for extensive open fractures of the tibia and fibula. A Thomas splint with Pearson attachment or a Böhler-Braun frame may be used to support the extremity.

DISTAL TIBIA AND FIBULA. The preferred site for insertion is 1¼ inches proximal to the tip of the medial malleolus and 1¾ inches proximal to the lateral malleolus. Insertion is from the medial side. This site is useful for open tibial fractures if the skin wound is not too close to the pin and for some tibial plateau fractures.

PROXIMAL TIBIA. The preferred site for insertion is 1 inch posterior and 1 inch distal to the most prominent point of the tibial tubercle. In children the distances are less, but care must be taken to stay away from the epiphyseal plate of the tubercle. The pin is inserted from the lateral side to avoid damage to the peroneal nerve. This site may be used for all femoral fractures, hip dislocations, and pelvic fractures where skeletal traction is indicated.

DISTAL FEMUR. The preferred site for insertion is the level of the adductor tubercle. Insertion should be from the medial side. Care must be taken to avoid entering the knee joint. This site may be used for the supracondylar and subtrochanteric fractures which are difficult to control with proximal tibial traction and when injuries preclude use of the proximal tibia. The disadvantages are the danger of entering the knee joint and scarring of the quadriceps or ligaments secondary to pin tract infection.

PROXIMAL ULNA. The preferred site is 1½ inches distal to the tip of the olecranon—less in children. The site is just distal to the level of the coronoid process of the ulna. It is inserted from the medial side with care taken to avoid injury to the ulnar nerve. Ulnar traction may be used for most fractures of the humerus and when combined with overhead traction is preferable for most displaced supracondylar fractures.

OTHER LOCATIONS. Skeletal traction may be used through the distal radius and ulna or the metacarpals for forearm fractures. This is seldom indicated and must be carefully applied to avoid compromising hand function.

Uses of Skeletal Traction

Straight skeletal traction and skeletal splint Russell's traction may be used with traction through the os calcis or distal tibia and fibula (Fig. 12-5). Other types of traction are usually preferable.

The Böhler-Braun frame may be used for tibial fractures and, in skilled hands, for some femoral fractures. A felt pad the length of

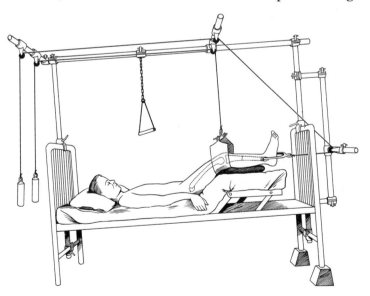

Fig. 12-5. Skeletal splint Russell's traction. (From Schmeisser [7].)

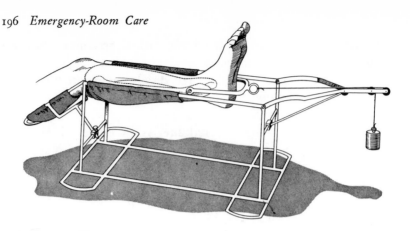

Fig. 12-6. Böhler-Braun frame. Knee flexion can be altered by raising or lowering the frame.

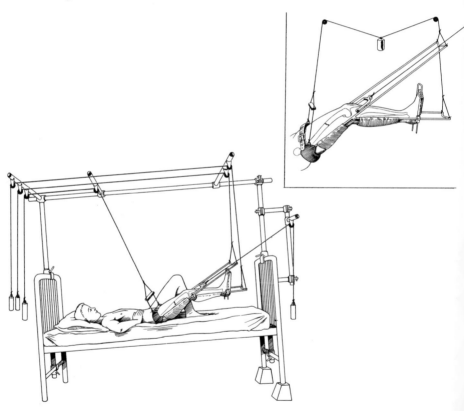

Fig. 12-7. Balanced suspension. The Thomas splint and Pearson attachment are balanced with multiple weights. The splint moves with the leg and provides support when the patient moves in bed. The inset shows the single-weight method of balanced suspension. The single-weight method is slightly faster to apply but is less flexible. (From Schmeisser [7].)

the frame in tubular stockinette should be placed between the leg and the supports of the frame (Fig. 12-6).

Balanced suspension with a Thomas splint and Pearson attachment is the most versatile method of support (Fig. 12-7) and is suitable for most fractures of the femur. It is also the most difficult to apply. The Pearson attachment is usually at the level of the knee. Muslin or canvas is pinned about the proximal portion of the Thomas splint and the Pearson attachment to support the leg. A felt pad in stockinette is placed between the leg and the splint. The splint is then suspended by three weights. The distal end of the attachment may be tied to the distal end of the Thomas splint when a fixed degree of knee flexion is desired. A modified single-weight suspension may also be used.

Ninety degrees-ninety degrees traction (Fig. 12-8) is occasionally necessary for subtrochanteric and supracondylar fractures of the femur.

Upper extremity traction through the proximal ulna may be used with lateral skeletal traction combined with skin traction on the forearm or overhead traction (Fig. 12-9). Rotation is easier to control with lateral traction. Overhead traction is usually preferable for supracondylar fractures of the humerus because the elevation aids in decreasing the amount of swelling associated with this injury.

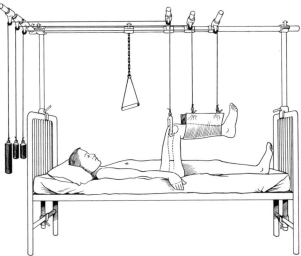

Fig. 12-8. Ninety degrees-ninety degrees traction. Skeletal traction may be applied through the femur as shown or through the proximal tibia. The leg is supported on a padded sling. (From Schmeisser [7].)

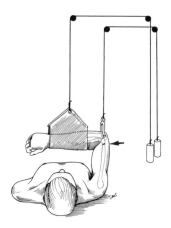

Fig. 12-9. Overhead skeletal olecranon traction. The forearm and hand are supported on a sling. Lateral traction may be applied to the humerus proximal to the fracture similar to that used in Dunlop's traction by adding a bar and pulley on the side of the bed.

Countertraction for all methods is provided by elevating the side of the bed to which the traction is pulling.

Precautions with Traction

The use of all traction requires close supervision if it is to be effective. The complications are similar for both skin and skeletal traction. The most frequent complications are the following:

1. *Skin blisters* can be prevented by avoiding wrinkles in the moleskin, avoiding excessive traction (10 pounds is maximum and 5 pounds is safer for skin traction), and replacing the skin tapes when they start to slip.

2. *Pin tract infection* is less likely to occur with meticulous aseptic technique when inserting the pin for skeletal traction, cutting the skin sufficiently to prevent pressure from the pin, and using a threaded wire. Pain at the pin site usually is minimal; if present, it is likely to indicate infection. Erythema and purulent drainage necessitate removal of the pin.

3. *Pressure necrosis* occurs because of pressure against a bony prominence by skin tapes, traction apparatus, or the bed. It can be

prevented by avoiding pressure against any area, most frequently the heel.

4. *Circulatory embarrassment* is usually due to an excessively tight elastic bandage or pressure against the popliteal area by the muslin or canvas on a splint. If the digits are swollen, pale, cyanotic, or cool, the elastic bandage should be reapplied. Pressure in the popliteal area can be avoided by applying the muslin carefully and by maintaining the leg in the proper position on the splint.

5. *Nerve palsy* may be a complication with traction. The peroneal nerve, where it crosses the fibula, and the ulnar nerve, behind the medial epicondyle, are both susceptible to pressure injury. Nerve palsy may be caused by a tight bandage, by pressure from the appliance supporting the extremity, or from pressure against the nerve while maintaining the elbow in acute flexion in individuals whose ulnar nerve subfluxes onto the epicondyle with elbow flexion.

HOSPITAL ADMISSION VERSUS AMBULATORY TREATMENT

The problem of disposition of the patient is most easily approached by determining the need for hospital admission.

Admission is necessary:

1. For all seriously injured patients.
2. For all patients requiring anesthesia.
3. If marked swelling, infection, or severe pain is anticipated.
4. If the necessary care cannot be carried out at home.
5. If there is no responsible person to note signs of impending difficulty and to return the patient for further care.
6. If the patient's home is too distant or inaccessible to permit prompt return if complications develop.
7. For observation even when the initial findings are negative if the trauma was such that occult injury is suspected.
8. For all neck and back injuries in which the findings on initial examination are equivocal.

If none of the indications for admission is present and if the injury is relatively minor with few, if any, anticipated problems, the patient may be treated on an outpatient basis.

PRECAUTIONS IN OUTPATIENT CARE

Injuries to Extremities

The instructions to the patient in outpatient care should be explicit. Care of the injured extremity is the same as in inpatient care.

The following instructions should be routine:

1. The injured part should be elevated above the level of the heart for the first 48 to 72 hours.

2. An ice bag next to the injured area will help minimize swelling.

3. The digits must be observed carefully and frequently for swelling, cyanosis, pallor, coolness, numbness, and localized pressure pain. The patient should be seen immediately if any of these findings occurs.

4. The patient should be seen the following day even if none of the signs of difficulty occurs.

5. Medications for pain should be prescribed if necessary. Narcotics of greater potency than codeine should usually not be given on an outpatient basis.

6. If the patient has an open wound with danger of infection, the temperature should be taken and recorded at least twice a day. If the temperature becomes elevated or pain increases, the patient should be seen immediately.

Injuries to the Back and Neck

Back and neck injuries without fracture, dislocation, or neurological deficit may often be treated on an outpatient basis. The primary objective is to rest the part.

The following instructions should be routine:

Low Back Pain
1. Bed rest with bathroom privileges is prescribed.

2. Two pillows are placed under the knees to flex the knees and hips when the patient is supine. The knees and hips should be flexed if the patient is on his side.

3. A heating pad turned on low may be used for 20 to 30 minutes three times a day if desired.

4. An analgesic and muscle relaxant may be prescribed.

5. The bed should be firm. Plywood can be placed between the mattress and springs if necessary.

6. The patient should be reevaluated in 5 to 7 days or admitted to the hospital at any time if the symptoms increase or do not subside.

CERVICAL PAIN

1. A rolled towel should be used behind the neck to support the cervical lordotic curve in a comfortable position.

2. The other directions are the same as for low back pain except that the heating pad is not used in the cervical area.

SPECIFIC INJURIES

Hand and Wrist

These injuries are discussed in Chapter 13.

Radius and Ulna

DISTAL RADIUS AND ULNA.   Fractures without displacement may be immobilized in a long arm cast or sugar tong splint and followed on an outpatient basis. Many of the distal radial and ulnar fractures in which shortening and dorsal angulation occur in adults, or only angulation in the child, can be reduced in the emergency room and treated on an outpatient basis.

Adequate pain relief may be obtained by the administration of intramuscular meperidine (Demerol) or by the injection of lidocaine or procaine into the fracture hematoma. Because the latter method converts a closed fracture to an open one with the attendant risk of infection, thorough skin preparation and draping, sterile gloves, and a mask must be used.

Other forms of anesthesia such as nerve block or intravenous injection of procaine or lidocaine distally to a pneumatic tourniquet can be used by surgeons experienced in these techniques.

After there is adequate analgesia, the patient's elbow is flexed 90 degrees and counteraction provided by an assistant holding the arm above the elbow. Traction is exerted on the patient's forearm. The operator can then disengage the fragments by controlling the distal fragment and hand with one hand and the proximal frag-

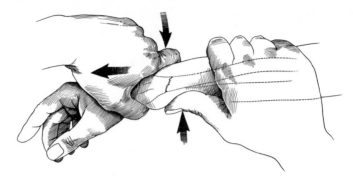

Fig. 12-10. Reduction of a distal radial fracture. Traction, pronation, slight flexion, ulnar deviation, and downward pressure on the distal radial fragment are applied with one hand while the proximal fragment is stabilized with the other hand.

ment with the other. The distal fragment and hand are then brought into slight flexion, moderate pronation, and moderate ulnar deviation (Fig. 12-10). By palpation of the anterior and posterior articular surfaces of the radius, one can determine whether the normal volar angle of the articular surface has been restored, and restoration of normal length can be determined by comparing the distal radius and ulna. A cast or splint is applied in this position and care-

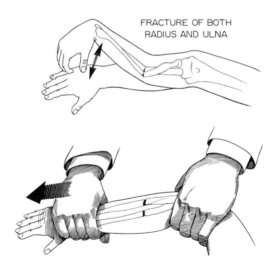

Fig. 12-11. Reduction of angulated fractures in children. One hand stabilizes the proximal fragment while traction and force to correct the angulation is applied with the other.

fully molded. Postreduction roentgenograms are necessary to confirm adequacy of reduction.

Angulated fractures in children can usually be reduced by manual correction of the angulation (Fig. 12-11).

If the reduction is unsatisfactory, the second attempt should usually be made in the operating room with regional block or general anesthesia.

Fractures with complete displacement and overriding should be reduced in the operating room and with regional or general anesthesia.

SHAFTS OF THE RADIUS AND ULNA. Fractures without displacement should be immobilized in a long arm cast and followed closely for subsequent displacement as the swelling subsides. Ulnar shaft fractures are frequently slow in healing and nonunion is common.

Fractures with angulation but without displacement in children can usually be reduced under meperidine analgesia by manipulatively correcting the angulation. The angulation tends to recur and requires close follow-up until there is sufficient callus to provide stability. Unacceptable angulation must be corrected and usually requires inpatient care.

Displaced fractures of the shaft of the radius, ulna, or both should be treated in the operating room by closed reduction in children and either closed or open reduction in adults. If the patient's condition contraindicates definitive treatment, alignment can be obtained by suspending the forearm by the fingers with the elbow flexed 90 degrees and applying countertraction to the upper arm. A plaster cast is then applied and the traction removed. Usually little analgesia is required if the extremity is handled with care.

RADIAL HEAD

DISLOCATION. Subluxation of the radial head is common in small children and is the result of a longitudinal jerk on the arm. The child refuses to use the arm. Examination reveals marked limitation of supination. Roentgenograms are negative. Reduction is accomplished by flexing the elbow to 90 degrees and quickly but gently supinating the forearm. A click or pop accompanies the reduction. The arm is then immobilized for 10 days in a posterior splint with the elbow flexed 90 degrees and the forearm in supination.

Dislocation of the radial head is usually associated with a fracture of the shaft of the ulna (Monteggia's fracture), and the patient should be admitted for treatment.

FRACTURE. A fracture of the radial head should be suspected when there is tenderness to palpation over the radial head and pain with elbow motion. If the anteroposterior and lateral roentgenograms do not show a fracture, further films at varying angles must be obtained to rule out a nondisplaced linear fracture.

Nondisplaced linear fractures should be immobilized for a few days in supination with the elbow flexed 90 degrees. Active motion can be started as pain subsides.

Displaced radial head fractures are treated on an inpatient basis by reduction in children, and either reduction or excision in adults.

OLECRANON. Nondisplaced fractures are treated by immobilization in a cast or splint with the elbow flexed 90 degrees.

Fractures with separation require admission for open reduction and internal fixation.

Elbow

Dislocations are surgical emergencies and usually require anesthesia; patients should be admitted. Fracture dislocations are common. The dislocation should be reduced and the fracture then treated appropriately. Again, admission and anesthesia are necessary.

Humerus

DISTAL HUMERUS. All persons with displaced fractures should be admitted for treatment. Nondisplaced fractures may be treated on an outpatient basis in a long arm cast with the elbow flexed slightly more than 90 degrees; however, the combination of a cast and swelling with the danger of ischemic contracture requires close surveillance. Hospitalization of 24 hours' duration, for observation, is justifiable.

SHAFT OF THE HUMERUS. Nondisplaced humeral shaft fractures can be treated without admission by a coaptation splint with sling and swathe (Fig. 12-12). If there is overriding and displacement, the fracture can be treated by manipulative alignment and a coaptation splint, by a hanging cast, or by skeletal traction. The splint, cast, or traction can be applied in the emergency room. Usu-

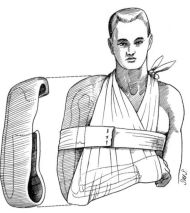

Fig. 12-12. Coaptation splint with sling and swathe. After reduction of the humeral fracture the arm or splint is padded with sheet wadding. The splint begins near the axilla and extends distally around the olecranon and then proximally over the lateral surface of the arm and over the shoulder. Wet roller gauze is then wrapped around the arm and splint, and the plaster about the elbow is molded to avoid pressure on the distal humerus and olecranon. The sling and swathe are then applied.

ally there is considerable swelling distal to the fracture. Radial nerve injuries are not uncommon. Patients with radial nerve injury secondary to fracture of the humeral shaft should be admitted.

PROXIMAL HUMERUS

SURGICAL NECK. Impacted fractures in the aged and those with little angulation in the younger adult should be treated with a sling and swathe. Circumduction exercises should be started as soon as pain permits, usually in 4 to 7 days. Impacted fractures in poor position in young adults may require admission for manipulation.

Patients having displaced fractures with no bone contact should be admitted and reduction obtained by closed manipulation, traction, or open reduction.

ANATOMICAL NECK. Impacted and nondisplaced fractures should be treated by sling and swathe and early motion. Displaced fractures require admission for closed or open reduction.

In children, fractures in this area usually occur in the metaphysis and extend to the epiphyseal plate, crossing it in the natural line of cleavage. If there is little displacement, the fracture may be treated with a hanging cast and swathe or a sling and swathe. Displacement requires admission for treatment by manipulation and shoulder spica or skeletal traction.

TUBEROSITIES.   Fractures with little or no displacement are treated the same as anatomical neck fractures. Displacement sufficient to impinge on the acromion with abduction usually requires open reduction, and the patient should be admitted.

Fracture Dislocation of the Shoulder

This is a very serious injury and requires admission for either closed or open reduction with anesthesia.

Dislocation of the Shoulder

In general, dislocations without fracture or nerve injury that are only an hour or two old, and recurrent dislocations, can be reduced in the emergency room with meperidine analgesia.

Dislocations with associated fractures or nerve injuries, older dislocations up to 3 weeks' duration, and, frequently, subglenoid dislocations require general anesthesia and muscle relaxation. The old dislocations will require open reduction if gentle closed methods fail.

Roentgenograms are always necessary prior to reduction even though a dislocation is clinically obvious. These are taken to demonstrate associated fractures and the position of the humeral head. An axillary view should be taken to rule out a posterior dislocation when the anteroposterior view fails to show a fracture or anterior dislocation.

Before beginning treatment the surgeon must know:

1. Whether it is the first dislocation or recurrent.
2. The duration of dislocation.
3. The position of the humeral head.
4. Whether there are associated fractures.
5. Whether there are concomitant nerve injuries.

ANTERIOR DISLOCATION.   The most common dislocations are subcoracoid and subglenoid. One gentle attempt at reduction in the emergency room with meperidine analgesia may be made. If it is unsuccessful, rather than use strenuous force, the reduction should be done under general anesthesia.

The Stimson method of reduction (Fig. 12-13) is most useful and carries little hazard if done with care. (Two other methods, the longitudinal traction method and the Kocher method, may also be

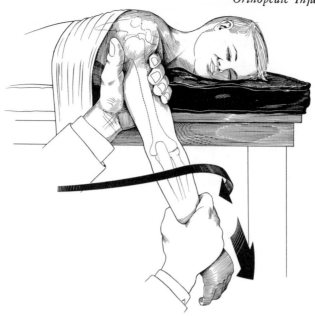

Fig. 12-13. Stimson method of reduction of anterior dislocation of the shoulder. The patient is prone on a table with the dislocated extremity hanging over the side. Traction, either manual or a weight hung over the wrist, is applied. The proximal humerus is controlled by the other hand. When the muscles relax, the proximal humerus is lifted laterally and posteriorly as the arm is gently rotated and adducted.

used. The reader is referred to the standard texts for descriptions of the latter two methods.) The patient is prone on a table or cart with the dislocated arm hanging over the side. Downward traction is applied until the muscles begin to relax. The humeral head is then lifted laterally and posteriorly into place as the arm is adducted toward the cart. Reduction is accompanied by an audible and palpable click, and the patient is immediately more comfortable. The arm is brought across the patient's chest as he is rolled onto his back.

Roentgenograms should always be taken after reduction and the peripheral nerves reexamined. The arm is held across the chest with a Velpeau bandage for 3 weeks.

Scapular Fractures

Scapular fractures rarely have significant displacement and may be treated on an outpatient basis with a sling and swathe followed by active exercises. A markedly displaced fracture of the acromion should be admitted for open reduction.

Acromioclavicular Dislocations

Acromioclavicular injuries produce swelling and local tenderness over the acromioclavicular joint. With complete dislocation the distal clavicle is visually prominent when the patient's arm is hanging at his side. Roentgenograms of acromioclavicular injuries should include an anteroposterior view of both shoulders with the patient standing and holding 5 to 10 pounds in each hand. This procedure demonstrates complete tears of the coracoclavicular ligaments when the displacement cannot be determined on physical examination. The dislocation tends to reduce when the patient is supine so that films taken in this position are often misleading; however, supine films will rule out a fracture of the distal clavicle and hence should be taken and read prior to taking the standing films. Dislocation of the acromioclavicular joint can be treated with an inelastic strapping which passes over the shoulder and under the flexed elbow. The top of the shoulder and elbow should both be padded prior to strapping. Care must be taken to avoid injury to the ulnar nerve at the elbow, and the strapping is discontinued or removed if ulnar nerve symptoms develop.

Reduction of a complete acromioclavicular separation can frequently not be maintained with strapping. If this is the case, the patient should be admitted for open repair.

Clavicular Fractures

Most fractures of the clavicle are obvious on examination. Occasionally a nondisplaced fracture in a child is not radiographically visible. If there is point tenderness over the clavicle, it should be treated as if fractured for 7 to 10 days, by which time callus will be palpable if a fracture is present.

Fractures of the clavicle are best treated by closed reduction and immobilization. Usually satisfactory alignment is obtained by elevation and extension of the shoulder. It is maintained with a well-padded stockinette or plaster figure-of-eight to hold the shoulders extended and a sling to elevate the shoulder. A well-molded Velpeau-type plaster jacket may be used in small children to provide better immobilization. Care must be taken to avoid compression of the neurovascular bundle in the axilla. These injuries can usually be treated on an outpatient basis.

Occasionally, with a very comminuted fracture or when the maximum cosmetic result is desired, the patient should be admitted and treated by bed rest with the shoulder elevated and extended. Open reduction is seldom warranted except when the fracture compromises neurovascular structures. Admission to the hospital for care is necessary.

Sternoclavicular Dislocation

Anterior dislocation must be differentiated from a prominent proximal clavicle and from degenerative arthritis, both of which have stable joints. With dislocation, the proximal clavicle is prominent, there is local tenderness and swelling, and frequently abnormal motion is palpable. Radiographic diagnosis is difficult and requires special views. This injury may be treated with a plaster figure-of-eight and a sling or a plaster Velpeau with the shoulder elevated and extended. Open reduction is seldom indicated.

Posterior dislocations are rare and may exert pressure on the structures of the anterior mediastinum. Patients with posterior dislocations should be admitted for care and the pressure relieved.

Pelvic Fractures

Considerable force is required to produce pelvic fractures and dislocations. Visceral injuries, particularly to the bladder and urethra, are common. The status of these structures must be determined promptly. Intrapelvic hemorrhage may also be sufficient to produce shock. Associated injury of iliac artery or vein may necessitate immediate surgical intervention. All patients with pelvic fractures, including acetabular fractures, should be admitted for treatment.

Hip Dislocations

Hip dislocations are usually posterior. Fractures of the posterior rim of the acetabulum and injury to the sciatic nerve, usually the lateral (popliteal) portion, are common. Roentgenograms must be taken of the hip and of the ipsilateral femur—the latter to avoid missing an associated femoral shaft fracture. The patient should be admitted for reduction of the dislocation under adequate anesthesia as soon as possible. Open reduction should be done if closed reduction is unsuccessful or unstable.

Fracture of the Hip

In *femoral neck fractures,* the injured extremity must be handled gently while adequate anteroposterior and lateral roentgenograms are obtained. With the possible exception of a valgus impacted fracture, surgical treatment is indicated for these injuries. Buck's traction will immobilize the leg sufficiently to provide some pain relief until definitive treatment is undertaken. All patients should be admitted.

Intertrochanteric and Subtrochanteric Fractures

Admission for treatment of these fractures is necessary. If operative treatment is planned, Buck's traction should be applied. These fractures can be treated by closed methods with skeletal traction. If surgical treatment must be delayed more than 2 to 3 days because of other injuries or medical problems, or if closed treatment is elected, balanced skeletal traction through the proximal tibia or distal femur should be applied in the emergency room.

In children, balanced skeletal traction in the older child and Russell's or Bryant's traction in the smaller child can be applied in the emergency room prior to admission (see earlier section on Traction in this chapter).

Femoral Shaft Fractures

A femoral shaft fracture is a serious injury, and admission is always indicated. Blood loss into the thigh in the adult may be 1000 ml or more and require replacement. Traction is usually used to obtain and maintain reduction until there is sufficient callus to apply a hip spica cast. Traction is usually applied in the emergency room. When other injuries require emergency surgery, traction can be applied in the operating room.

Skeletal traction through the proximal tibia with the leg in balanced suspension is preferable for adults and older children. Small children may be treated in Russell's traction and infants in Bryant's, Russell's, or Buck's traction (see section on Traction).

Open reduction and internal fixation, usually with a Küntscher or Hanson-Street nail, is an acceptable method of treating some femoral shaft fractures in adults. It is rarely indicated as an emergency procedure.

Supracondylar and Condylar Fractures

These fractures all require admission. Because the popliteal vessels are immediately behind the distal femur, the vascular status must be ascertained and therapeutic measures instituted promptly if they are injured.

There is wide variation in this type of fracture. Most supracondylar fractures can be treated satisfactorily by skeletal traction though more knee flexion is required than for shaft fractures. Open reduction is indicated in selected cases, particularly single condylar fractures and T-condylar fractures.

Dislocations of the Knee

This is a rare and extremely severe injury with a strong possibility of damage to the vessels and nerves. Immediate reduction under anesthesia is indicated. Admission is always necessary.

Fractures of the Patella

A bipartite patella should not be mistaken for a fracture. Its margins are smooth, it is usually the upper outer portion of the patella, and it is often bilateral.

Nondisplaced fractures may be treated with a cylinder cast for 4 to 6 weeks on an outpatient basis. Marked hemarthrosis may require aspiration prior to application of the cast.

Fracture of the patella with separation of the fragments or comminuted fractures require admission for operative repair. A cylinder cast or posterior splint may be applied in the emergency room for immobilization when operation must be delayed.

Dislocation of the Patella

The patella usually dislocates laterally as the knee is actively extended from a flexed position. Reduction can be accomplished by pulling the patella medially as the knee is extended. Anesthesia is not usually necessary but meperidine analgesia is desirable. After reduction the patella is immobilized in its normal location with a well-molded cylinder cast for 4 or 6 weeks to permit the medial retinacula to heal. Active quadriceps and knee flexion exercises are then started.

Tibial Plateau Fractures

These injuries require admission. If there is little or no displacement, the leg should be immobilized in a cast for about 4 weeks and then mobilized by protected active motion. Weight-bearing should be deferred until healing is complete, usually 12 to 15 weeks.

Skin traction or skeletal traction on a Böhler-Braun frame will often improve position and permit early active motion. Open reduction is frequently necessary for displaced fractures. A long leg cast or posterior splint provides immobilization until operation can be done.

Tibial Spine Fractures

All patients with tibial spine fractures should be admitted. Undisplaced fractures of the tibial spine are treated by immobilization in a cylinder cast with the knee extended. Open reduction is required if there is displacement which interferes with motion.

Tibial Shaft Fractures

Undisplaced shaft fractures in children are immobilized in a long leg cast with the knee flexed 20 degrees and may be treated on an outpatient basis. Unstable oblique fractures of the tibia and fibula can often be satisfactorily reduced in the emergency room with meperidine analgesia, and the patients should be admitted.

The technique for reduction is shown in Figure 12-14. The patient is supine with the buttock on the injured side on the edge of the cart. The thigh is abducted and extended so the leg hangs over the cart. The knee is flexed. An assistant stabilizes the thigh, and reduction is accomplished by traction on the foot and gentle manipulation of the fracture to obtain alignment, apposition, and length. A shortening of one-half inch is permissible in the adult. A well-molded long leg cast is then applied and postreduction roentgenograms are obtained. If the reduction is unacceptable, anesthesia is usually necessary for remanipulation.

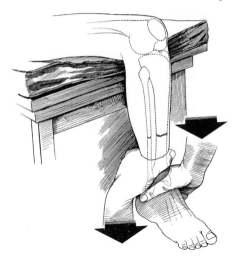

Fig. 12-14. Closed reduction of tibial shaft fracture. Manual traction is applied to the leg, which is hung over the edge of the table. Alignment and apposition are accomplished by gentle manipulation. A long leg cast is then applied.

Displaced transverse fractures with overriding usually require anesthesia for reduction.

Fractures of the Fibula

Isolated fractures of the fibula proximal to the distal 3 inches usually require only symptomatic treatment with an elastic bandage or cast. Injury to the peroneal nerve can occur when the fracture involves the proximal 2 to 3 inches of the fibula.

Ankle Fractures

Ankle fractures comprise a number of injuries to bone and ligaments. The following points are helpful in making a correct diagnosis and plan for treatment.

1. All ankle injuries are fractures until adequate roentgenograms prove otherwise. Films of the entire fibula must be made when there is a fracture of the medial malleolus and an intact lateral malleolus.
2. In general, fracture of a single bone implies ligamentous injury on the other side of the joint.
3. A fracture of the shaft of the fibula above the distal tibiofibu-

lar articulation with an associated injury to the medial side of the ankle implies disruption of the distal tibiofibular ligaments.

LATERAL MALLEOLUS. Solitary undisplaced or minimally displaced fractures can be reduced with meperidine analgesia by internal rotation (not inversion) of the foot. A long leg cast will give better immobilization and is more comfortable, though many physicians use short leg casts for this fracture.

FRACTURE OF FIBULA WITH TEAR OF DELTOID LIGAMENT. Fracture of the fibula above the ankle joint with a tear of the deltoid ligament implies a tear of the distal tibiofibular ligaments and instability of the ankle mortise.

General anesthesia is usually required for closed reduction. The ankle mortise and distal tibiofibular joint must be anatomically restored. Open reduction with repair of the deltoid ligament and a screw or bolt to hold the distal tibiofibular joint is usually necessary. Admission is necessary for both closed and open treatment.

BIMALLEOLAR AND TRIMALLEOLAR FRACTURES. Undisplaced fractures can be treated by either a long or a short leg cast. The former provides better fixation and is preferable for the first 3 weeks. The foot is immobilized in as neutral a position as possible. The major problem is swelling sufficient to necessitate splitting the cast. Roentgenograms should be taken after 10 days, for the position may be lost as the swelling subsides.

Displaced fractures will require admission. When the foot is displaced laterally the medial skin becomes stretched over the fracture and ischemic necrosis may result. Alignment should be obtained immediately to avoid this. The foot is splinted with a pillow or cardboard splint prior to obtaining the initial roentgenograms. The ankle mortise must be restored, and this requires an anatomical reduction. Reduction may be attempted in the emergency room when there are skin blisters or abrasions or the patient's condition does not permit anesthesia. Usually the position is sufficiently accurate so that further closed or open procedures may be postponed until more nearly optimum conditions exist.

The patient is supine with hip extended, knee flexed, and leg hanging over the cart. Traction is applied by grasping the heel in one hand and the foot in the other and pulling downward. The talus can then be brought under the tibia by pulling downward and forward on the heel while an assistant stabilizes the tibia. The malleoli are then molded to complete the reduction and a long leg cast is applied.

FRACTURE OF THE DISTAL TIBIA WITH ANKLE JOINT INVOLVEMENT. This fracture, with the exception of the posterior lip or malleolus as part of a trimalleolar fracture, is fortunately uncommon. Solitary fractures are usually comminuted in adults. In children they are likely to involve the lateral portion of the epiphysis. Nondisplaced fractures with minimal swelling are treated with a plaster cast and may be treated on an outpatient basis. All patients who require reduction must be admitted.

Fracture of the Talus

Talar fractures may be osteochondral fractures of the body, fractures of the talar head, neck, or body, or fracture dislocations. Patients with these injuries should be admitted. Fracture dislocations require prompt reduction under anesthesia. If displaced, the other fractures require reduction or excision of the small osteochondral fragment.

Fractures of the Calcaneus

Undisplaced fractures of the anterior promontory of the calcaneus (Fig. 12-15) may be treated on an outpatient basis with a short leg cast. All other fractures of the calcaneus require admission. A bulky compression bandage should be applied and the foot elevated. Definitive treatment depends on the type of fracture and the preference and experience of the surgeon.

Fractures of the Other Tarsal Bones

These fractures are uncommon as isolated injuries and are usually compression fractures. Some improvement can occasionally be obtained by manipulation. Open reduction is seldom indicated. Plaster cast immobilization is required. An accessory scaphoid should not be mistaken for a fracture. It is smooth, round, and commonly bilateral.

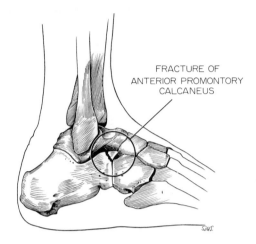

FRACTURE OF
ANTERIOR PROMONTORY
CALCANEUS

Fig. 12-15. Fracture of the anterior promontory of the calcaneus. Since this fracture is frequently difficult to visualize, anteroposterior, lateral, and oblique views may be necessary.

Tarsometatarsal Dislocations and Fracture Dislocations

These injuries may be missed because the swelling has obliterated the deformity and the displacement is not detected on the roentgenograms. Comparison views of the other foot should be taken if there is any question. Admission is necessary for anesthesia and reduction.

Metatarsal Fractures

Undisplaced fractures should be treated with a well-molded short leg cast with no weight-bearing allowed for 3 weeks. A molded rubber or cork arch support is then used in the shoe until healing is complete. The fractures are usually treated on an outpatient basis. Displaced fractures may require open reduction, in which case inpatient care is necessary.

Phalanges

Closed fractures of the phalanges of the lateral four toes and nondisplaced fractures of the great toe can usually be treated by taping the injured toe to the adjacent toes. Cotton or gauze should be placed between the toes to prevent maceration. The taping should not be tight enough to compromise circulation to the toes.

Displaced fractures of the great toe can usually be reduced and immobilized in a plaster cast. Occasionally traction as described for finger fractures or fixation with a Kirschner wire is necessary.

Knee Injuries

Examination of the injured knee, and fractures and dislocations about the knee, have been discussed. The most frequently injured structures at the knee are the ligaments and the menisci.

MEDIAL COLLATERAL LIGAMENT SPRAIN. Incomplete tears should be treated with a cylinder cast for 3 to 6 weeks depending on the severity of the sprain. Quadriceps-setting exercises should be done in the cylinder. Unprotected weight-bearing is permitted when good quadriceps strength has been obtained.

Complete tears as evidenced by a palpable defect in the ligament, or instability of the knee, should be surgically repaired.

MENISCUS INJURIES. It is difficult to make the diagnosis of a tear of a meniscus immediately after an injury except in those cases in which the knee is "locked." If the knee is "locked," admission is necessary and extension must be obtained by manipulation, traction, · or meniscectomy. If a tear of the meniscus is suspected but the knee is not "locked," it should be treated conservatively with immobilization with a bulky dressing or cylinder cast and no weight-bearing allowed until the symptoms subside. Repeated examination is mandatory after the acute symptoms subside.

Ankle Sprains

Roentgenograms should be taken to rule out fractures in all ankle injuries. Minimal sprains with little swelling and tenderness may be treated by adhesive strapping and protected weight-bearing. Moderate and severe sprains with marked swelling should be treated with a compression bandage, elevation, and no weight-bearing. After 24 to 48 hours a short-leg walking cast can be applied. This will permit ambulation and provide sufficient stability for ligamentous healing. Stress films of the ankle taken after the injection of a local anesthetic are occasionally necessary to determine the degree of injury. If a complete tear of the ligament is demonstrated, open repair may be desirable.

Ruptured Achilles Tendon

The physical findings have been discussed. This injury requires admission for open repair.

Spinal Fractures

The physical and roentgenographic examinations of patients with spinal injuries have been discussed. Neurosurgical consultation should be obtained when there is neurological deficit. The primary goal in the emergency-room care of patients with spinal injuries is to do no harm.

Cervical Spine Fractures

Head halter traction with the neck in neutral position and a collar or sandbag should be applied to stabilize the neck whenever a fracture is suspected. This should be done before the patient is moved or roentgenograms are taken. If a fracture is present, skull traction should be applied, with skull tongs under local anesthesia if facilities permit. The patient is then moved to a Stryker or Foster frame.

Dorsal and Lumbar Fractures

Patients with these fractures should be admitted. Neurosurgical consultation should be obtained if there is neurological deficit. If the fracture is of a stable type, a firm bed will be satisfactory. If it is unstable, the patient should be placed on a Stryker or Foster frame. The best method of moving the patient is to place three or four assistants on each side of the stretcher. Each grasps the under-sheet with about 1 foot between the hands. Each rolls the sheet in his hands to the edge of the patient's body. They then pull the sheet taut and move the patient to the bed or frame.

Acute Back Strain and Discogenic Back Pain

The patients may be treated conservatively at home or in the hospital, depending on the severity of their symptoms and their ability to carry out conservative care at home. Roentgenograms should always be obtained and, depending upon neurological findings, further investigation may be necessary.

GENERAL REFERENCES

Blount, W. P. *Fractures in Children*. Baltimore: Williams & Wilkins, 1955.

Boyes, J. H. *Bunnell's Surgery of the Hand* (5th ed.). Philadelphia: Lippincott, 1970.

Cave, E. F. *Fractures and Other Injuries*. Chicago: Year Book, 1961.

Committee on Trauma, American College of Surgeons. *The Management of Fractures and Soft Tissue Injuries* (2d ed.). Philadelphia: Saunders, 1965.

Flatt, A. E. *The Care of Minor Hand Injuries*. St. Louis: Mosby, 1959.

Rank, B. K., and Wakefield, A. R. *Surgery of Repair as Applied to Hand Injuries*. Baltimore: Williams & Wilkins, 1960.

Schmeisser, G., Jr. *A Clinical Manual of Orthopedic Traction Techniques*. Philadelphia: Saunders, 1963.

Watson-Jones, Sir R. *Fractures and Joint Injuries* (4th ed.). Baltimore: Williams & Wilkins, 1955.

The Hand

13

MARK K. WANG
W. BRANDON MACOMBER
DONALD B. KETTELKAMP
CHARLES ECKERT

United States Department of Labor statistics indicate that of approximately two million disabling work injuries, 75 percent involve some permanent impairment of hand function. While industrial accidents represent less than one-fourth of all accidents, they are responsible for more than one-half of all hand injuries. Home accidents constitute another significant cause of hand injuries, to which each new household innovation or mechanical gadget adds its toll.

The personal suffering and hardship of the victim of a hand injury are bad enough, but the total economic loss to the nation in terms of man-hours lost to production, permanent loss of skilled workers, and monetary payment for medical care and compensation is staggering in magnitude.

The first responsibility of the medical profession is to help and encourage both industrial management and the workers to devise and use protective safety devices. Once the hand has been injured, treatment is directed toward maximal recovery of function and minimal duration of disability. The best opportunity to achieve this is in the emergency room—and the responsibility lies with the surgeon who first treats the patient.

HISTORY

Age

Age often helps to determine the choice of operative procedure. Children, with greater vascularity of tissue, require more conservative débridement and they are better candidates than adults for primary tendon repairs, since they are not prone to adhesions. In older patients surgical procedures requiring prolonged immobilization should be avoided if possible because of the fear of permanent stiffness of the joints.

Sex

The sex of the patient is an important factor, also. While a deformed but stable, serviceable finger is readily accepted by a male laborer, a deformity can cause anxiety and distress in a female patient, to whom cosmetic effect is usually important.

Previous Injury of the Hand

Any previous injuries of the hand may result in malfunction and malformation unrelated to the present injury. Unless clearly noted and explained, the findings of local examination can be confusing if not misleading.

Duration

The amount of time that has elapsed since the accident affects the degree of contamination and growth of bacteria in the wound. The 6-hour time limit formerly fixed to differentiate a contaminated from an infected wound has been modified by the use of antibiotics. Now, under favorable conditions, with minimal gross contamination and tissue damage, primary closure of the wound can be attempted as late as 12 hours after injury.

Nature and Circumstance of the Injury

The exact nature of the accident, the type of machinery involved, and any first-aid treatment received since the accident must be ascertained and evaluated. This information may give valuable clues to the extent and depth of the injury; the presence of crushing, compression, or avulsion injuries; the degree of gross contamination; or the retention of foreign bodies.

Position of the Hand at the Time of Injury

In tendon injuries, the exact position of the fingers and hand at the time of injury determines the amount of retraction of the proximal end of the severed tendon. The level of severance of the tendon moves distally in relation to the level of skin laceration in proportion to the degree of flexion of the injured finger or wrist at the time of the accident. This information is invaluable to the surgeon.

Occupation and Mentality of the Patient

There is no rule of thumb for the management of hand injuries. Each patient must be treated as an individual. His age, mentality, occupation, dominant hand, and the condition of the uninjured hand must be considered in determining the type of treatment. Patients of retirement age should not be subjected to prolonged, elaborate reconstructive surgery even though a more functional hand can thus be obtained. Patients of below-average intelligence do not fare well with surgical procedures which depend upon the intelligent cooperation of the patient for success. The problem of a musician or surgeon, whose occupation demands sensitive use of individual fingers, is different from that of an unskilled laborer. Injury to a dominant hand deserves every surgical procedure which can help achieve maximal recovery of function, while injury to the nondominant hand may be treated less extensively.

EXAMINATION

An acute injury of the hand should be examined in two stages: the essential examination preliminary to surgery and a detailed examination carried out during surgery under regional or general anesthesia. The preanesthetic examination, done in the emergency room, is concerned with the whole hand and its function. It must determine which structures are involved and which structures may be damaged. The continuity or functional activity of these structures is systematically established by simple clinical tests. The detailed examination of the wound and underlying structures is withheld for the second stage in the operating room.

Skin

The location, extent, depth, and direction of skin disruption usually pinpoint the site of impact by the traumatizing force. These factors alert the physician to possible damage to underlying deep structures, which must be individually evaluated.

In an avulsion injury, the extent of skin loss and structures exposed can be roughly determined and the viability of the partially detached skin estimated. Although final determination of the actual skin loss can be made only in the operating room, the preliminary examination prepares the surgeon and helps him to plan for the resurfacing procedure.

In burns, the extent and depth of injury must be estimated (for details see Chapter 15).

In a grease gun injury, the finger is injected by a pneumatic grease gun at a pressure of 600 pounds or more during the accident. The entrance is a small puncture wound often difficult to locate. The entire involved finger is markedly swollen and tense with the overlying skin pale. The pain is often intense. With a positive history, diagnosis is not difficult. The examiner must estimate the extent of grease diffusion by observing the extent of local swelling.

FOREIGN BODY. In case of foreign body retention, such as a broken needle, the site of entrance must be located. Gentle palpation of the surrounding skin may help to locate the object, if it is superficially situated. If none is palpable, the functions of each of the deep structures along its pathway must be carefully and gently tested. A nonpalpable foreign body must be located by the use of roentgenography. Anteroposterior and lateral views of the involved part are needed. If practical, radiopaque skin markers can be of help.

FROSTBITE. In frostbite, the involved finger or hand appears white and frozen. More often, at the time of examination in the emergency room, the thawing has begun. The part appears hyperemic and edematous. Occasionally there is blister formation. Rarely is actual gangrene seen at this stage.

Tendon

Whenever a tendon injury is suspected, the examiner should note the following:

1. The position of the fingers and hand. An injured hand is held in a relaxed position in which the fingers are maintained in normal alignment. Besides the obvious deformity of fracture or dislocation, the relative position of the finger is altered when one of its tendons is severed. If a flexor tendon is cut, the finger lies extended from its normal position; if an extensor tendon is cut, the finger is abnor-

mally flexed. Abnormal posture is made even more evident by passive extension or flexion of the wrist.

2. The tendon tension in the fingers. If an examining fingertip is placed on the pulp of each finger of the injured hand and pressed lightly, the tension of the flexor tendon can be gauged. Reduced tension is the best objective test for a divided flexor tendon.

3. Active motion of the involved finger. This requires the active cooperation of the patient and should not be expected of children or of unconscious or disoriented patients.

FLEXOR TENDONS. Failure of active flexion of the interphalangeal joint of the thumb indicates division of the flexor pollicis longus tendon. Failure of active flexion of the distal interphalangeal joint of the finger demonstrates severance of the flexor digitorum profundus tendon. Failure of active flexion of both distal and proximal interphalangeal joints when the metacarpophalangeal joint is fixed by the examiner indicates severance of both flexor tendons of the finger.

EXTENSOR TENDONS. Mallet finger deformity and inability to extend actively the distal interphalangeal joint are the results of severance of the extensor tendon at this level or avulsion of the extensor tendon at its insertion to the distal phalangeal bone. If the central tendon of the extensor mechanism is severed at the level of the proximal interphalangeal joint, the latter is in flexion position and cannot be actively extended. If the extensor tendon is severed over the metacarpophalangeal joint, the patient cannot hyperextend the metacarpophalangeal joint with the interphalangeal joint semiflexed. His attempt to do so produces straightening of the finger and flexion of the metacarpophalangeal joint.

In performing these tests, the examiner will find that testing movements of a particular joint requires him to stabilize the proximal joint. An impaired range of motion is not of diagnostic significance. Only complete absence of movement is indicative of a severed tendon.

GLOSSARY OF TENDON INJURIES IN THE HAND

1. The *flexor digitorum sublimis* is a flexor of the metacarpophalangeal and proximal interphalangeal joints. It is tested by holding three fingers in extension and having the patient flex the remaining finger. If it is intact, the proximal interphalangeal joint

will flex acutely and the distal interphalangeal joint will be relaxed in extension.

2. The *flexor digitorum profundus* is a flexor of all three joints. It is tested by holding the proximal two joints in extension, while the patient attempts to flex the distal interphalangeal joint.

3. The *lumbricales and interosseous muscles* flex the metacarpophalangeal joints and extend the interphalangeal joints. They are rarely involved as a solitary injury.

4. The *flexor pollicis longus* flexes both joints in the thumb. If the metacarpophalangeal joint is held in extension, it flexes the interphalangeal joint.

5. The *intrinsic muscles of the thumb* provide opposition, adduction, flexion, and abduction of the thumb. Loss of any of these motions implies their injury.

6. The *extensor digitorum communis, extensor indicis proprius,* and *extensor digiti quinti* are extensors of the metacarpophalangeal joints and with the intrinsics are extensors of the proximal interphalangeal joints. The patient is unable to extend the metacarpophalangeal joints of the middle and ring fingers when the extensor digitorum communis is severed and of the little and index fingers only when both extensors to those digits are lacerated. It is extremely important to note the duel extensors to the index and little fingers.

7. The *extensor pollicis longus* extends the metacarpophalangeal joint and with the intrinsics the interphalangeal joint of the thumb. When it is severed, the patient is unable to extend the first metacarpal, the metacarpophalangeal joint, and usually the interphalangeal joint.

8. The *extensor pollicis brevis* is also an extensor of the metacarpophalangeal joint; however, it is weak and can be sacrificed without loss of function.

9. The *abductor pollicis longus* abducts the first metacarpal and stabilizes the carpometacarpal joint of the thumb. When it is severed, the patient cannot widely abduct or stabilize the base of the thumb.

Nerves

Tests of nerve function are usually subjective, and an upset patient may be unreliable. They are of little value in young children.

MEDIAN NERVE

MOTOR FUNCTION.　The thenar muscles are paralyzed by severance of the motor branch of the median nerve. The thumb loses its ability

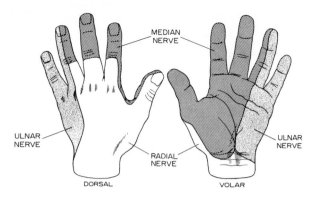

MEDIAN
NERVE

ULNAR
NERVE

ULNAR
NERVE

RADIAL
NERVE

DORSAL

VOLAR

Fig. 13-1. Sensory distribution of the median, ulnar, and radial nerves on the hand.

to oppose the fingers. The patient cannot lift the thumb directly forward at a right angle to the plane of the extended hand, nor can the tip of the thumb touch the tip of the little finger. The possible variations in innervation of the thenar musculature (by the ulnar nerve) must be kept in mind.

SENSORY FUNCTION. Light touch is tested with a wisp of cotton wool. The usual pattern of anesthesia subsequent to a median nerve injury is illustrated in Figure 13-1.

ULNAR NERVE

MOTOR FUNCTION. Injury of the ulnar nerve paralyzes interosseous muscles. With the fingers straight (no flexion or hyperextension), it can be seen that the power of adduction and abduction to and from the middle finger has been lost. Pinching between the tips of the index finger and thumb is weak, and the first interosseous muscle is flaccid under the examiner's finger during this action.

SENSORY FUNCTION. The usual pattern of anesthesia following severance of the ulnar nerve is illustrated in Figure 13-1. Variations are common. The dividing line of sensory distribution between the ulnar and median nerves is occasionally at the middle finger rather than the ring finger, as illustrated.

RADIAL NERVE

MOTOR FUNCTION. The radial nerve distal to the level of the wrist is purely sensory in nature. No motor disturbance is manifested by its severance at or distal to that level.

SENSORY FUNCTION. Anesthesia can be demonstrated on the dorsum of the hand over the area not innervated by the ulnar and median nerves (Fig. 13-1). The exact area is variable and of minimal surgical significance, as the nerve has already divided into a number of peripheral branches. It is unusual for all of these to be cut in cases of injuries of the wrist or the hand.

DIGITAL NERVE.   The digital nerve is also a purely sensory nerve. Its severance produces anesthesia on that half of the flexor surface of the finger distal to the level of injury.

Bones

The bones and joints of a hand are superficial. The exact site and nature of bony injuries can usually be observed from the wound in compound fractures. The usual signs of fracture, such as deformity, false motion, and crepitation can easily be demonstrated. Nevertheless, x-ray examination is necessary whenever fracture or dislocation of the injured hand is suspected. It offers additional information on the degree of displacement and, of particular importance, the involvement of joints by fracture lines. Other information affecting surgical repair, such as exposure of bone or joint, soft tissue coverage, or attachment of fractured fragments and viability of injured tissue, can be obtained only by careful examination of the wound in the operating room.

TREATMENT—GENERAL

After the general condition of the patient has been carefully evaluated to rule out concomitant injuries requiring more urgent treatment and after shock, if present, has been combated, a general plan is then made for the surgical treatment.

Selection of Anesthesia

All minor injuries of the hand for which surgical treatment can be performed in the emergency room require local anesthesia, either by local infiltration or regional block. Lidocaine (Xylocaine), 1 to 2%, is the preferred agent. No epinephrine is used for hand surgery.

All extensive injuries, especially those of children, need general anesthesia. When general anesthesia is indicated, surgery must be performed in the operating room. It is the responsibility of the emergency-room physician to contact the staff of the anesthesia department for preoperative medication.

In cases when general anesthesia is contraindicated because of a history of food intake within 6 hours or the pulmonary or cardiac condition of the patient, a brachial plexus block or local intravenous anesthesia may be selected.

If general anesthesia is necessary, a general physical examination and a routine urine and blood examination should be made in the emergency room. When required, blood for typing and cross matching is obtained and intravenous fluid therapy started.

Explanation to the Patient

Once the extent of injury is estimated in the emergency room, it is the responsibility of the surgeon to inform the patient of the extent of injury, its significance to him, and the general plan of treatment. This is especially important if amputation of one or more digits is unavoidable, if prolonged hospitalization is needed, or if a series of reconstructive procedures is anticipated.

Tetanus Prophylaxis

All open wounds of the hand, including burn and frostbite injuries, should receive tetanus prophylaxis (for details, see Chapter 11).

TREATMENT—LOCAL

Management of a Wound Being Prepared for Surgery in the Operating Room

After hemostasis has been secured, either by local pressure or by ligation of individual vessels in case the bleeding is arterial in nature, the wound is dressed with sterile gauze. No local cleansing of the wound is indicated. In general, it is best to carry out the entire wound toilet in the operating room including shaving the hair, washing the skin, and irrigating the wound.

Definitive Treatment

FOREIGN BODY IN HAND. Only superficial and palpable foreign bodies can be removed in the emergency room. All others should be removed in the operating room under general anesthesia.

BURNS OF THE HAND. If burn injury is limited to the hands and involves less than 5 percent of the total body surface, the first dressing, including local cleansing and minimal débridement, can be done in the emergency room. Primary excision of deeply burned skin is not indicated at this time owing to the lack of clear demarcation in depth and width (see Chapter 15).

FROSTBITE OF THE HAND. All constricting clothing must be gently removed. The injured hand is to be immersed in warm water (40 to 42°C) for rapid thawing. There must be enough water in the tank to maintain the desired temperature. The thawing should be completed in 20 minutes. The frostbitten hand must never be massaged. The local cleaning of gross contamination must be extremely gentle. The blisters are left intact. After complete thawing, the injured hand is left exposed or dressed as for burn injuries. The patient is then admitted.

LACERATIONS OF SKIN. Simple lacerations of the skin without damage to deep structures can be repaired under local anesthesia. The wound is thoroughly irrigated with sterile saline solution to remove all gross contamination. The skin edges are carefully debrided, all devitalized tissue being removed. After careful hemostasis and thorough examination of the depth of the wound to make sure there is no injury to deep structures, the laceration is closed in layers, using absorbable material, 4-0 catgut for the buried sutures and 5-0 silk or other nonabsorbable material for the skin sutures. A pressure dressing is then applied to the wound. If the laceration is extensive, the entire hand is included in the dressing with the fingers separated in functional position and their tips exposed when possible.

Dog bites of the hand should be treated as ordinary lacerations. Repair of the laceration should always be attempted. The police must be notified and the responsible dog observed for symptoms of rabies (see Chapter 11).

Human bites, however, should *never* be closed because of the virulent bacterial contamination from the oral cavity. The wound must be thoroughly cleansed with copious saline irrigation and hemostasis achieved. No attempt should be made to repair any damage of the deep structures if present. The wound is laid open for continuous saline compresses. The patient is admitted.

FINGERTIP INJURIES. The most common type of hand injury resulting from household accidents is the finger injury. It can be satisfactorily handled in the properly equipped emergency room if the patient is cooperative.

SLICING INJURIES WITH SOFT TISSUE LOSS. Glancing or tangential injuries by a knife blade or broken glass or by gouging, planing, chopping, or slicing machinery may produce clean-cut areas of skin and soft tissue loss uncomplicated by other tissue damage. The resulting defects generally involve either a finger pulp or the tip of a finger. The phalangeal bone may or may not be exposed. The bleeding, though profuse, is capillary in nature.

The aim of emergency treatment is primarily skin replacement. When no bone is exposed or when the area of exposed bone is small enough to be covered by surrounding soft tissue, a free skin graft is usually sufficient. In some instances the amputated portion of skin is not badly traumatized and is preserved by the patient. When it is available and not macerated or dried out, it should be placed in sterile saline solution to which penicillin has been added. Any retained fat on the undersurface is removed and the skin used as a full-thickness graft. No substitute for palmar or plantar skin will give results as satisfactory as the replantation of plantar or palmar skin.

1. Anesthesia in these cases is best obtained by block of the digital nerves at the base of the finger. Excessive volumes of fluid infiltrated at this site and the addition of epinephrine to the local anesthetic are both contraindicated because of the risk of obliterating the blood supply with resultant gangrene. For this reason not over 3 ml of solution should be injected. Lidocaine is the preferred agent. After thorough cleansing with saline solution and careful débridement, hemostasis is obtained. The wound is again carefully examined to assure a satisfactory base for a free skin graft. If a small area of bone is exposed, it must be covered by soft tissue without tension. If only the tip of the phalangeal bone is exposed, it may be rongeured slightly to permit soft tissue coverage.

2. When the amputated skin is not available or is unsuitable for replacement, if the defect is small and located at the tip of the finger, a thin split-thickness skin graft is preferred. This thin graft will contract after healing, reducing the scarred area, and being hidden beneath the fingernail will simultaneously prevent a tender fingertip. A thin skin graft can be obtained with a razor blade or Blair knife. The anterior surface of the upper thigh or the flexor surface of the forearm is the most commonly used donor site. Under local anesthesia, the skin of the donor site is stretched taut with two

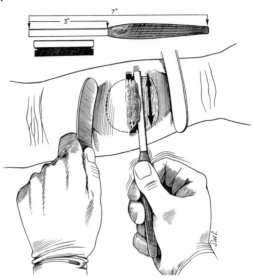

Fig. 13-2. Technique of taking a split-thickness skin graft with a razor blade attached to a Weck handle. Note that the donor site skin is stretched taut with two tongue blades.

tongue blades. By to-and-fro strokes with the razor blade at an acute tangential angle with the skin surface, a graft of the desired size is easily obtained. The desired thickness can be obtained by varying the pressure of the blade on the skin during the procedure. The donor site is covered by a single layer of nonadherent ointment muslin gauze. A pressure dressing is then applied (Fig. 13-2).

When the defect is large and occupies the pulp surface of the distal phalanx, a thicker graft is desirable. A thick graft is more durable, less deforming, and less likely to result in a tender tip. If contamination is not excessive and the elapsed time between injury and treatment is not prolonged, a full-thickness skin graft can be used. This is obtained from the flexor surface of the wrist or forearm. A transverse ellipse of full-thickness skin of suitable size is taken. The attached fat and a thin layer of dermis are carefully removed from its undersurface to assure a better "take" of the graft (Fig. 13-3). The donor site is closed primarily in layers, with sutures of 4-0 catgut for the subcuticle and 5-0 silk for the skin.

When a large area of bone, joint, or tendon is exposed, a pedicle graft will be needed for resurfacing. This procedure is best performed in the operating room.

3. The skin graft must be trimmed to fit the defect. It is carefully anchored in place using a continuous 4-0 catgut or 5-0 silk

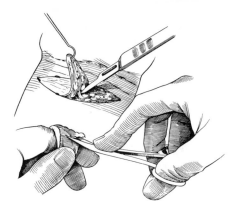

Fig. 13-3. Technique of taking a full-thickness skin graft. Note that the attached fat and a thin layer of dermis are removed from the undersurface of the graft.

suture. Pressure is then maintained over the graft by a dressing held by the long ends of interrupted sutures tied over it (Fig. 13-4).

GUILLOTINE AMPUTATION. This is usually the result of a chopping accident or injury by cutting machinery. An open bone section is characteristic. The aim of emergency treatment is to obtain a primary closure of the stump.

1. Shortening of the bone is often necessary. When the injury is on a nonessential finger such as the long, ring, or little finger and

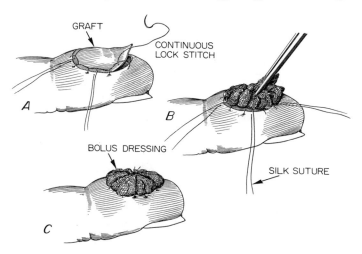

Fig. 13-4. "Stent" pressure dressing for a skin graft. Note that the interrupted sutures are left long and are tied over the gauze dressing to maintain uniform pressure on the graft.

the other fingers are unaffected, it is wise to achieve primary closure by further bone resection. This reduces convalescence to a minimum. After thorough cleansing by saline irrigation, and careful débridement, the availability of local viable soft tissue is determined. The bone should be shortened just enough to allow primary closure without tension. When the resection is at the level of the interphalangeal joint, the cartilage at the distal end of the remaining phalangeal bone must be carefully and completely removed to prevent chronic chondritis and a tender stump. The digital nerves should be identified and shortened beyond the level of amputation to minimize neuroma formation. The soft tissue is then closed in layers without tension. Complete hemostasis must be achieved, for a hematoma in the wound is the chief cause of secondary breakdown.

2. Maximal length of the stump should be retained. When injury occurs to the thumb or index finger, or when the patient's occupation is one in which the use of all fingers is of crucial importance, every attempt must be made to preserve the length of the finger. A pedicle flap is needed, and the procedure must be carried out in the operating room.

AVULSION. Massive avulsion or degloving of the skin of the finger or hand is usually caused by combined forceful compression and traction. It often results from accidents with a roller or other mobile machinery. Such injuries, as a rule, are too extensive to be handled in the emergency room.

COMPRESSION INJURIES. Compression injuries may vary in severity from a fingertip simply jammed in a car door to a whole hand flattened by a hot molding press. The most common household accident is the wringer injury. The strength of the compressing force and the duration of its application determine the severity of the injury.

JAMMED FINGER. Blood blister, pulp hematoma, and nail damage require only local cleansing and a simple dressing. A subungual hematoma may require trephining through the nail to release pressure and relieve pain. A split skin should be treated as a simple laceration. The closure, however, must be loose to allow for subsequent swelling. Roentgenographic examination is usually indicated to rule out fracture of the phalanx. A frequent sequela of car door injuries to digits is avulsion of the base of the nail. When present, this finding is indicative of a compound fracture of the distal phalanx. Treatment is carried out under digital nerve block anesthesia. The proximal half of the nail is excised, the fracture reduced by direct pressure, and the tip of the finger supported on a well-padded splint for 2 weeks.

WRINGER INJURY. This injury occurs among housewives and children when the hand and forearm are caught and drawn between the rollers. In adults it is the back of the hand that receives the maximal injury, while in children it is the forearm or arm that suffers. When the injury is seen early, the swelling may not be evident and the extent of skin necrosis may still be hidden. Therefore, even though preliminary examination does not reveal any open wound or skin damage, prompt medical attention is needed. Roentgenogram of the injured limb is taken to rule out possible fracture. The involved part is thoroughly cleansed and a pressure dressing applied (a single layer of xeroform gauze, topped by layers of soft absorbing roller gauze). Moderate and uniform pressure is applied with an elastic bandage. The fingers must be separately dressed, the hand maintained in a functional position, and the fingertips exposed for observation of the circulatory efficiency of the extremity. The limb must be elevated.

When split skin or necrosis is observed, conservation is the principle to be followed in emergency treatment. The wound is simply cleansed and a pressure dressing applied to the injured limb as described above. Closure of the skin laceration is sometimes inadvisable to prevent circulatory embarrassment by impending edema. Definitive treatment should be postponed for 5 to 7 days until the exact extent of damage is defined. While this treatment can be accomplished in the emergency room, hospitalization for observation is advisable.

GREASE GUN INJURIES. All injuries of this type require radical relaxation incisions of the involved part and thorough cleansing and removal of embedded grease. These measures should not be taken in the emergency room.

NERVE INJURIES. Severance of the median or ulnar nerve at the level of the wrist or in the palm is often associated with injuries of other deep structures. Because of the buried position of the nerve in the palm and often concomitant injuries of the tendon at wrist level, repair must be performed under general anesthesia with the use of a pneumatic tourniquet in the operating room.

Severance of the digital nerve, however, may occur with a simple laceration of the finger. In such cases, repair of the digital nerve can be carried out in the emergency room. Under regional block anesthesia, a bloodless field is obtained using a broad rubber band around the base of the injured finger. The digital nerve is identified and both distal and proximal severed ends are isolated. After conservative trimming of the nerve ends, end-to-end anastomosis can be performed. Interrupted 6-0 silk sutures on a fine atraumatic needle are used for approximating the nerve sheath around the periphery of the severed nerve bundle. As a rule three or four sutures are sufficient. The tourniquet is then released and hemostasis secured. The skin laceration is repaired in layers.

TENDON INJURIES. The indications for the treatment of tendon lacerations in the emergency room are limited. The emergency-room care will be discussed separately for flexor and extensor tendon injuries.

FLEXOR TENDON INJURIES. These should never be repaired in the emergency room. However, the decision for primary versus late repair must be made, and when late repair is elected, simple suture of the laceration can be done in the emergency room.

The laceration must be clean with minimal tissue damage and contamination if primary repair is to be considered. Primary repair, if decided upon, must be performed in the operating room. It may be considered for the following conditions:

1. Incomplete lacerations.
2. Laceration of the flexor digitorum profundus tendon distal to the insertion of the flexor digitorum sublimis.
3. Laceration of both tendons proximal to the distal palmar crease.
4. Laceration of the flexor pollicis longus.
5. Laceration of the intrinsic muscles and tendons to the thumb and little finger.
6. Laceration of tendons at the wrist level.

Late repair should be considered for the following:

1. All tendon injuries when contamination of the wound is great or the skin is devitalized so that primary healing is questionable.
2. All lacerations of both flexor tendons between the distal

palmar crease and the insertion of the flexor digitorum sub-limis.

The goal in these injuries is to obtain primary healing of the overlying tissue and skin. Many of the wounds may be treated by careful cleansing, débridement, and suture in the emergency room. The part should be immobilized in the functional position until healing is complete.

EXTENSOR TENDON INJURIES. The extensor tendons are subcutaneous and accessible. Repair in the emergency room may be justifiable when adequate facilities are available.

Injuries to the insertion of the extensor tendon to the distal phalanx may be repaired in the emergency room (Fig. 13-5).

1. Tendon laceration can be repaired by end-to-end suture or a Bunnell pull-out wire depending on the length of the distal stump. The finger should be immobilized with a splint, cast, or Kirschner wire with the distal interphalangeal joint in extension, but not hyperextension.

2. Tendon avulsion, with or without a flake of bone, can usually be treated satisfactorily with immobilization as for laceration for at least 4 weeks.

3. The articular fracture requires accurate reduction. If this is accomplished by extending the joint, immobilization is carried out as described above. If not, an open reduction in the operating room should be done.

Small lacerations of the extensor aponeurosis can be repaired by end-to-end suture with fine silk or chromic catgut sutures.

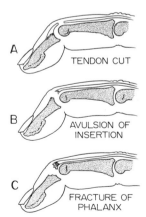

A TENDON CUT

B AVULSION OF INSERTION

C FRACTURE OF PHALANX

Fig. 13-5. Injuries to the insertion of the extensor tendon.

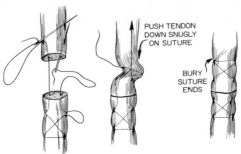

Fig. 13-6.   Buried Bunnell suture for tendon anastomosis. A Bunnell or small Keith needle is attached to each end of the suture. The suture is then placed as shown. After the suture is tied, both ends of the suture are passed through the tendon, drawn tight, and cut. This permits the ends of the wire to retract into the tendon as shown.

Laceration of an extensor tendon on the back of the hand can be repaired in the emergency room.

The technique of repair in the emergency room is as follows: Local infiltration with procaine or lidocaine, 1% or 2%, will provide adequate anesthesia. The proximal end of the tendon is then drawn into the wound and held there by transfixing it at right angles with a small Keith needle. The technique of Bunnell with a buried 5-0 braided wire suture is then used to approximate the tendon (Fig. 13-6). Placing the suture in the proximal end first and extending the finger facilitates suture.

A bulky compression dressing and a light plaster splint are used to immobilize all of the fingers in a functional position. Active motion may be started after 3 weeks and full use after 5 weeks.

The injuries which should not be repaired in the emergency room are as follows:

1. Lacerations which completely sever the extensor aponeurosis.
2. Lacerations of the central slip of the extensor tendon over the proximal interphalangeal joint.
3. Lacerations of the extensor pollicis longus and abductor pollicis longus when there is appreciable retraction of the proximal stump.

JOINT INJURIES

SPRAINS.   A sprain is a torn ligament. It may be minimal, with only a few fibers torn, or complete, with all the fibers torn, or any degree in between.

The diagnosis of a *sprained wrist* after an injury is based on tenderness about the joint capsule, pain with motion, and normal roentgenograms. The treatment consists of support with an elastic bandage or a cast, depending on the degree of injury. Avulsion fractures of the triquetrum are treated in a similar manner. The major pitfall in making the diagnosis of a "sprained" wrist is a fracture of the navicular. If there is tenderness over the anatomical snuffbox, and pain on the radial side of the wrist when the first metacarpal is pushed toward the radius, a fracture of the navicular must be suspected. Special roentgenograms of the navicular must be obtained if these findings are present and the usual roentgenograms fail to show a fracture. Failure to demonstrate a fracture even with special views does not exclude fracture of the navicular. Plaster immobilization should be used for 2 to 3 weeks and the roentgenographic examination repeated when fracture of the navicular is suspected.

Incomplete tears of the collateral ligaments of *thumb* and *fingers,* as evidenced by local tenderness with stability of the joint, may be treated on an outpatient basis with an adhesive tape spica about the thenar eminence and proximal phalanx or by immobilizing the finger in the position of function on a padded aluminum splint. Complete tears of the collateral ligaments and avulsion fractures of the collateral ligaments with displacement should be repaired in the operating room. Hyperextension injuries may result in damage to the volar capsule with local tenderness and limited, painful motion. Treatment consists of immobilizing the finger in a functional position on a padded aluminum splint.

DISLOCATIONS. Dislocations represent severe soft tissue injuries. There is usually moderate to severe swelling in the immediate post-reduction period and frequently some residual loss of motion secondary to scarring.

Dislocations of the *wrist* and *carpometacarpal joints* are usually dorsal and often associated with fractures. Roentgenograms should always be taken prior to and after reduction. Usually anesthesia will be required for the reduction, and the extremity should be observed in the hospital until the danger of excessive swelling and cast pressure is past.

Metacarpophalangeal dislocation is most common at the thumb, index, or little finger. Roentgenograms should always be taken. One attempt at closed reduction in the emergency room is warranted, and if it is successful, the patient may be treated on an outpatient basis. If it fails, the patient should be admitted for open reduction.

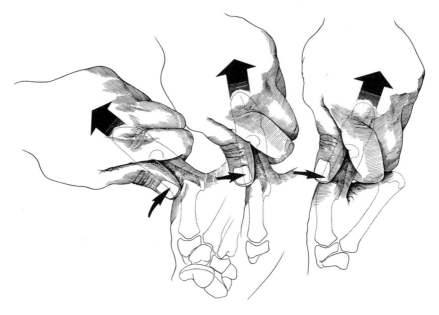

Fig. 13-7. Technique of closed reduction of a dislocation of the metacarpo-phalangeal joint. The base of the proximal phalanx is pushed around the metacarpal head. Moderate traction is maintained during the reduction.

The technique for closed reduction is as follows: The hand is prepared as for an open procedure. Approximately 5 ml of 1% lidocaine is injected into the dislocated joint and infiltrated about the area. Gentle traction is then applied in the direction of deformity, and, while the metacarpal is being stabilized with the other hand, the base of the proximal phalanx is pushed around the metacarpal head and the thumb flexed (Fig. 13-7). Tincture of benzoin on the digit and wearing gloves improve ability to control the digit. After reduction, the joint should be immobilized in moderate flexion for 3 weeks.

The *interphalangeal joints* can be reduced by traction and flexion. They should be immobilized for 3 weeks before active exercises are begun. When anesthesia is necessary, a metacarpal block rather than local infiltration should be used.

FRACTURES.   All displaced open fractures in the hand with the exception of the open pulp injury with a tuft fracture of the distal phalanx should be treated in the operating room on an inpatient basis. Closed fractures without displacement or displaced fractures which can be satisfactorily reduced and are stable without internal fixation can be treated in the emergency room.

THE PROXIMAL METACARPAL. Fracture of the base of a metacarpal without dislocation usually has minimal displacement and may be treated with a short arm plaster cast that extends to the metacarpal head.

Intracapsular fractures of the base of the first metacarpal (Bennett's fracture) are often easy to reduce but difficult to immobilize by closed methods. Closed treatment can be attempted in the emergency room after infiltration of the joint and hematoma with a local anesthetic agent.

Reduction is accomplished by longitudinal traction on the thumb as the base of the metacarpal is pushed onto the greater multangular bone (Fig. 13-8). Longitudinal skin or skeletal traction and a well-molded cast are then used to maintain reduction. A Kirschner wire through the metacarpal which is incorporated into the cast is another method of immobilization.

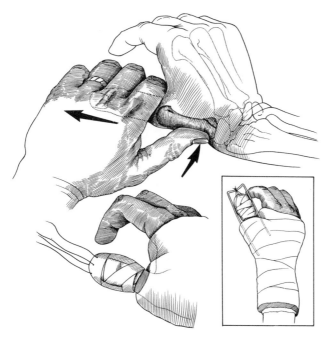

Fig. 13-8. Closed treatment of Bennett's fracture. Reduction is by traction, abduction, and pressure on the base of the metacarpal. Immobilization is accomplished with plaster cast and traction. Open reduction and Kirschner wire fixation are usually necessary.

Open reduction and fixation with Kirschner wires is a very satisfactory method of treatment, but it requires hospital admission and should be done in the operating room. The method of treatment must be determined by the surgeon on an individual basis.

THE METACARPAL SHAFT. Fractures of the metacarpal shaft usually present with dorsal angulation. If the fracture is oblique, minimal overriding may be accepted. Immobilization for 3 weeks in a well-molded short arm cast that extends to the metacarpophalangeal level is usually sufficient for fractures of the inner metacarpals. The border metacarpals may be treated in a similar manner, but it is more difficult to maintain the reduction and frequently the finger must be immobilized as well. The cast should extend to the interphalangeal joint for the first metacarpal while the thumb is abducted and the metacarpophalangeal joint slightly flexed.

Internal fixation with one or two Kirschner wires is also a satisfactory method of treatment; however, this should not be done in the emergency room.

THE METACARPAL NECK. This fracture is reduced by flexing the proximal phalanx 90 degrees, pushing dorsally with the finger and palmarward on the metacarpal shaft (Fig. 13-9). Care must be taken to maintain correct rotation of the finger. After reduction a well-padded short arm plaster cast is applied with the finger in the position of reduction. It is extremely important to *avoid pressure over*

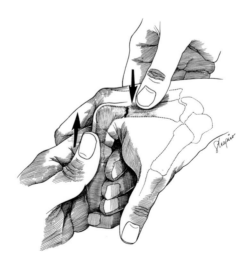

Fig. 13-9. Technique of closed reduction of metacarpal neck fracture. Care must be taken when applying the cast to avoid pressure necrosis over the metacarpophalangeal and proximal interphalangeal joints.

the dorsum of the metacarpophalangeal and proximal interphalangeal joints because of the danger of pressure necrosis of skin and tendons. The finger should not be immobilized in maximum flexion.

If the reduction is unstable, admission for internal fixation with a Kirschner wire is indicated.

THE PHALANGES. Most closed phalangeal fractures can be treated satisfactorily by closed methods. Accurate reduction is essential. A metacarpal block provides adequate anesthesia when it is needed.

A molded short arm cast is applied into which a prebent aluminum splint has been incorporated. The splint must be carefully bent to hold the finger in semiflexion at all joints without angulation. Tube gauze is placed over the finger and reduction accomplished with traction and manipulation. The finger is then taped to the splint. If swelling is excessive, the tape can easily be cut and reapplied (Fig. 13-10).

If traction is needed to maintain the reduction, a long piece of tube gauze is held to the sides of the finger with collodion and the free ends are tied about a rubber band which is fastened to a safety pin in the cast. Traction can also be applied in a similar manner by attaching it to a wire or silkworm gut suture, or Kirschner wire placed through the pulp.

Internal fixation of an unstable fracture with a Kirschner wire should be done in the operating room and the patient admitted to the hospital. Active exercises can usually be started after 3 or 4 weeks of immobilization.

Phalangeal fractures distal to the tendinous insertions require

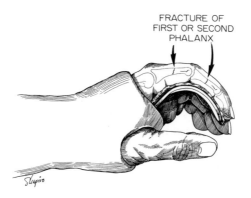

FRACTURE OF
FIRST OR SECOND
PHALANX

Fig. 13-10. Reduction and immobilization of phalangeal fractures with a padded aluminum splint incorporated into a short plaster cast. Minimal corrections in angulation of the fracture can be made by appropriately bending the splint.

protection until tenderness disappears. Avulsion fractures of the extensor insertion have been discussed with tendon injuries. Those of the flexor profundus insertion require patient admission and open repair in the operating room.

INFECTIONS. Disability resulting from infections of the major fascial spaces and synovial sheaths of the hand is potentially even greater than that following injury. Fortunately, as a result of effective antimicrobial therapy, the frequency of serious hand infections has declined in recent years. Prompt recognition and treatment continue to be important in the preservation of manual function, for even the most trivial infection if mistreated can cause severe crippling.

The more superficial lesions, involving skin primarily, can be treated in most instances without recourse to hospitalization and in this sense can be considered minor. If the principles of treatment are understood and followed and the cooperation of the patient is enlisted, the end results will be uniformly excellent. Abrogation of the principles, or lack of cooperation by the patient, can lead to serious complications. Patients with infections of tendon sheaths and fascial spaces are admitted to the hospital for treatment, but recognition is the responsibility of the emergency-room physician.

MINOR INFECTIONS

1. Furuncles are infections of hair follicles, which on the fingers and hand are limited to the dorsum. They begin as folliculitis which usually subsides with rest, the application of local heat, and avoidance of trauma. When resistance is low, as in patients with systemic disease such as diabetes, or the virulence of the organism is great, a furuncle or carbuncle may eventuate. Most furuncles, however, develop as a result of traumatizing the initial follicle infection. They are usually located in the skin over the proximal phalanx. Central necrosis occurs with suppuration beneath. In some cases there is associated lymphangitis and lymphadenitis with systemic signs of infection.

Antibiotics are not indicated except when the furuncle is complicated by lymphangitis and lymphadenitis, or deep spread in the finger occurs. The patient is instructed to avoid squeezing the lesion or otherwise traumatizing it. The affected part is placed at rest with the application of local heat. When the central necrotic plug loosens, it frequently can be lifted out with a pointed forcep. This may provide adequate drainage, but sometimes further drainage is required.

It is best accomplished under general anesthesia, since both local infiltration and conduction anesthesia hazard spread of infection.

The carbuncle consists of a confluent group of furuncles. Antimicrobial therapy should be given after culture of the wound and the determination of bacterial sensitivity to the various antimicrobial agents. Adequate incision and drainage are accomplished when suppuration occurs. Patients with carbuncles should be hospitalized. Carbuncles are particularly common in diabetics under poor control.

2. Paronychia is a staphylococcal infection of the skin at the margin of the nail often caused by infection in a hangnail. A small abscess forms, which if opened at the proper time will promptly subside. If neglected, the infection tends to spread to the base of the nail, then around the cuticle to the opposite side. This tendency led to the name *run around,* a common synonym for paronychia. In neglected cases, an abscess forms beneath the base of the nail, elevating it.

The diagnosis is apparent with the observation of inflammation in the skin at the margin of a nail. A subungual abscess is suspected when the cuticle is involved and point pressure on the base of the nail evokes pain. There is also pain when slight dorsal pressure is applied on the end of the nail.

The uncomplicated paronychia is treated by rest and the application of local heat. When an abscess forms, it frequently can be drained using a pointed scalpel blade without anesthesia. If necessary, conduction anesthesia can be induced by infiltration around the digital nerves in the region of the proximal phalanx. Three ml of 2% lidocaine or less is used for this purpose; no epinephrine is used.

Subungual abscess is drained by making parallel incisions extending from the skin fold at each margin of the base of the nail proximally for 4 to 5 mm. A flap is elevated exposing the base of the nail, which is excised with sharp-pointed scissors. Removal of the distal portion of the nail is unnecessary for drainage, so it should be left in place to protect the sensitive nail bed. A small piece of the fine-mesh gauze is inserted beneath the flap for several days.

3. A felon is an infection of the volar closed space over the distal phalanx. Anatomically this is in reality a series of closed spaces formed by connective tissue septa which course from the periosteum of the phalanx, distal to the epiphysis, to the dense dermis of the volar skin. Enclosed within the septa are areolar tissue, numerous

sensory nerve fibers, and the nutrient arteries to the shaft of the phalanx. Infection is introduced by a puncture wound, which may be trivial and at times is related to occupation. The responsible organism is the staphylococcus. Infection is heralded by slight throbbing discomfort, which rapidly progresses to intense throbbing pain. On examination there is slight swelling and the volar pad is tense and tender.

If the patient is seen within 6 hours of the onset of symptoms, the infection may be aborted by rest, elevation, the application of local heat, and the use of large doses of parenteral penicillin. In most cases, however, early incision and drainage are indicated, and these can be done in the emergency room under digital nerve block anesthesia providing analgesia is complete. This is important because it will be impossible to open the space properly without complete analgesia. A single incision is made along the lateral or medial margin of the distal closed space using a pointed knife blade. The incision is carried to the dermis on the opposite side completely transecting all of the fibrous septa. On the thumb and small finger the incision is made on the lateral (radial) side while on the other three fingers it is made on the medial (ulnar) side. This selection is based on keeping the resultant scar as far as possible from the side that is used the most in grasping, writing, and so forth (Fig. 13-11).

Only a small amount of pus will be found in early cases. Culture and antimicrobial sensitivities should be obtained, and pending the results of these studies penicillin is given. A small piece of rubber

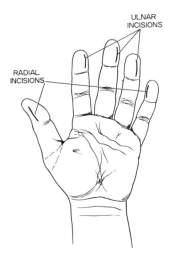

Fig. 13-11. Incisions for opening of a felon on the various digits.

dam is inserted to keep the wound open, and a dry dressing is applied. The wound is dressed daily with precaution to prevent premature closure of any portion. Pain relief is usually rapid following drainage, but the patient should be given codeine and aspirin to cover residual discomfort.

Delay in drainage results in osteomyelitis of the distal phalanx, usually not including the epiphysis, which has a separate nutrient blood supply not affected by the rise in pressure in the distal closed space. With the development of osteomyelitis, sequestration of part or all of the phalanx may occur. Treatment should be expectant after drainage has been provided.

4. The name *collar-button abscess* is descriptive of any abscess having a superficial and a deep component connected by a narrow isthmus. It is important because the deeper component may go unrecognized at the time of drainage, necessitating a second procedure when the patient fails to show the expected improvement after the first incision. Two varieties are seen in the hand. In one, an intraepidermal abscess develops in the horny calloused hand of a laborer with the main pocket lying subcutaneously connected to the epidermal abscess by a small opening in the dermis. In the second, typically located in the web space between the index and middle finger, there are volar and dorsal components separated by the dividing fibers of the palmar aponeurosis. In both instances the signs of inflammation are evident; appreciation of the possibility of the presence of the deeper abscess is usually sufficient for its demonstration at the time of operative drainage. The first-mentioned variety can be conveniently handled in the emergency room, whereas the web space infection is preferably drained in the operating room under general anesthesia.

MAJOR INFECTIONS. Patients with the following infections of the hand should be admitted to the hospital for definitive treatment. Operation is best done under general anesthesia using a pneumatic tourniquet to provide a bloodless field, otherwise, it is likely that important structures will be damaged.

1. *Streptococcal gangrene* is fortunately seldom seen today; it is mentioned both for the sake of completeness and because its early recognition and appropriate treatment are necessary for maximum salvage of tissue. As the name implies, the lesion is basically a streptococcal infection, but careful bacteriological study will sometimes show other organisms growing in symbiosis with the streptococcus.

In our experience the lesion has been seen most frequently among laboratory technicians and personnel working in autopsy rooms or in similar circumstances in which there is exposure to highly virulent organisms. The incubation period is short and the clinical evolution of the inflammatory process fulminant, so that when the patient is first seen, evidence of loss of viabilty of tissue is likely to be present.

Massive antimicrobial therapy should be started in the emergency room with penicillin G in the non-penicillin-sensitive patient. If exudate is present, a culture should also be obtained prior to admission to the hospital.

2. *Suppurative tenosynovitis* is a true surgical emergency in which prompt and proper care are necessary to prevent necrosis of tendons. Knowledge of the anatomy of the synovial sheaths is essential for accurate diagnosis. The flexor tendons of all digits are enveloped in sheaths as shown in Fig. 13-12. The tendon sheaths of the flexor tendons of the thumb and small finger extend into the palm and forearm as the radial and ulnar bursae, and since the radial and ulnar bursae communicate with each other in most instances, infection involving one will usually involve the other. The flexor sheaths of the index, middle, and ring fingers do not commonly communicate with each other or with the radial or ulnar bursae. They begin in the palm just proximal to the metacarpophalangeal joints and extend distally close to the insertion of the flexor digitorum profundus tendons.

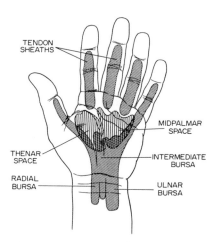

Fig. 13-12. Synovial sheaths and deep fascial spaces on the volar surface of the hand. (From E. Lampe. Surgical anatomy of the hand. *Clin. Sympos.* 9:3, 1957. © 1957 CIBA Corporation, adapted from and reproduced with permission from the *Clinical Symposia* by Frank H. Netter, M.D.)

The clinical manifestations of suppurative tenosynovitis are pain, swelling, and tenderness in the anatomical distribution of the tendon sheath. The finger is held in slight flexion, and great pain is experienced when the examiner attempts to extend it.

The causative organism is either the streptococcus or the staphylococcus. Aqueous penicillin G should be given in the emergency room while arranging for admission of the patient to the hospital. Definitive treatment should never be attempted in the emergency room.

In neglected cases infection spreads to the middle palmar space from the sheaths of the middle and ring fingers, and to the thenar space from the sheath of the index finger.

Infection of the radial and ulnar bursae usually follows infection of the flexor synovial sheath of the thumb and small finger. Because the bursae frequently communicate with each other, infection in one is usually soon followed by infection in the other. Seldom is the volume of pus formed sufficiently great to obliterate the palmar concavity. Diffuse swelling of the digit occurs with pain and tenderness over the sheath and its proximal extension. Swelling is likely to be greatest on the dorsum of the hand due to the rapid accumulation of edema fluid in the loose tissues of the dorsal subcutaneous space. This should not be mistaken for suppuration. The signs of tenosynovitis involving the thumb and small finger are otherwise similar to signs of infection in the flexor sheaths of the other digits.

If treatment is delayed, necrosis of the sheath occurs followed by spread of infection to the middle palmar and thenar spaces and the major forearm space.

3. *The major fascial spaces* include the middle palmar space, the thenar space, the major forearm space, the dorsal subcutaneous space, and the dorsal subaponeurotic space. Lesser fascial spaces also are present along the lumbrical tendons and between the muscles of the thenar and hypothenar eminences. For the detailed anatomy of these spaces, the reader is referred to the classic studies of Kanavel. Suffice it to say that infection can occur in any of these spaces by direct implantation, by the spread of infection through lymphatics, by spread from infection within synovial sheaths, or by osteomyelitis of adjacent bones.

The middle palmar space lies beneath the flexor tendons of the middle, ring, and small fingers; it is bounded medially by the hypothenar muscles and laterally it is separated from the thenar space by a fascial band attaching to the periosteum of the middle metacarpal bone. The thenar space lies lateral to this septum in the same anteroposterior plane extending to the web between the index finger and thumb. Infection in the middle palmar space tends to obliterate the palmar concavity, the swelling extends to the thenar space, but pain and tenderness are limited to the midpalmar space. As swelling increases, the pain and tenderness, which in early stages are severe, tend to lessen. Extension into the lumbrical spaces of the ring and small fingers occurs with swelling in the web spaces along the lumbrical canals.

Infection in the *thenar space* produces marked swelling which is rather sharply and strikingly limited to the distribution of the thenar space; thus it is easily recognizable. Pain and tenderness are also present.

The major forearm space, although not in the hand, is included because of its frequent involvement from the spread of infection within the radial and ulnar bursae. It lies deep to the flexor digitorum profundus tendons on the fascia covering the pronator quadratus muscle. When it is involved by infection, pus rapidly spreads upward as far as the elbow.

The dorsal subaponeurotic space lies between the fascia covering the dorsal interosseous muscles and the aponeurosis joining the extensor tendons. Infection generally arises by direct implantation, but lymphatic spread also occurs. When infected there is marked swelling, pain, and tenderness throughout the dorsum of the hand.

Emergency-room management of major fascial space infections of the hand is limited to arranging for prompt admission to the hospital. Antimicrobial treatment, usually with penicillin G, may be started while the above arrangements are in process.

GENERAL REFERENCES

Boyes, J. H.   *Bunnell's Surgery of the Hand* (4th ed.). Philadelphia: Lippincott, 1964.

Cave, E. F.   *Fractures and Other Injuries*. Chicago: Year Book, 1961.

Converse, J. M.   *Reconstructive and Plastic Surgery*. Philadelphia: Saunders, 1964.

Kanavel, A. B.   *Infections of the Hand* (7th ed.). Philadelphia: Lea & Febiger, 1939.

Rank, B. K., and Wakefield, A. R.   *Surgery of Repair as Applied to Hand Injuries*. Baltimore: Williams & Wilkins, 1960.

Maxillofacial Injuries 14

MARK K. WANG
W. BRANDON MACOMBER

Automobile accidents, contact sports, explosions, and falls account for most facial bone fractures. Braunstein [1], in a survey of 1000 automobile accidents involving 1678 persons, reported head injuries in 72.3 percent, of which 7.2 percent had sustained fractures of the facial bones. Kuloski [4] has pointed out that mandibular fractures are more common in crash injuries than fractures of either the maxilla or the zygomatic arch, in a ratio of 4:1. Gerrie [3], in a review of 150 facial fractures in contact sports, found that the mandible was involved in 25 percent, the malar bone in 21 percent, the zygomatic arches in 3 percent, and the maxilla in 21 percent. Approximately half of contact sport fractures are nasal. McCoy et al. [5] found that midfacial fractures account for approximately 40 percent of all facial fractures, with one-third of these also involving the orbital bone.

Rowe and Killey [6] in analyzing 500 cases of facial fractures, stated that the majority of fractures occur in the 20 to 39 year age group (53.4%). Only 1.2% were sustained before the age of five. After the age of 60 years, the mandible becomes brittle and thin due to alveolar absorption. It can be fractured very easily.

HISTORY

A detailed history should be obtained from the patient if he is conscious and able to recollect the details of the accident. If not, a reliable witness may be able to give an excellent account of the injury.

Date and Time of Injury

This information is important in relation to physical findings such as the amount of local swelling or the degree of wound infection in late cases. From a medicolegal viewpoint, date and time are crucial.

Nature of the Accident

AUTOMOBILE ACCIDENTS. The driver catapults forward against the steering wheel through a short arc and usually suffers injuries of the mandibular region, while the front seat passenger is usually thrown forward through a wider arc hitting the windshield and dashboard and is more likely to damage the maxilla, malar bones, nose, and zygomatic arch.

FALLS. The patient who falls forward on the point of the chin commonly sustains a midline fracture of the mandible with bilateral fractures of the condylar necks. If he falls on the side of his face, the prominence of the malar bone usually produces a zygomatic fracture.

BLUNT TRAUMA. A direct blow by a blunt object, such as a fist, usually produces a fracture at the site of impact. Such trauma on the side of the mandible, however, can cause a condylar fracture on the contralateral side in addition to the isolateral body fracture due to the transmission of the traumatic force.

PENETRATING INJURIES. The nature of the wound depends upon the type of missile and its velocity. The entry wound of a bullet is generally small and comparatively clean, whereas a fragmentation missile usually produces a ragged, contused wound. A bullet fired from a distance travels at a low velocity and is often retained in the tissue after penetrating the skin and fracturing the bone. A fast-traveling bullet at close range, however, is more likely to penetrate beyond the bone and produces a large explosive type of exit wound.

Loss of Consciousness

The depth and duration of loss of consciousness is a valuable indication of the severity of any concomitant cerebral damage. When a patient is brought in unconscious with fracture of a facial bone, it must be assumed that the cerebral condition is due to trauma until proved otherwise. Sudden loss of consciousness may follow epileptic fits, cerebral or cardiovascular accident, hypoglycemia, diabetic coma, and so forth. The level of consciousness may be affected by ingestion of alcohol or other drugs.

Symptoms Suggestive of Other Injuries

As facial fractures are often accompanied by other injuries, a careful evaluation of symptoms related to other systems of the body is necessary.

EXAMINATION

General Examination

STATE OF CONSCIOUSNESS. Restlessness and disorientation may be the result of cerebral damage, severe hemorrhage, or excessive alcohol or drug intake. One should always smell the patient's breath. Coma or convulsions resulting from trauma usually indicate severe brain damage. The patient's neurological status must be closely and repeatedly observed. Failure to recognize a developing epidural, subdural, or subarachnoid hemorrhage or signs of spinal cord compression from a fractured or displaced cervical vertebra is indefensible.

HEMORRHAGE AND SHOCK. In nonpenetrating facial injuries, hemorrhage, as a rule, is not a severe problem. In gunshot wounds, however, bleeding can be massive and often demands immediate attention. A patient in shock without evidence of significant bleeding from the facial wound is usually suffering from other concomitant injuries, and a meticulous search for the cause is mandatory. The chest should be carefully evaluated for rib fractures, hemothorax, pneumothorax, and hemopericardium; the abdomen for splenic, hepatic, kidney, or gastrointestinal injury; and the extremities and pelvis for fractures.

AIRWAY. The rate, depth, and rhythm of respiration, and the patency of the airway should be carefully observed. Respiration may be irregular or labored owing to severe intracranial injury, coma, or alcoholic intoxication. The airway may be partially blocked by the following: (1) intranasal or pharyngeal blood clots; (2) the tongue, fallen back due to a bilateral displaced mandibular fracture, comminution of symphysis of mandible, or comatose state of the patient; (3) swelling of the floor of the mouth, secondary to mandibular fracture; or (4) downward and backward displacement of the palate secondary to a bilateral maxillary fracture.

Local Examination

INSPECTION

SOFT TISSUE INJURY. Areas of contusion and abrasion usually indicate blows by a blunt object. Swelling and ecchymosis are often suggestive of deep injuries, perhaps a fracture of the underlying bone. The degree of gross contamination, especially the extent of ground-in dirt, must be noted. When laceration of the skin occurs, the depth of the injury, the extent of undermining of skin edges, and the viability of the injured soft tissue must be carefully determined. Deep lacerations over the pathway of vital structures such as the facial nerve, Stensen's duct, or lacrimal duct, call attention to possible damage of these underlying structures and warrant further investigation.

BLEEDING. The oral and nasal cavities, the external ear canal, and the orbit should be inspected for active bleeding, ecchymosis, presence of blood clots, or leakage of cerebrospinal fluid. Positive findings suggestive of basal skull fractures require further study, and, quite often, will modify the treatment.

SYMMETRY OF FACE. Asymmetry of the face can be detected if the patient is seen immediately after the accident before local swelling develops. The deformity after a fracture of nasal bone may range from a slight depression to marked deviation and tilting of the entire nose. The nasal septum must be carefully observed for deviation or distortion. A depressed malar prominence invariably follows a zygomatic fracture. In bilateral maxillary fracture of the Le Fort III type,* the midportion of the face may appear markedly elongated

---

* Le Fort I is a transverse fracture of the maxilla above the apices of the teeth detaching the tooth-bearing portion from the rest of the maxilla. Le Fort II is a pyramidal type of fracture affecting the central region of the middle third of the facial bones over an area extending from the glabella to the alveolar margin. Le Fort III is a high-level suprazygomatic fracture. The line of fracture, transversely situated, extends across the glabella and above the zygomatic bones on both sides.

and flattened because of downward displacement of the fractured segment.

MOVEMENT OF JAW AND OCCLUSION OF TEETH. A patient who has incurred a severe facial injury should be asked to open and close his mouth. Pain and trismus during motion are indicative of a mandibular fracture, usually at the condylar level. Deviation of the mandible occurs toward the side of fracture because of pull by the unopposed contralateral external pterygoid muscle. The occlusion of the teeth can be markedly altered in severe fractures of maxilla or mandible. Even in simple fractures with minimal displacement, the patient often can detect such minor alterations by experiencing changed pressure distribution on the teeth during occlusion.

PALPATION. Palpation of facial bones with both hands is the most reliable method of detecting fractures of facial bones. The examination must be gentle, bimanual, systematic, and simultaneous on both sides. The examiner aims to determine the following:

SYMMETRY OF THE FACIAL BONES. The palpating finger should start at the forehead and move downward over the frontal bone, the supraorbital ridge, the bony orbital rim, especially the lateral and infraorbital borders, the zygomatic arch, the malar prominence, the nasal bone, and the mandibular ramus, in that order. One often can detect displaced fractures by noticing asymmetry of the palpating fingertips over corresponding bony structures, in spite of swelling of the overlying soft tissue. In zygomatic fractures, the malar prominence and the lateral portion of the orbital floor are often displaced downward and medially, producing a flat deformity on the fractured side. In nasal fractures, the fractured bone gives on gentle pressure and is usually displaced medially at the site of impact and laterally on the contralateral side.

POINT OF TENDERNESS. A localized point of tenderness usually represents the exact site of fracture. Often some bony irregularity, unusual mobility, or occasionally crepitus can be detected, especially in fracture of the orbital rim or nasal bones.

OCULAR GLOBE AND VISION. For injuries of the ocular globe and ophthalmic nerve see Chapter 16. There are, however, frequent visual disturbances secondary to fractures of neighboring bones with which the examiner must be familiar.

DIPLOPIA. Diplopia often occurs following zygomatic or maxillary fractures. Marked downward displacement of the infraorbital floor in association with zygomatic fracture lowers the eye on the affected side. This is the most common cause of double vision. Retro-bulbar hemorrhage pushing the eyeball forward, injury of the third and sixth cranial nerves impairing the movement of the ocular globe, or "blowout" fractures of the orbital floor with herniation and immobilization of the inferior rectus and inferior oblique muscles are also occasionally responsible [2].

MOVEMENT OF THE OCULAR GLOBE. When diplopia is present, its extent must be determined. The patient is instructed to follow the examiner's finger, gazing upward, downward, laterally, and medially and stating the presence and degree of double vision. The range, ease, and symmetry of movement of the eyes must be carefully observed and recorded.

TRACTION TEST. When diplopia and limitation of eyeball movements, especially upward and laterally, are present in association with a suspected maxillary fracture, the traction test must be performed to rule out a blowout fracture, in which the globe is herniated through the orbital floor and the inferior ocular muscles are caught by the fractured bony fragments.

After induction of local anesthesia along the inferior sulcus of the affected ocular globe, traction is applied to the tendon of the inferior rectus muscle by a fine forceps. If the muscle is caught in a blowout fracture, the ocular globe cannot be rotated upward. This simple procedure can differentiate adhesion of the inferior rectus muscle from weakness or paralysis of the superior rectus, which can produce a similar clinical picture.

LOCAL NEUROLOGICAL DISTURBANCE. Even without intracranial or spinal injuries, any localized neurological disturbance secondary to facial bone fracture must be recognized. Positive findings often alert the examiner to a fracture although no displacement of the involved bone is obvious.

SENSATION. Anesthesia of the frontal and anterior scalp area is indicative of supraorbital nerve injury. When no skin laceration is present, fracture of the supraorbital rim must be suspected. Fracture of the maxilla at the infraorbital foramen invariably damages the infraorbital nerve and causes anesthesia of the cheek, nose, and upper lip on the fractured side. A fracture of the mandible anterior to the angle can damage the mental nerve and produce anesthesia of the lower lip.

MOTOR POWER OF FACIAL MUSCLES. In facial injuries with deep lacerations of the preauricular area, the possibility of facial nerve injury must be kept in mind. The patient must be instructed to wrinkle his forehead, close his eyelids, and contract his lips by whistling to rule out possible damage to the various branches of the facial nerve. One must be very cautious in interpreting findings when there is marked local swelling.

LACERATION OF LACRIMAL OR PAROTID DUCT. Deep lacerations along the pathway of the lacrimal duct or of Stensen's duct along the cheek require further examination. The lacrimal canaliculus, through its punctum, and Stensen's duct, through its intra-oral opening, can be investigated by gently introducing a probe of suitable size into either orifice. The appearance of the probe in the wound is indicative of injury of the duct.

TONGUE-DEPRESSOR TEST. This test is useful when little or no external signs of fracture are present, and when the occlusion of teeth appears satisfactory. The patient is instructed to maintain a closed bite on a single wooden tongue blade while the examiner attempts to pry open his jaws by twisting it. When no fracture is present, the blade will break; when there is a fracture, even slight pressure on the blade will produce pain and cause the patient to open his mouth. During this test the presence or absence of teeth should be carefully noted [7].

ROENTGENOGRAM. Most fractures of facial bones can be diagnosed without roentgenograms. Particularly in nasal fractures, clinical examination alone can provide a diagnosis because the bony structure is superficial. However, the exact extent and site of fracture can be determined only by roentgenographic examination. The roentgenogram also provides a permanent record of the injury in medicolegal cases. Therefore, whenever a fracture of a facial bone is suspected, roentgenographic examination is in order. It is done *after* a thorough clinical examination and evaluation, and after the institution of the necessary emergency therapy for maintenance of the airway and control of shock. Water's view in stereoroentgenograms is most useful for the study of maxillas, maxillary sinuses, orbital rims, zygomatic complexes, and nasal bones. The right and left lateral profile views with the mandible in open and closed positions are used for study of the mandible, temporomandibular joints, and existing dentition. Occasionally a lateral oblique view of the mandible is taken to obtain more information on mandibular body, angle, or ascending ramus. Study of the mandibular symphysis may require a posteroanterior view of the mandible.

CLINICAL PICTURE OF INDIVIDUAL BONE FRACTURES

1. Nasal bone.
    a. Local ecchymosis and swelling.
    b. Bleeding and obstruction of the nasal cavity on the fractured side.
    c. Asymmetry of the nose; depression at the site of impact by the traumatizing force; lateral displacement on the opposite side if this fracture is bilateral.
    d. Crepitation and "give" under mild pressure on the fractured bone.
    e. Deviation of the septum in bilateral fractures.
2. Zygomatic complex.
    a. Ecchymosis and swelling of the malar and periorbital region.
    b. Flatness of the malar prominence.
    c. Tenderness along the zygomatic arch and lateral and inferior orbital rim.
    d. Anesthesia of the cheek, nose, and upper lip on the injured side.
    e. A lowered inferior orbital rim with possible diplopia.
    f. A negative traction test.
3. Maxilla.
    a. Local swelling and ecchymosis.
    b. Positive tongue-blade test.
    c. Altered dental occlusion.
    d. Unusual mobility of the fractured fragment. The fragment may involve only the dento-alveolar arch (Le Fort I) or up to both maxillae (Le Fort III).
    e. Anesthesia at the infraorbital nerve distribution.
    f. Elongation of the face (Le Fort III fracture).
4. Blowout fracture.
    a. Signs of maxillary fracture.
    b. Diplopia.
    c. Deepened supratarsal sulcus.
    d. Backward and downward displacement of ocular globe.
    e. Limitation of ocular movement on upward rotation, occasionally on downward and lateral movement.
    f. Positive traction test.

5. Mandible.
    a. Local swelling and ecchymosis.
    b. Local tenderness.
    c. Positive tongue-blade test.
    d. Trismus in condylar fractures.
    e. Altered dental occlusion.
    f. Anesthesia of lower lip (in transverse ramus fracture with mental nerve damage.

TREATMENT

General Treatment

CONTROL OF HEMORRHAGE. Usually hemorrhage is not severe and can be controlled by local pressure. When branches of the facial artery, greater palatine artery, or internal maxillary artery are severed, the bleeding can be severe enough to threaten exsanguination. In such cases, if the bleeding vessel can be visualized and isolated, it should be clamped and ligated immediately. When bleeding points cannot be located, the wound should be packed temporarily and the patient transported to the operating room. Occasionally, posterior nasal tamponade may be used to control bleeding from the posterior pharyngeal region. Ligation of the external carotid artery to control bleeding in a major gunshot or avulsion wound of the maxillary region should be performed in the operating room. The bleeding in such cases can be temporarily controlled by finger pressure on the transverse process of the 6th cervical vertebra.

TREATMENT OF SHOCK. See Chapter 2.

AIRWAY. An adequate airway must be maintained while the patient is waiting for operation. Prompt control of hemorrhage and thorough cleansing of the nasal, oral, and pharyngeal cavities of blood clots, loose teeth, bone fragments, broken dentures, or other foreign materials are usually adequate to provide a free airway. Airway obstruction may also result from the tongue's falling backward in bilateral mandibular fractures, especially when the patient is unconscious. A tongue suture using 3-0 silk is needed to hold the tongue in a forward position.

Indications for tracheostomy include:

1. Fracture of maxilla and/or mandible associated with severe injury to the soft palate, tongue, or pharynx, when massive swelling has or will obstruct the upper air passage.

2. Fracture of jaw bones requiring intermaxillary wiring associated with severe nasal injuries obstructing nasal passage.

3. Fracture of jaw bones requiring intermaxillary wiring in a comatose patient.

4. Fracture of jaw bones associated with thoracic injuries affecting the respiratory function of the patient.

TETANUS PROPHYLAXIS. All facial or intra-oral lacerations will require tetanus prophylaxis. All fractures of the maxilla or mandible with the fracture line extending into dental sockets are considered compound fractures and require similar treatment (for details, see Chapter 11).

ANTIBIOTICS. All compound fractures of the maxillofacial bones should be given prophylactic antibiotic treatment. Broad-spectrum antibiotics, usually penicillin and streptomycin, are given intramuscularly in the emergency room.

Local Treatment

SOFT TISSUE INJURY

1. *Deep abrasion wound with ground-in dirt.* This type of wound on the face, if not treated properly, results in pigmentation and tattooing marks quite deforming and difficult to correct. The wound must be thoroughly irrigated with sterile normal saline solution. The embedded dirt particles must be carefully removed with a soft, fine toothbrush. Large granules can be picked off by a pair of fine-tip forceps or a large straight needle. It requires a careful, gentle, meticulous, and thorough job, aiming to remove *all* embedded foreign bodies. After completion, the wound is dressed with a single layer of xeroform ointment gauze and multiple layers of flat absorbing gauze. A pressure dressing is then applied using Ace bandage or broad adhesive strips to prevent edema of the tissue.

2. *Lacerations and avulsions* (for details, see Chapter 11). Facial scars are exposed. During primary repair, therefore, the aim should be to achieve not only primary healing, but to prevent deforming scars. The débridement must be thorough but conservative. The hemostasis must be complete. All dead space should be obliterated.

Approximation of tissue layers must be accurate, and fine suturing material used. As a rule 4-0 plain catgut is used for buried sutures and 6-0 silk for the skin sutures. A narrow, long avulsed skin flap, even if viable, is best excised if the defect can be closed without tension. An avulsed partial-thickness skin flap attached on one side should also be excised, to prevent the formation of a raised indurated scar. Any localized loss of skin, the defect of which cannot be closed without tension, is best treated with free skin graft or neighboring skin flaps if available. Such wounds should be treated in the operating room.

Injury to deep structures such as facial nerve, Stensen's duct, or lacrimal duct must be repaired. Surgery should be performed in the operating room.

Facial Bone Injuries

Emergency care of maxillofacial injuries is usually limited to diagnosis of the extent of injury and preparation of the patient for specific surgical treatment. Practically all surgical treatment for facial bone fractures should be performed in the operating room.

1. *Fracture of maxilla.* Immediate surgery is indicated when a blowout fracture is diagnosed or suspected. The herniated orbital content and incarcerated ocular muscles must be reduced promptly to avoid further damage or adhesion formation. A compound fracture or a severe displaced comminuted fracture of the maxillary sinus wall requiring antral packing for reduction should also be treated as early as possible and the local swelling disregarded if the general condition of the patient permits. This should be done in the operating room. The application of intermaxillary or suspension wiring or other dental appliances can be postponed until the general and local condition of the patient becomes more favorable.

Compound Fracture of Maxilla or Mandible.

Definitive treatment of compound fractures must sometimes be delayed because of associated injuries, or in late cases when severe local ecchymosis and swelling prevent accurate manipulation and reduction of the fractured fragments. In such cases attempts must be made to convert all compound fractures into simple ones unless clear evidence of local infection is already present. The soft tissue wounds of the skin and mucous membrane must be thoroughly irrigated, carefully debrided, and closed in layers under local anesthesia. This can be done in the emergency room if the wound is not too extensive.

Definitive treatment of fractured facial bones can be delayed for a maximum of 3 weeks. Beyond that time, healing by fibrous union makes reduction of bony fragments difficult, if not impossible.

FRACTURES OF THE NOSE. Most nasal fractures seen before the onset of edema can easily be reduced in the emergency room, and the patient can be sent home. Late-arriving cases in which edema has masked the local deformity, or those complicated by comminuted nasal fractures, or any nasal fractures in children do not belong in this category.

ANESTHESIA. Local anesthesia is used. Cotton pledgets soaked with lidocaine (Xylocaine) 5% and epinephrine 1:100,000 in equal amounts are used as intranasal packing under the fracture site for both anesthetic and vasoconstricting effect. These packs are left in place for 10 to 15 minutes. With marked intranasal edema, it may be necessary to repack the nose two or three times. Occasionally supplementary injection with procaine (Novocain) 2% may be required.

MANIPULATION. The exact site of nasal fracture and the presence of septal displacement can be determined by careful external examination and intranasal inspection. Almost all nasal fractures can be reduced by upward and outward force. A Kelly clamp is convenient for this purpose. It must be put directly under the fracture site and not too high in the nose, lest it impinge on the nasal portion of the frontal bone and cause damage to the mucosa without reducing the fracture. As the fractured bones are manipulated upward and forward with the instrument in one hand, the other hand is used to apply external pressure to mold the bones into position (Fig. 14-1). The displaced nasal septum can often be replaced by simple elevation of the depressed fractured nasal bones. If this maneuver is not successful, the fractured septum must be reduced to normal position by a Kelly clamp. In rare cases in which the septal cartilage is severely comminuted and telescoped, submucous reduction with a fine-tip forceps to replace individual fragments in position may be necessary.

IMMOBILIZATION. After satisfactory reduction, the fractures are held in position by means of intranasal packing and external splinting. A long strip of narrow xeroform or petroleum jelly gauze is used for the intranasal packing. It should be carefully packed into

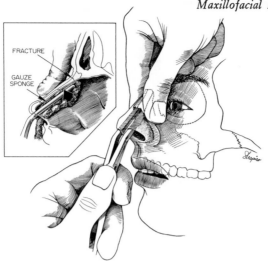

FRACTURE

GAUZE
SPONGE

Fig. 14-1. Manual reduction of nasal fracture. The tip of the clamp lies directly under the fracture site but does not extend beyond the fracture level.

the nose under the fracture site to maintain the reduced position. Gentle finger pressure applied externally over the fracture site is maintained during the entire procedure to prevent overcorrection. Whenever the nasal septum is fractured, bilateral intranasal packing is needed to maintain correct alignment.

Dental compound should be used for an external splint. Flat gauze, three or four layers thick, makes a padding underneath the splint. Dental compound should be softened to a malleable consistency in hot water, molded over the nose, trimmed to fit, and allowed to harden. The splint is then held in position with strips of adhesive (Fig. 14-2). Packing the nose should not be done if there is a concomitant basal fracture with leakage of cerebrospinal fluid.

FRACTURE OF ZYGOMA. When the patient is seen early, before local edema sets in, emergency reduction is indicated. It is preferable to use Gillies' approach under general anesthesia and in the operating room.

When marked edema is present, reduction must be postponed until it has completely subsided. The patient should be admitted to a hospital.

FRACTURE OF THE MANDIBLE. A simple fracture of the mandible with full dentition can be reduced and immobilized by intermaxil-

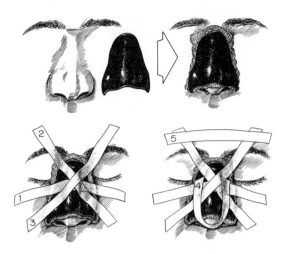

Fig. 14-2. Immobilization of nasal fracture. The molded dental compound is fixed over the nose as a splint. Half-inch-wide adhesive strips used for fixation are applied in the order indicated. The pressure over the nose must be symmetrical and uniform.

lary wiring alone. Complicated fractures, such as fracture at the angle or ascending ramus, or fracture with insufficient dentition for firm intermaxillary wiring, may require open reduction and direct wiring of the fractured fragments. It is preferable to have arch bars for the upper and lower teeth in place before the open reduction, so that immobilization can be effected immediately after operation. As a rule, no emergency surgery is needed in mandibular fracture except for closure of soft tissue wounds to prevent infection.

REFERENCES

1. Braunstein, P. W. Medical aspects of automobile crash injury research. *J.A.M.A.* 163:249, 1957.
2. Converse, J. M., and Smith, B. Blowout fracture of floor of orbit. *Trans. Amer. Acad. Ophthal. Otolaryng.* 64:676, 1960.
3. Gerrie, J. Face injury in sport. *Plast. Reconstr. Surg.* 14:225, 1954.
4. Kuloski, J. *Crash Injuries.* Springfield, Ill.: Thomas, 1960.
5. McCoy, F. J., Chandler, R. A., Magnan, C. G., Jr., More, J. R., and Siemson, G. An analysis of facial fractures and their complication. *Plast. Reconstr. Surg.* 29:381, 1962.
6. Rowe, W. L., and Killey, H. C. *Fracture of the Facial Skeleton.* Baltimore: Williams & Wilkins, 1955.
7. Wang, M. K. H., and Polayes, I. M. Management of facial fractures. *Med. Times* 92:957, Oct. 1964.

Burns 15

MARK K. WANG
W. BRANDON MACOMBER

The death rate for extensive burns remains high despite the greater understanding of burn physiology and improved measures to cope with burn shock. The improved measures are evidenced by an increase in average survival time during the past 20 years from 4.6 days to 15.7 days. Control of infection in burns by the topical application of mafenide (Sulfamylon) 0.5% [7], silver nitrate [8], or gentamicin (Garamycin) [6] gives promise of further decline in mortality risk, particularly in patients with 30 to 60 percent body-surface burns.

The care of seriously burned patients is primarily conducted after admission to the hospital. In this chapter we propose to discuss the care of patients with minor burns who do not require hospitalization, as well as the responsibilities of the emergency-room physician for the initial evaluation of the more seriously burned patient and for the institution of therapy.

Upon arrival in the emergency room the seriously burned patient should be examined for evidence of airway obstruction or pulmonary edema and for manifestations of shock, for if present they will require immediate action. In their absence the history and physical examination, including examination of the burned part, may proceed in a more leisurely fashion.

HISTORY

The history should be obtained while the patient is checked for evidence of respiratory obstruction and shock.

Nature of Injury

Both the nature of the injurious agent and the environment in which the accident occurred provide helpful clues to the expected seriousness of tissue damage. Burns following an automobile accident are often compounded by other injuries. The patient who has been burned by fire in an enclosed room will be more likely to evidence upper respiratory injury. Hot oil or metal produces a deeper injury than does hot water. Hot air or flames produce a dry burn while hot fluid often produces a moist one. The area of burn visible immediately after an electric burn is always smaller than the actual extent of tissue damage. The amount of tissue damage by a chemical agent, either acid or alkaline, can be mitigated by prompt irrigation with copious amounts of 0.85% sodium chloride solution.

Duration

The time interval between burning and the first examination often affects the general condition of the patient as well as the local appearance of the burn. The patient seen within half an hour after an accident may not yet show evidence of shock or of respiratory obstruction. Even blister formation of a second-degree burn may not yet be apparent, but it may develop subsequently.

Previous Treatment

In acute cases, there should be an inquiry into the nature of treatment previously received—whether any irrigation has been undertaken in the case of a chemical burn, or whether an analgesic has been administered. In late-arriving cases, transferred from another hospital, the nature and frequency of previously applied dressings, the quality and quantity of parenteral fluids, and the presence of concomitant injuries must be ascertained.

Tetanus Immunization

In all patients, a history should be obtained of previous active or passive immunization against tetanus, including the dates and reactions to antitoxin.

Significant Symptoms

Besides symptoms directly related to the burn injury, such as anxiety and pain, a careful review of systems and past history is important to rule out complications or other injuries. Vomiting, common in the early stages of extensive burns, should never be bloody or projectile. A history of hypertension or liver or kidney disease may modify vital signs or the validity of blood and urine studies.

PHYSICAL EXAMINATION

The examination room should be warm and free from drafts. There should be a good direct light, either natural or artificial. The patient should be completely undressed and laid on a sterile sheet if the burn is extensive, so that the entire burn can be exposed.

Local Examination

The examination of the burn wound must be done under aseptic conditions. A cap and gown and sterile gloves should be worn.

Location of Burn Area and Total Extent of Area Involved. The "rule of nines" is used to estimate the total percentage of body surface involved (Fig. 15-1). While this is not entirely accurate and can be difficult to apply, it is easy to remember and is the most common method [1].

Depth of Burn. A simple erythema with redness, swelling, and tenderness but with no death of epithelium represents a *first-degree burn*. The presence of blisters in the area of erythema indicates a *superficial second-degree burn*. Unfortunately, *deep second-degree burns* and *third-degree burns* present a similar clinical appearance and are not easily differentiated. The involved skin appears to be dry; it is brown or white; and it is anesthetic to pinprick. When charring and evident thrombosis of small vessels is present, the burn is almost always full-thickness. To make differential diagnosis even more difficult, the majority of deep burns are mixed. The deeper burn areas are usually surrounded by concentric zones of more superficial involvement, and the demarcation between them is

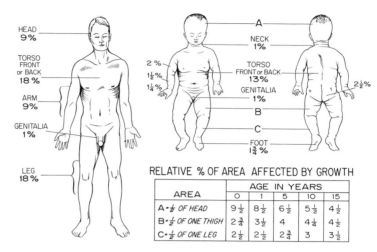

HEAD
9%

TORSO
FRONT
or BACK
18%

ARM
9%

GENITALIA
1%

LEG
18%

A

NECK
1%

2%

1½%

1¼%

TORSO
FRONT or BACK
13%

GENITALIA
1%

B

C

FOOT
1¾%

2½%

RELATIVE % OF AREA AFFECTED BY GROWTH

AREA	AGE IN YEARS				
	0	1	5	10	15
A = ½ OF HEAD	9½	8½	6½	5½	4½
B = ½ OF ONE THIGH	2¾	3½	4	4¼	4½
C = ½ OF ONE LEG	2½	2½	2¾	3	3½

Fig. 15-1. The "rule of nines," including conversion chart for adaptation for infants and children.

not always clear. It may take weeks before an accurate assessment of the depth of burns can be made.

DEGREE OF CONTAMINATION. Contamination includes dirt, clothing, and any local medications that have been applied under unsterile conditions.

CIRCULATORY EMBARRASSMENT. A deep circumferential burn of the extremity can produce a constricting effect that impairs circulation distal to the burn site. Nonelastic burned skin, acting as a tight envelope, combines with increasing edema and tension of the underlying soft tissue to produce progressive constriction, all the more dangerous since it may not be immediately evident.

It is advisable in extensive burns to diagram the areas involved, indicating the various depths of injury, estimated by clinical examination, as an adjunct to calculating the total percentage of burned body surface.

General Examination

MENTAL STATE. In the early stages, even in extensive burns, the patient is usually conscious and oriented, though occasionally restless and sluggish in response. This, however, may not be his condition if there has been excessive alcohol intake, inhalation of toxic gas during the accident, or concomitant brain damage. The examiner should always smell the breath of a disoriented patient.

PRESENCE OF SHOCK. The blood pressure and pulse rate are taken routinely as soon as the patient is brought to the emergency room, providing an unburned extremity is available for application of the cuff. Burn shock is manifested by diminished sensorium; a rapid, thready pulse; hypotension; and pallor, sweating, and coldness of the skin in unburned areas. Even if the manifestations of shock are absent at the time of examination, persistent vomiting, involvement of more than 30 percent of total body surface, or the concomitant presence of other major injuries such as a fracture of a long bone points to impending shock.

RESPIRATORY TRACT INVOLVEMENT. In all burns, but particularly those involving the head and neck, the patency of the respiratory tract should be carefully determined. The respiratory rate should be taken repeatedly. The lungs should be examined for evidence of congestion or consolidation. The respiratory sounds should be noted. Examination of the oral and pharyngeal mucosa may show direct evidence of injury. Hoarseness of voice and stridor are indicative of obstruction. It must be emphasized that one single examination with normal findings in the early stage of the burn injury does not rule out respiratory tract involvement. Edema, congestion, and exudation in the respiratory tract take time to develop. Therefore, repeated periodic examinations in suspicious cases are of utmost importance.

URINARY OUTPUT. Urinary output is indicative of the kidney function and the state of hydration of the patient. In extensive burns, when there is a massive fluid shift into injured tissue and marked reduction of the circulating blood volume, the exact recording of hourly urinary output is essential. For this purpose an indwelling catheter is necessary.

EMERGENCY TREATMENT

The following are general guide lines to determine whether a patient should be hospitalized:

Ambulatory Patient

Superficial burns not involving the lower extremity and constituting less than 5 percent of total body surface can be treated in the emergency room. The patient can be permitted to return to his home.

Hospitalization

Hospitalization is definitely indicated when any of the following is present:

1. Extensive burns involving more than 15 percent of body surface.
2. Burns of head and neck with a history suggestive of heat damage or smoke inhalation with possible respiratory tract involvement.
3. Deep burns involving the lower extremity.
4. Late infected burns.

Borderline Cases

The age and mentality of the patient must be weighed carefully, as well as whether he can be adequately cared for at home. When in doubt, it is wise to admit the patient for observation for at least several days.

PROGNOSIS

Discussion of the burned patient's prognosis with his family in the emergency room can be much more realistic if the following determining factors are kept in mind:

Extent of Burns

Burns involving less than 15 percent of total body surface are considered minor burns and carry minimal mortality. Burns involving more than 20 percent of total body surface are considered extensive. Burns involving 50 percent of the total body surface have a mortality of 50 percent, burns involving 75 percent of the total body surface have a mortality of 90 percent, and burns involving 90 percent of the body surface have a mortality of 100 percent. To estimate the percentage of body surface involved, the "rule of nines," as illustrated in Figure 15-1, is used.

Following burn injury there is rapid passage of extracellular fluid containing protein into the wound. When extensive, the great loss of extracellular fluid leads to depletion of the plasma volume and is the main cause of burn shock.

Depth of Burns

The deeper the destruction of skin due to burns, the slower the healing and consequently the greater the chance of bacterial invasion. Phillips and Cope [9] found wound infection responsible for 20 percent of burn deaths. Wartman [12] reported that in the first week after burn injury the most common cause of death is respiratory obstruction and shock; in the second week, shock and sepsis play equal parts; and in the third week, sepsis becomes the most important factor. The significance of the depth factor, directly affecting the incidence of sepsis, cannot be overemphasized.

Location of Burns

Phillips and Cope [9, 10] reported that respiratory tract damage with or without superimposed sepsis is responsible for 42 percent of burn deaths. Burns of the face and neck, especially those inflicted by fire in an enclosed room, are often accompanied by upper respiratory tract damage, as previously noted.

Age

The very young and the very old do not fare well with burn injuries. Children under 5 and adults over 60 years of age carry a significantly higher mortality. In a series of 283 burn cases in the Albany Medical Center Hospital, the average death rate is below 10 percent for adults under 60, as contrasted with 60 percent for those above that age. Pruitt [11], in a review of 1100 burn cases, found that the overall mortality for those under 4 years of age was 18.07 percent; for young adults, 15 to 49 years, 15.38 percent; and for those 50 years and over, 39.29 percent.

LOCAL TREATMENT

1. All burns involving more than 15 percent of total body surface should be treated in the operating room. Only minor burns involving less than 15 percent of body surface should be treated in the emergency room.

2. Strict asepsis is to be observed. Cap, mask, and sterile gloves are to be used by all personnel in contact with the patient.

3. The burned area should be thoroughly and gently cleansed with soap and water and irrigated with sterile saline solution. All gross contamination should be meticulously removed. Grease or ointment on the burn surface can be cleansed with ether. Intact blisters should be left alone; those which are broken should be thoroughly debrided of all loose tissue. The surface is first covered by a single layer of fine-mesh gauze impregnated with Xeroform ointment. Then comes flat, absorbing gauze, 10 to 15 layers thick on the trunk or buttock and fixed in place with adhesive tape strips. On the extremity, 5-yard gauze rolls are placed over the gauze flats and fixed with an elastic bandage. In burns of the hand, all fingers are separately dressed and maintained in a semiflexed position. The thumb is kept in a position of opposition.

GENERAL TREATMENT

Obstruction of the Airway

Burns involving the head and neck may also involve the upper respiratory tract with resultant signs of obstruction. When signs of obstruction are present such as stridor, air hunger, retraction of the intercostal spaces, or cyanosis, immediate treatment is indicated. Relief of obstruction is best accomplished by passing an endotracheal tube under local anesthesia, which permits the subsequent tracheostomy to be carried out at leisure in the operating room [3].

The inhalation of smoke or toxic gases can damage both upper and lower respiratory tract with resulting pulmonary edema, atelectasis, or pneumonia. If pulmonary edema is present which is not on a cardiogenic basis, we believe it is best treated by means of continuous positive-pressure breathing through a cuffed endotracheal tube (or tracheostomy tube) and a volume-cycled respirator.

Tetanus Prophylaxis

All burn injuries are considered open wounds, irrespective of site, depth, or total area involved. Prophylaxis against tetanus is therefore mandatory and should be given to all patients while in the emergency room. An accurate record of treatment given should be kept. (See Chapter 11 for tetanus prophylaxis.)

Antibiotics

Antibiotics are not recommended for routine use in patients with burns treated on an ambulatory basis. The decision for or against the use of antibiotics in patients with extensive burns should be left to the surgeon who will be responsible for definitive care.

Pain Therapy

Most minor burns do not require significant medication for relief of pain during or after the initial treatment. Extensive burns occasionally require analgesic drugs, although deep burns are usually not painful because of the local destruction of the nerve endings in the burned skin. When medication is indicated in extensive burns, it should always be given in small doses by the intravenous route, since shock-impaired circulation can delay absorption of a drug given by subcutaneous or intramuscular injection.

Fluid Therapy

Extensive burn injuries will require fluid therapy to correct the quantitative and qualitative alterations of the extracellular fluid volume. Treatment should be started immediately, in the emergency room, before local treatment of the burn wound. In extensive burns involving more than one extremity, extreme care is needed to avoid unnecessary trauma to the undamaged superficial veins. The most distal vein should be used, by surgical cutdown if necessary. A plastic catheter No. 16 or No. 18 French, is inserted. A sample of blood is obtained for typing and cross matching and for base line levels of hematocrit, sodium, potassium, chloride, urea nitrogen, and carbon dioxide content. An infusion of Ringer's lactate or normal saline solution is then started [4, 5].

Kidney Function

In extensive burns, some impairment of renal function should be anticipated. An incidence of acute renal failure in patients suffering burn shock of 5.1% was reported by Casen [2]. A fixed specific gravity of the urine around 1.010 or low urine osmolarity with oliguria in the early postburn period (48 to 72 hours) is an ominous sign. Since the hourly urine output is a reliable guide for fluid therapy, a retention catheter should be passed in all patients with extensive burns while they are in the emergency room. The urine initially removed after passage of the catheter is saved for analysis, and the hourly output is thereafter recorded.

REFERENCES

1. Berkow, S. A.   A method of estimating the extensiveness of lesions (burns and scalds) based on surface area proportion. *Arch. Surg.* (Chicago) 8:138, 1924.
2. Casen, J. S.   Treatment of Renal Failure. In Wallace, A. B., and Wilkinson, A. W. (Eds.), Second International Congress on *Research in Burns.* Edinburgh and London: Livingston, 1966. P. 12.
3. Connell, J. F., Jr.   Successful Therapy of Patients with Pulmonary Burns, In Artz, C. P. (Ed.), First International Congress on *Research in Burns.* Philadelphia: Davis, 1962. P. 19.
4. Cope, O., and Moore, F. D.   The redistribution of body water and the fluid therapy in the burn patient. *Ann. Surg.* 126:1010, 1947.
5. Evans, E. I., and Bigger, I. A.   The rationale of whole blood therapy in severe burns: A clinical study. *Ann. Surg.* 112:693, 1945.
6. MacMillan, B. G., Hill, E. O., and Altmeier, W. A.   Use of topical silver nitrate mafenide and gentamycin in the burn patient. *Arch. Surg.* (Chicago) 95:472, 1967.
7. Moncrief, J. A., Lindberg, R. B., Switzer, W. E., and Pruitt, B. A.   Use of topical antibacterial therapy in the treatment of burn wounds. *Arch. Surg.* (Chicago) 92:558, 1966.
8. Moyer, C. A., Brentano, L., Gravens, D. L., Margraf, H. W., and Monafo, W. W.   Treatment of large human burns with 0.5% silver nitrate solution. *Arch. Surg.* (Chicago) 90:812, 1965.
9. Phillips, A. W., and Cope, O.   An Analysis of the Effect of Burn Therapy on Burn Mortality. In Wallace, A. B., and Wilkinson, A. W. (Eds.), Second International Congress on *Research in Burns.* Edinburgh and London: Livingston, 1962, P. 1.
10. Phillips, A. W., and Cope, O.   Burn therapy: II. The revelation of respiratory damage as a principal killer in the burn patient. *Ann. Surg.* 155:1, 1962.

11. Pruitt, B. A., Turnbusch, W. T., Mason, A. D., and Pearson, E. Mortality in 1100 consecutive burns treated at a burn unit. *Ann. Surg.* 159: 396, 1964.

12. Wartman, W. B. Mechanism of Death in Severe Burn Injury: The Need for Planned Autopsy. In Wallace, A. B., and Wilkinson, A. W. (Eds.), Second International Congress on *Research in Burns*. Edinburgh and London: Livingston, 1962. P. 6.

Ocular Emergencies

16

ROBERT D. REINECKE

Patients appearing at general emergency rooms with eye complaints comprise 15 to 30 percent of all patients. The closer the emergency room is to an industrial center, the closer the percentage will be to 30 percent. Since the patient's chief complaint will determine the urgency of treatment, the items for consideration will be organized in that fashion, with exceptions noted. The carefully documented medical history is as important here as in any other medical problem. Paralleling the history's importance is documentation of every finding of the examination with exact notation of the hour. Careful notation of all medications given is mandatory. The visual acuity of each eye should be taken as soon as feasible during the examination.

OCULAR TRAUMA

Chemical Trauma

Typically, there is a report by phone that a chemical has been splashed into an eye. The nurse answering such calls *must* be aware that treatment on the spot is necessary. The nurse should instruct the patient to hold his open eye under a steady stream of water from any available source. The *open* eye should be emphasized. The medical and nursing staff should be fully aware that water is the irrigat-

277

ing fluid of choice, and promptness of such irrigation can save an eye. When the patient arrives in the emergency room with a history of a chemical in his eye, prompt irrigation is essential—prior to taking the patient's history, address, or any other steps. A flexible hose attached to a low-pressure faucet is ideal. The patient should lie down with his head over a sink. The eyelids should be held open and, if the patient is in severe discomfort, a drop of proparacaine should be instilled. pH paper should be used to test the patient's cul-de-sac from time to time. If the chemical was acid, as soon as the pH returns to normal the irrigation may be stopped. If alkali, the pH must remain normal for at least 7 minutes after stopping the irrigation. Hours of irrigation may be necessary for alkali injuries (Fig. 16-1).

After the irrigation procedure has been initiated and the general condition of the patient stabilized, the ophthalmic resident or ophthalmologist should be called. The eye may look surprisingly good shortly after the injury, but subsequently may reveal severe damage.

Tear gas and Mace injuries are chemical injuries and should be so treated. The pocket tear gas guns are dangerous and can cause

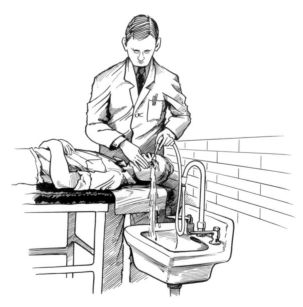

Fig. 16-1. Emergency irrigation of eye after a chemical injury. A steady stream of water flushes the eye as the lids are held open. If the chemical is alkali, this procedure may necessarily be continued for several hours.

permanent visual loss if fired at close range because the high velocity helps the material penetrate the eye.

If large numbers of patients appear after a riot where tear gas was used, a triage unit should be assembled with an ophthalmologist as part of the team to determine who should have ocular irrigations.

Blunt Ocular Trauma

Snowballs, baseballs, hockey pucks, squash balls, handballs, tennis balls, champagne corks, and almost every other conceivable missile seem to strike the orbit with regularity. Irrespective of the missile, the general type of injury is the same and the complications identical.

The blow may drive varying contents of the orbit into the maxillary sinus, producing the blow-out fracture. Limitation of eye movement, diplopia, and anesthesia of the cheek in the area supplied by the infraorbital branch of the first division of the 5th cranial nerve are clues to this complication. X-rays are necessary to confirm the diagnosis.

The eye itself may be injured by blunt trauma. The eyeball may be ruptured with expulsion of the ocular contents either out of the eye or out of the sclera to lie beneath the conjunctiva. Less severe blows may produce bleeding into the anterior chamber. The blood settles out, producing a typical hyphema. If the bleeding is more severe, the entire anterior chamber may be filled with blood, producing an "eight-ball hyphema" (Fig. 16-2). Often a fine dust of blood

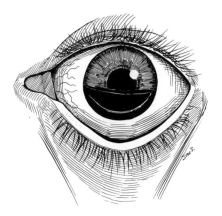

Fig. 16-2. Hyphema. If the bleeding continues, the entire anterior chamber may be filled with blood, producing the "eight-ball hyphema."

in the anterior chamber can be identified only with a slit-lamp examination by an ophthalmologist. Hospital admission is needed for any intraocular bleeding, because the bleeding may recur and cause extremely high ocular pressure. Surgical intervention is occasionally necessary.

Other late complications such as glaucoma or retinal detachment may follow blunt trauma. Hence, follow-up care by an ophthalmologist is mandatory.

Sharp Ocular Trauma

Small foreign bodies in the eye, an injury experienced by most persons, usually are washed from the eye by the increased tear flow. If the foreign body has a sharp jagged edge, or is sticky, it will adhere to the cornea or conjunctiva. The foreign body usually adheres to the conjunctival surface of the upper lid. Thus, it is important to evert the lid and remove foreign bodies with a moistened cotton-tipped applicator. To evert the lid, the lashes are grasped, the lid is pulled (down for the upper lid and up for the lower lid) so that it can be folded over a small rounded rod or stick. Since the foreign body may be tiny, some magnification is helpful.

If no foreign body is found on the conjunctiva, the cornea should be examined next. If a foreign body is seen on the cornea, place a drop of proparacaine in the conjunctival cul-de-sac, wait 15 seconds, and try to remove the foreign body with a moistened cotton-tipped applicator. If the foreign body refuses to budge, the patient should be referred to an ophthalmologist.

Although tears may wash the foreign body from the eye, the symptoms may persist due to a corneal abrasion. To ascertain this, the conjunctiva should be touched with a moistened fluorescein strip. A corneal abrasion will stain bright green (Fig. 16-3). Corneal abrasions may also result from anything striking the eye, such as a fingernail or paper edge.

A corneal abrasion should be treated with a drop of antibiotic to prevent bacterial invasion and a drop of scopolamine, 2%, to avoid severe pain of ciliary spasm. The eye should be securely patched.

When patching an eye, a folded single eye pad is placed on the closed upper lid, this followed by a full eye pad and secured in place with Scotch tape, or M&M plastic tape. Avoid adhesive tape, if possible.

Sharp missiles may penetrate the eye causing serious damage.

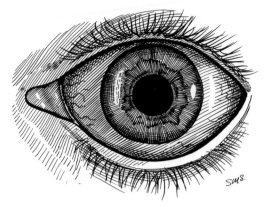

Fig. 16-3. The light vertical area represents the green-staining area of a corneal abrasion after fluorescein has been applied. Local antibiotics and mydriatics usually constitute adequate treatment.

Little need be said about such injuries except to caution the emergency room personnel to avoid manipulation of such patients and to prepare such patients for hospital admission. Other penetrating eye injuries, although serious, may cause few eye signs or symptoms immediately after the injury. Since a sharp knife or a fine projectile can penetrate an eye with few immediate eye signs, it is imperative that patients be examined carefully who give a history of possible ocular penetration. Note irregularities of the pupil, opacities of the media, or signs of ocular bleeding. If the history suggests that a flying projectile entered the eye, x-rays for ocular foreign bodies should be obtained. When the clinical examination and x-rays fail to reveal any sign of foreign body or ocular penetration, it is well to refer the patient to an ophthalmologist for a follow-up examination within a few days.

A special form of corneal abrasion is caused by wearing a contact lens too long. If the patient has worn his contact lenses twice his usual wearing time, approximately 4 hours after removing his lenses a severe pain will develop in both eyes. A drop of local anesthesia is necessary before he can open his eyes. Fluorescein reveals diffuse staining over the lower half of both corneas. Patches should be applied to both eyes after a drop of antibiotic has been placed in each eye; systemic narcotics should be given, and the patient assured that he will be better in 24 hours, at which time he should see his ophthalmologist before using his contact lenses again.

Ultraviolet radiation produces the same signs and symptoms as wearing contact lenses too long. Typically, the patient is exposed to ultraviolet irradiation from a welder's arc or a sunlamp. Approximately 8 hours later he experiences severe eye pain and cannot open his eyes until some local anesthetic solution is instilled. The topical anesthesia relieves all discomfort and fluorescein reveals the damaged corneal epithelium. Severe demands are usually made upon the physician to give the patient a topical anesthetic for home use, but local anesthetics should *never* be given to patients, since they prevent corneal healing and can lead to intractable pain and resistant corneal ulcers.

LOSS OF VISION

The complaint "loss of vision" is an emergency until proved otherwise. This holds true even if the complaint is transient, for the amblyopia fugax may be the precursor to an occlusion of a central retinal artery.

Occlusion of the central retinal artery causes the patient to lose vision, the completeness of which depends on the amount of collateral circulation to the retina via the cilioretinal artery. Occasionally, a patent cilioretinal artery will preserve central vision, and conversely, occasionally an isolated occlusion of a cilioretinal artery will destroy central vision, leaving the remainder of the visual field intact. The retinal picture caused by an occluded central retinal artery is striking. The retina becomes edematous a few minutes after the occlusion. The edema makes the retina relatively opaque and, hence, gray-white everywhere except in the foveal area, where the retina is normally thin. There, a cherry-red spot is seen. The arteries show clumping of the blood giving the slowly moving "box car" effect—often in the wrong direction. If flow can be re-started, the changed picture is obvious. Promptly upon making the diagnosis the eye should be massaged intermittently to produce a pumping effect and to lower the intraocular pressure. Lowering the intraocular pressure gives a favorable arterial pressure differential on the two sides of the occlusion which may dislodge the embolus. A 90% oxygen: 10% carbon dioxide inhalation is started promptly in an effort to dilate the blood vessels. Acetazolamide (Diamox) is given intravenously to lower the ocular pressure further and, if the ophthalmologist deems it necessary, a bit of aqueous may be drained to lower the pressure further. The latter is a dangerous procedure in inexperienced hands and should not be attempted by anyone other than the ophthalmologist. A blood sample should be drawn as soon as possible for an erythrocytic sedimentation test to rule out temporal arteritis as a cause of the occlusion. Steroids should be started promptly, if temporal arteritis is the diagnosis, thereby possibly avoiding a similar retinal artery occlusion in the second eye.

Sudden loss of vision accompanied by a cloud floating up and over the field of vision often indicates a hemorrhage within the eye. The ophthalmoscope will confirm the diagnosis. An ophthalmologist should see such a patient to determine if a break in the retina caused the hemorrhage. Such breaks must be treated surgically to prevent a retinal detachment.

Failing vision following experiencing a flash of light within the eye usually means a detached retina. While the diagnosis can often be confirmed with a direct ophthalmoscope, it often cannot; and more detailed examination with other instruments is necessary. If the patient experiences a flash of light repeatedly with each sudden movement of the eye, the condition is probably benign, but should be followed closely. The latter symptoms are that of a detached vitreous—a condition which requires no treatment and is compatible with good vision.

Intermittent loss of vision may be the aura of a migraine headache. The aura of a hemianopia may disturb the patient more than the headache itself. A detailed history will establish the diagnosis. Uniocular intermittent loss of vision should be regarded as a symptom of an impending carotid occlusion until proved otherwise. Ophthalmodynamometry will aid in establishing this diagnosis.

Chronic loss of vision may be a complaint related to an increasing neurological field deficit—hence, visual fields will aid in establishing the diagnosis, but are seldom indicated as part of the emergency room work-up unless other symptoms make the diagnosis an acute problem. Most frequently the chronic loss of vision (aside from the need for different glasses) is related to macular disease, a disturbance easily seen with the ophthalmoscope. A patient suddenly may note poor vision in one eye although the poor vision actually has been present for years. A uniocular cataract causing the poor vision suddenly noted by the patient exemplifies such a case. Most people seldom compare the vision of one eye with the other and do not note failing vision in one eye unless one eye has a chance occlusion.

PAINFUL EYE(S)

Severe eye pain associated with decreased vision typifies acute narrow-angle glaucoma. The prompt and accurate diagnosis of this condition mandates the presence and use of a tonometer in all emergency rooms. The Schiøtz tonometer is used easily and should be mastered by anyone doing emergency-room care. A drop of proparacaine in both eyes allows the tonometer to be held by the sleeve and lowered to the corneal surface. The patient should lie down, hold his hand at arm's length directly over his other eye, and look at his thumb. The lids are separated by the thumb and forefinger of the examiner and the tonometer held between thumb and forefinger of the examiner's other hand (Fig. 16-4). (Relaxation of the patient will prevent spurious high-pressure readings.) The tonometer's needle indicates the scale reading. A conversion table in the tonometer case indicates the pressure in the eye. The lower the tonometer scale reading, the higher the intraocular pressure.

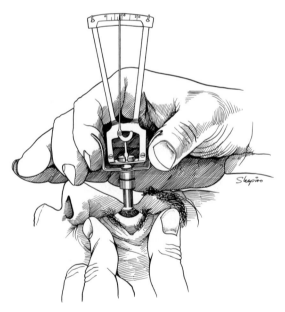

Fig. 16-4. Proper application of a Schiøtz tonometer to the eye. The lids are pulled away from the eye so that the intraocular tension will not be artifactually elevated. As the tonometer is lowered onto the eye, the sliding collar will be at the middle of the shaft and the entire weight of the tonometer will rest on the eye. Local anesthetic has been applied.

A pressure greater than 20 is considered abnormal, but no emergency exists unless the pressure is above 35. If the pressure is greater than 35, then the patient should be seen by an ophthalmologist without delay. Elevated intraocular pressure can cause such severe nausea and vomiting that the patient may be treated for those symptoms rather than the true problem.

If the patient has a red, painful eye with decreased vision and a small pupil, he probably has iritis rather than glaucoma. In either instance, the intraocular pressure should be measured and the patient referred to an ophthalmologist for treatment and follow-up.

The red, painful eye with a purulent discharge usually has bacterial conjunctivitis. Appropriate bacterial identification is as important here as elsewhere—smears, culture, and sensitivity studies should be initiated. A local ophthalmic antibiotic can be started while the bacterial identification is underway. Local antibiotics should be continued for at least 5 days. The condition of the cornea should be carefully noted and fluorescein staining done. Bacterial corneal ulcers can progress rapidly; perforation may occur; and the eye may be lost. This disastrous series of events is particularly prone to happen in the severely debilitated patient.

The red, painful eye which exhibits no discharge other than clear tears probably has a viral infection. Some of the viruses produce a preauricular adenopathy as well as a pebblelike pattern of the tarsal conjunctiva. These infections are self-limiting and disappear in about 14 days. Herpes simplex virus, on the other hand, causes more ocular damage than any single infection in the United States and should constantly be kept in mind. The two diagnostic signs are (1) hypesthesia of the cornea and (2) a dendritic pattern. The dendritic pattern (treelike) is recognized easily with fluorescein staining (Fig. 16-5).

Cortisone-like drugs usually are contraindicated in herpes simplex, for they accelerate the virus growth. Iododesoxyuridine (IDU), an antiviral drug, is the drug of choice and, in the ointment form, can be given every 4 hours. Ocular complications of herpes simplex are sufficiently common that ophthalmological consultation should be obtained the same or following day. If the dendritic figure has progressed to a corneal ulcer, the patient (as with all corneal ulcer patients) constitutes an emergency which should be handled by ophthalmological consultation and usually with hospital admission.

Shingles (herpes zoster) of the first division of the 5th cranial nerve is a simple diagnosis. Particularly important is the presence or

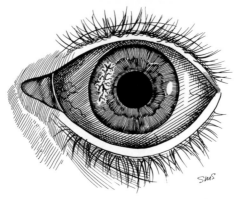

Fig. 16-5. The typical dendritic ulcer stains with fluorescein, corneal sensitivity is reduced, and often the eye is not severely inflamed. Cortisone treatment may be disastrous.

absence of ocular involvement. The ocular complications may cause ultimate blindness on the affected side. Accordingly, whenever the diagnosis of shingles of the first division of the 5th cranial nerve is made, an ophthalmological consultation and follow-up is in order.

PROPTOSIS

The infant with a bulging eye is an emergency. If the patient shows signs of sepsis, the most likely diagnosis is ethmoiditis with a cellulitis of the orbit. If signs of sepsis are absent, a malignant tumor (rhabdomyosarcoma) should be suspected.

Proptosis in an adult comes on more slowly in most cases and seldom constitutes an emergency. The exceptions to the previous statement are two: First, relatively sudden proptosis, with engorged conjunctival vessels, and a bruit heard about the head indicates an arteriovenous aneurysm and an admission to neurosurgery. Second, proptosis with engorged conjunctival vessels accompanied by signs of sepsis indicates a septic thrombosis of the cavernous sinus, another serious emergency admission, this time to the ophthalmological service.

Proptosis of sudden onset and associated with recent trauma, evidencing tight lids without dilated conjunctival vessels, signifies a retrobulbar hemorrhage. Such a patient, although having a frightening appearance, usually recovers completely without treatment. Reports, however, have indicated that such patients at times have permanent damage and thus need careful evaluation. If the intra-orbital pressure is too great, the retrobulbar blood can be drained. The drainage must be done by an experienced physician who is cognizant of the orbital structures and will not damage them while aspirating the blood.

BRIGHT RED EYE

The common complaint of "blood in my eye" typically means that the patient has had a subconjunctival hemorrhage. Unless the bleeding recurs several times, no hematologic work-up is indicated. Reassurance should be given the patient that the blood will be absorbed in about 2 weeks and that his vision is not threatened.

TEARING AND PAIN

Tears flowing down the cheek of the patient are annoying but do not constitute an emergency unless pain is present. If the eye is involved with any disease, excess tears are the problem. If no eye disease is present, tearing, and severe pain just lateral to the bridge of the nose, mean acute dacryocystitis. Although antibiotics and hot compresses may slowly alleviate the problem, an ophthalmologist can often introduce a fine probe through the lacrimal canaliculus, relieve the pressure, and allow the patient to go home in comfort.

Otorhinolaryngological Emergencies

17

FLOYD B. GOFFIN

EAR

Acute Otitis Externa

After swimming in fresh water or after self-inflicted trauma from such objects as bobby pins or toothpicks, inflammatory edema may occur in the external auditory canal. This may be sufficient to produce local tenderness, otalgia, trismus, and at times regional lymphadenitis.

A sterile wick of cotton or gauze* impregnated with an astringent ointment (Ergophene), allowed to remain in place in the canal for 24 to 36 hours, is a satisfactory way of reducing cellulitis to the point that the canal is "open" enough for local meticulous cleansing with such agents as 70% alcohol saturated with boric acid or 5% Burow's solution. The canal is then ready for instillation of topical medication at home (e.g., 2% acetic acid or Burow's solution). Dry heat, analgesics, and at times antibiotics are necessary adjuncts.

The possibility of a coexisting otitis media must always be kept in mind. In some cases visualization of the drum may be very difficult, but every attempt at inspection must be made.

---

* The wick may be prepared from a narrow strip of gauze folded on itself to provide a moderately firm segment about 3 mm in width and about 2 to 3 cm in length, depending upon the degree of occlusion of the canal. A wick is readily inserted with delicate Hartman or Noyes ear forceps.

Acute Otitis Media

Acute infection of the middle ear space is usually an extension of or associated with an acute upper respiratory infection. Exudate collects from occlusion of the eustachian tube and accumulates behind the tympanic membrane.

With distortion or loss of the landmarks on the tympanic membrane, or bulging, the cardinal surgical principle of incision and drainage of a closed space abscess is in order. The operation may be carried out on cooperative adults without anesthesia but will usually require general anesthesia or sedation with narcosis in children. It is the writer's habit to "bundle" infants rather than resort to general anesthesia.

After the canal has been meticulously cleaned and swabbed with alcohol, an incision with a myringotomy knife is made in the posterior-inferior quadrant of the tympanic membrane, just medial to the margin (annulus) of the drum (see Fig. 17-1). A simple stab incision is not sufficient to produce adequate drainage.

To promote drainage, negative pressure may be applied through a pneumatic otoscope or by direct suction from a sterile No. 5 French Baron suction tip. A culture and bacterial sensitivities should be obtained, and antimicrobial therapy instituted. Penicillin is used initially, but this may require modification when the bacterial sensitivity to various agents has been determined.

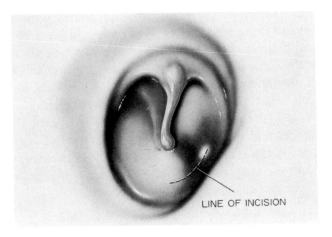

LINE OF INCISION

Fig. 17-1. Proper location of myringotomy incision on the eardrum.

A dry sterile cotton plug is then inserted into the orifice of the canal and is changed as necessary.

Nasal decongestants systemically and by drops are prescribed in all instances to reduce edema and congestion of the eustachian tube.

Acute Mastoiditis

Acute mastoiditis is not a condition to be treated in the emergency room, but its recognition is mandatory. This complication may occur in the second or third week of the course of acute otitis media. Persisting discharge, pain, fever, mastoid tenderness, prolapse of the posterior canal wall, or "nipple-like" protrusions of middle ear mucosa through a perforation should alert the examining physician. Mastoid x-rays including Law's, Towne's, and Owen's projections should be ordered. The reader is referred to standard texts on otology for a complete discussion of this complication.

Foreign Bodies

Wood particles, cotton, or insects in the external auditory canal usually produce considerable tissue reaction. Hearing loss, pain, or both will be the presenting complaint. The possibility of underlying preexistent otitis externa or otitis media as the cause of insertion of a foreign object (e.g., cotton applicator with loss of cotton by impaction) must be kept in mind and searched for.

Loose objects may be removed by irrigation. Flat objects may be removed by Hartman or Blake forceps (see Fig. 17-2).

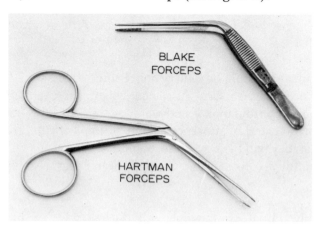

BLAKE
FORCEPS

HARTMAN
FORCEPS

Fig. 17-2. Types of forceps for removing foreign bodies from the ear.

A small cerumen hook or loop inserted just beyond the object may be positioned to deliver it in a forward motion. In some instances it will be necessary to admit the patient for extraction through endaural or postaural incision.

In all cases attempted removal should be made only by a physician intimately familiar with the anatomy and techniques, as canal wall skin or even drum with ossicles may be delivered by the unwary and inexperienced. Impacted or ossicular dislocation is a hazard without proper instruments.

External Trauma

The compression of air in the external canal due to a slap from the open hand or a blast of air, as well as the insertion of a sharp object in the canal, may produce rupture of the tympanic membrane. No attempt at repair should be made immediately. Most simple lacerations heal spontaneously. A culture of the external canal should be obtained and antibiotics instituted if signs of suppuration supervene.

NOSE

Epistaxis

The sine qua non of the management of the patient with epistaxis is intimate knowledge of nasal anatomy as well as a good light source assuring binocular vision of the field.

Since any epistaxis may be difficult to control, the ingenuity of the rhinologist will be strained, but several general principles are applicable to all cases:

1. Stop the bleeding by cautery or pressure.
2. If necessary, replace the blood which has been lost. Do a hemoglobin determination if in doubt.
3. Sedation and reassurance are in order. Patients are usually afraid that they will bleed to death. Some do!
4. Carefully consider the etiology. Search for clotting abnormalities.

Usually the initial examination will disclose whether bleeding is coming anteriorly in the nasal fossa or more posteriorly, as evidenced by blood dripping down the posterior oropharyngeal pillars. In severe epistaxis, the gushing of blood anteriorly and posteriorly may make it impossible to determine the site.

It is necessary to use suction to evacuate the nose and nasopharynx of blood and mucus. A flattened piece of long-fiber cotton, moistened with cocaine and epinephrine,* is inserted in the bleeding nasal fossa (see Fig. 17-3). Continued bleeding posteriorly with this cotton in place is usually indicative of a source in the nasopharynx or adjacent choana and posterior nasal fossa.

While the cotton pledgets remain in place, attention is paid to the preparation of the cautery. A wire loop is heated "red hot" in open flame and plunged into chromic acid crystals to form a "bead" about 2 × 2 mm in size (see Fig. 17-4). After a full 5 minutes the pledgets are removed. It is usually possible to determine the site of an anterior ooze, to which the chromic acid "bead" is gently applied. No attempt should be made to "smear" the area with the acid nor should the cautery be held for more than a few moments. Overcauterization may result in excessive tissue necrosis and even nasal septal perforation. Alternate methods include use of electrocautery. In the author's experience, silver nitrate is useful only for extremely minor capillary bleeding.

An additional expedient to "seal" the cauterized area is the plac-

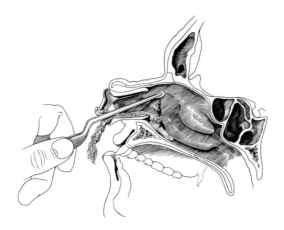

Fig. 17-3. Initial step in localization of bleeding point in the nose. A cotton pledget moistened with cocaine and epinephrine has been inserted.

* The author employs epinephrine 1:1000 mixed with 4% cocaine HCl solution in ratio of 1:5. No more than 100 mg of cocaine should be used at any one time. Possible sensitivity should be ascertained by careful questioning before use.

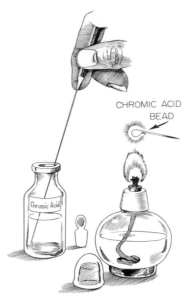

CHROMIC ACID
BEAD

Chromic Acid

Fig. 17-4.   Preparation of a chromic acid bead on a wire loop.

ing of a small piece of oxidized cellulose gauze over the treated area.

When cauterization fails, it becomes necessary to "pack" the nose, using bayonet forceps and half-inch strips of gauze impregnated with petroleum jelly. First along the floor of the nasal fossa, thence superiorly, the chamber is packed so that the gauze sits in an accordion fashion (see Fig. 17-5).

When there is posterior bleeding it is necessary to draw a pack* up into the nasopharynx. A urethral catheter (No. 10 or No. 12 French) is passed into each nasal fossa so as to present in the oropharynx. The ends are grasped with a Kelly clamp, and the strings on the ends of the pack are affixed, one to each catheter, and then drawn out through the nose. When pulled through, the two strings are tied over gauze placed in front of the columella; this prevents cutting of the skin by the string. The pack may be placed on only one side posteriorly when it is certain that bleeding is coming from one choana or one side of the nasopharynx. The oral strings are held loosely in place beyond the mouth by adhesive on the cheek.

When epistaxis is known to be secondary to hematological defects, it is preferable not to cauterize the nasal mucosa. Local tissue

---

* A convenient posterior pack may be prepared by folding a 4 × 4 gauze on itself and tying it in the center so that a long double string hangs from both sides.

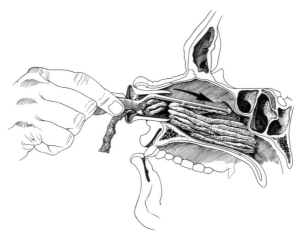

Fig. 17-5. Packing the nose to control bleeding. It is essential that the pack be in firm contact with the actual bleeding point; otherwise it will be ineffectual.

necrosis from cauterization in such cases readily leads to wider areas of oozing. Absorbable gelatin sponge or oxidized cellulose gauze moistened with epinephrine may be placed over the bleeding point and left undisturbed. At other times it is, of course, necessary to resort to packing.

Acute Infections of the Nose and Sinuses

Generally speaking, acute rhinitis or sinusitis is not treated in the emergency room. In some instances, however, it may be deemed advisable to initiate treatment of acute sinusitis by packing the appropriate meatus with a cotton pledget moistened with 4% cocaine to initiate drainage and acquire secretions for cultures.

Foreign Bodies

Persistent unilateral nasal discharge in the young should be considered the classic manifestation of either a foreign body or a tumor. The odor is usually foul. At times the object, if it has been present for a long time, is encased in crustings.

Paper, cloth, small toys, parts of jewelry, and so forth, may be inserted in one or both nostrils. There may be two or more objects in the same nasal fossa. Roentgenograms will reveal radiopaque

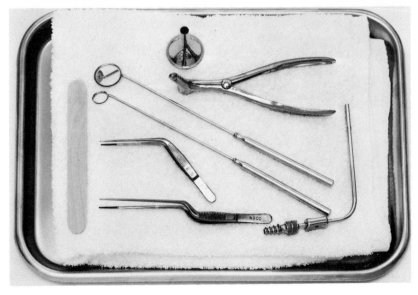

Fig. 17-6. Instruments commonly used for otolaryngological examination.

foreign bodies but radiolucent objects may be present and will not be visualized.

A cerumen curet or cupped forceps are useful for removal. Care should be exercised not to lacerate the mucosa, lest epistaxis compound the problem. Caution must be taken not to dislodge the foreign body posteriorly. It would be embarrassing to wind up doing a bronchoscopy for a nasal foreign body!

PHARYNX AND LARYNX

Trauma

The emergency treatment of pharyngeal or laryngeal trauma is usually not in the province of emergency-room care. In all cases, however, with history suggestive of this trauma, careful inspection of the pharynx and larynx is necessary to ascertain the presence and degree of damage, particularly to the airway. Any ecchymosis of jaw or neck should alert the examiner to possible coexisting laryngeal damage. Indirect mirror examination may disclose hematoma, edema, fracture, or dislocation. Arrangements for emergency admission and operation may be indicated.

Foreign Bodies

A common Friday night occurrence is the search for fish bones in the pharynx or larynx.

Foreign bodies in the pharynx or larynx are more common in edentulous patients and may lodge in the base of the tongue, vallecula, pyriform sinus, or acutely obstruct the glottis. The term *restaurant coronary* has been used to describe the acute strangulation seen in individuals wearing dental plates who have imbibed a number of alcoholic drinks and are talking while eating. Incompletely masticated food, usually meat, is aspirated, with resulting obstruction of the airway. If life is to be saved, immediate tracheostomy is necessary.

In less urgent situations removal of foreign material by indirect or direct laryngoscopy can be done by physicians skilled in these techniques. Local anesthesia is induced by spraying the hypopharynx and larynx with cocaine or tetracaine. With an assistant or the patient holding the tongue forward, an attempt can be made to remove the foreign object, using the laryngeal mirror and appropriate forceps. One should always be alert to the presence of more than one foreign body. Translucent bones may be very difficult to find and require diligent search. If the search is unsuccessful, direct laryngoscopy is then carried out. Frequently bronchoscopy is also indicated, in which case admission to the hospital is usually necessary when complete removal of foreign objects is not accomplished by indirect laryngoscopy.

Acute Infection

Acute pharyngitis or laryngitis is not treated in the emergency room. However, in severe tracheobronchitis it may be advisable to give rapidly acting steroids, which may obviate the need for tracheotomy. Careful observation of the patient should be maintained after hospitalization in such cases. In children it is important not to carry out repeated local examinations. They should be placed in a high-humidity room and closely observed for increasing respiratory obstruction.

Acute tonsillar and peritonsillar abscess may be seen at times in the emergency room. Cultures should be obtained and generally the antibiotic of choice is penicillin. When toxic manifestations and an impending airway obstruction are present with peritonsillar abscess, or if there is fluctuation of the anterior pillar or soft palate, the patient should be admitted for observation and definitive therapy; the latter usually includes incision and drainage.

Poisoning 18

PAUL R. PATTERSON

Accidental acute poisoning as well as the purposeful ingestion of poisons with suicidal intent is increasing yearly. With the establishment of poison-control centers in almost every major city in the United States, over 800,000 poisonings a year have been reported. While mortality has been reduced in young children to approximately 2400 cases per year, adolescents and adults have succumbed to accidental poisoning and suicide by poisoning in numbers many times greater. In addition to a rising mortality, the permanent ill effects of poisons on brain, liver, kidney, and other organ systems are also increasing. Physicians and hospitals can help to reduce the harmful effects of poisoning by alerting the public to the toxicity of common household products; and by establishing poison-control centers staffed by experienced personnel who have ready access to cross references on the more than 350,000 poisonous substances to which the public may be exposed in their houses, garages, stores, and factories.

This chapter will describe the staff organization, necessary supplies and equipment, general plan of operation, and management of cases requisite for an efficient poison-treatment service in a general hospital. We will not attempt to review the details of signs, symptoms, and extended management of individual poisons, but from the information contained herein it should be possible to provide intelligent care in the emergency room for the victims of exposure to the more common poisons.

It is recommended that a physician on the staff of the hospital who is interested in toxicology be appointed poison-control director. In this position he should have direct responsibility for all aspects of emergency-room care of the victims of poisoning. If management is not available in the emergency room, he should make certain that a well-equipped, properly indexed poison-treatment cabinet is provided. This should contain appropriate detoxifying agents, antidotes, and all other equipment necessary for management of the more common emergencies. Once organized, the poison-treatment cabinet must be maintained properly by the replacement of drugs and equipment as used. This is the responsibility of the nursing service under direction of the poison-control director.

A library containing reference texts and an index card reference file should be provided in the poison-control area of the emergency room. Suitable texts are listed at the end of this chapter. For the development of the index-card file, the hospital should be registered with the National Clearinghouse for Poison Control Centers of the United States Department of Health, Education, and Welfare, which will provide the initial reference file and, as new toxic materials are found, will add cards to the file. The name, address, and telephone number of the nearest poison-control center should be placed in several strategic areas in order to afford ready access to consultation as needed.

The following list of equipment and medications which should be available in the poison-treatment cabinet is from our own facility. It will provide for management of 95 percent of patients seen in the emergency room with actual or possible poisoning. The poison-control director should also determine common toxic products used by major industry in his area in order to supplement the list as found necessary from the information thereby obtained.

Equipment for Emergency-Room Treatment

Airways (sizes 1, 3, 5) and endotracheal tubes (cuffed)
Blunt scissors
Can opener and ampule knife
Cardiac resuscitation equipment
Catheters, No. 10, No. 12, and No. 20 French
Chemically clean and sealed specimen bottles for toxicological analysis of
    vomitus, urine, blood, and stools

Ewald aspirating bulb
Gastric lavage: Gastric tubes, sizes 20 and 30, and Asepto syringes to fit. Levin tubes, sizes 12 and 14, with adapting 20- and 50-ml hypodermic syringes. Moss tubes for lavage, small, medium, and large
Ice packs
Laryngoscope
Lumbar puncture trays
Restraints and restraining boards
Resuscitation equipment including oxygen and respirator
Suction pump and equipment
Tourniquets
Tracheostomy set
Venous cutdown trays

MEDICATIONS NECESSARY TO TREAT POISONING

Drug	Purpose
Activated charcoal, 500 gm	Adsorption inactivation
Aluminum hydroxide gel, 500 ml	Antacid
Ammonium carbonate, 1-lb can	Formaldehyde
Amyl nitrite ampules, 1 doz	Cyanide
Antisnakebite (polyvalent 15-ml ampules) serum	North American snakes
Atropine sulfate ampules	Phosphate ester, insecticides
Caffeine sodium benzoate, 2-ml ampules	Stimulant
Calcium gluconate, 10-ml ampules	Fluoride, black widow spider bite
Calcium lactate, 400 gm (1-lb can)	Phenol
Castor oil, 1 pint	Fluoride, tetany
Chloral hydrate, 0.6 gm, 5-ml ampules	Anticonvulsant, sedative
Dextrose 50%, 10- and 50-ml ampules	Cerebral edema
Dimercaprol (BAL), 5-ml ampules, 10% in oil	Arsenic and mercury
Diphenhydramine hydrochloride (Benadryl), 10-ml ampules	Bee stings and other anaphylactic episodes
Ephedrine sulfate, 25-mg ampules	Hypotension
Epinephrine, 1 mg, 1-ml ampules	Allergic reactions
Ether, ¼-lb can	Anticonvulsant
Glycerine, 1 pint	Fluorine
Lemon juice concentrate in cans	Lye
Lorfan tartrate, 1 mg, 1-ml ampules	Morphine, opium derivates
Menadiol sodium diphosphate, 75 mg, 2-ml ampules	Bishydroxycoumarin, warfarin
Methylene blue, 0.5 gm, 50-ml ampules	Methemoglobin
Milk, evaporated, can	Acids
Milk of magnesia, 1 quart	Acids

Drug	Purpose
Mineral oil, 500 ml	Demulcent
Morphine sulfate, 10-mg ampules	Shock, pain
Nalorphine hydrochloride (Nalline), 10 mg, 2-ml ampules	Morphine, opium derivates
Olive oil in pint cans	Demulcent activity
Paraldehyde, 2- and 5-ml ampules, 1-gm capsules	Ethyl alcohol
Pentobarbital sodium, 0.5-gm ampules	Seizure
Pentothal, 500-mg ampules	Seizure
Phenobarbital sodium, 0.3 gm, 2-ml ampules	Seizure
Potassium permanganate 1%, 500 ml for dilution—1 tsp to 1 pint water	Alkaloids and selected compounds
Pralidoxine chloride (Protopam), 3 gm	Phosphate ester, insecticides
Sodium bicarbonate, 1-lb boxes	Bleaches
Sodium chloride, 1-lb boxes	Emetic
Sodium nitrite 3%, 10-ml ampules	Cyanide
Sodium thiosulfate 25%, 50-ml ampules	Cyanide
Solutions for intravenous use, all available hospital preparations; renew yearly	Acidosis, alkalosis, flushing
Starch, corn, 1-lb boxes	Iodine
Syrup of ipecac, 120 ml	Emetic
Urea solution	Cerebral edema
Vitamin K, 50 mg, 1-ml ampules	Warfarin, bishydroxycoumarin

GENERAL CONSIDERATIONS

A telephone call from a frantic parent of a poison victim, or from a relative or friend of the victim, for advice from the emergency-room physician necessitates quick, positive, and decisive thinking on his part. He should have readily available, preferably at the telephone, a general chart of emergency measures to which he can refer. If a given compound is not included in his chart, it is better to take the time to consult the index file than to guess at the compostion or properties of the compound. Giving the correct advice, even at the expense of several minutes' delay, may be life-saving in directing the best course of management.

When corrosives such as strong alkalies or acids have been ingested, vomiting should be avoided because it may cause esophageal rupture. The best initial treatment is directed toward neutralization, dilution, or inactivation. For strong acids, milk of magnesia, milk, egg albumin, or flour in water can be used. Alkaline carbonates which release carbon dioxide when in contact with acids are contraindicated. For strong alkalies, a mixture of equal parts of vinegar and water or diluted citrus fruit juice is a satisfactory neutralizer.

Irritant hydrocarbons such as kerosene, turpentine, and gasoline frequently induce vomiting. These substances are very irritating to to the lungs, and the danger of aspiration during vomiting is great. Therefore, induced vomiting in this instance is also contraindicated.

For practically all other ingested poisons, prompt emptying of the stomach is of great importance. Studies indicate that vomiting is probably the most efficient means of accomplishing this. The American Academy of Pediatrics, accordingly, has recommended that in every home with small children a supply of syrup of ipecac and activated charcoal be kept on hand for use in case of accidental ingestion of poisons. A pharmaceutical company has now marketed a "Poison Control Kit" containing 30 ml of syrup of ipecac and 30 ml of an aqueous suspension of activated charcoal. The accompanying literature contains instructions to use the material only upon the direction of a physician or a poison-control center. With this advice we agree.

Syrup of ipecac is an emetic; the dose is one tablespoon followed by several glasses of water or milk. If vomiting fails to occur within 20 minutes, the dose should be repeated. If this fails, gastric lavage in the emergency room is indicated and the patient should be promptly transported to the hospital.

Activated charcoal is an antidote which has the capacity to adsorb many harmful compounds, thereby inactivating them. (If given with the syrup of ipecac it will inactivate it.) Subsequent to vomiting, however, it will be useful in binding the residual poison.

If an emetic is not available in the home, emesis can usually be induced by inserting a finger in the back of the throat. When vomiting cannot be induced, a demulcent such as flour in water, evaporated milk, or whole milk should be given. In any case, following completion of the above, the patient should be promptly seen in the emergency room for examination and further treatment as indicated.

For patients seen in the emergency room who have not been previously treated the basic management is as follows:

1. Except where corrosives or irritant hydrocarbons are involved, the stomach is emptied by induced emesis or gastric lavage. Acids

or alkalies are neutralized. Lavage is permissible for irritant hydrocarbons, but if emesis occurs as the tube is passed, precautions are necessary to avoid aspiration.

2. An antidote is given to neutralize residual toxic material. The antidote may be specific or nonspecific, depending upon the nature of the poison.

3. Laxatives may be given to accelerate elimination from the intestinal tract. In heavy metal poisoning, nausea, vomiting, and extreme diarrhea occur; obviously in such cases laxatives are not indicated.

4. Further treatment is symptomatic, based upon the systemic manifestations of the specific poison.

5. Application of hemodialysis to the patient manifesting extreme toxicity can save his life if the physician knows which substances can be dialyzed from blood when absorbed in high concentrations. Included in this group are barbiturates, chlorates, salicylates, diphenylhydantoin (Dilantin), thiocyanates, bromides, and ammonia.

TREATMENT OF POISONING FROM UNKNOWN SUBSTANCES

It is always difficult to treat poisoning from an unknown substance, but it should be remembered that the symptoms resulting from poisoning are often sufficiently characteristic to permit a reasonably accurate estimate of the nature of the offending agent.

1. Caustic compounds, such as lye and sink-drain clearing products, produce lesions of the mucous membranes of the mouth, burns of the skin, and excessive drooling if ingested.

2. Central nervous system depressants—barbiturates, chloral hydrate, and so forth—after causing an initial brief stage of hyperactivity, result in sleep, coma, and respiratory depression.

3. Stimulants such as nicotine or strychnine cause hyperactivity, frequently followed by convulsions. Unfortunately convulsions occur with many other substances as well.

4. Pinpoint pupils may result from codeine in cough syrup, nicotine, some insecticides, or simply smoking Daddy's pipe.

5. Dilated pupils accompany belladonna intoxication, and ephedrine and cocaine ingestion, and are a late response to nicotine.

6. A characteristic odor to the breath is imparted by cyanide, turpentine, and oil of eucalyptus (used in some mosquito repel-

lents). Perfume is of course also recognizable and is usually harmless.

7. The cherry-red mucous membranes of carbon monoxide poisoning may be recognizable.

8. Heavy metals characteristically produce nausea, vomiting, severe abdominal cramps, and diarrhea. Later their nephrotoxicity is evidenced by oliguria.

IDENTIFICATION OF POISONS

In some cases the poison can be identified only by analysis of gastric contents, feces, blood, or urine. This is a laborious and time-consuming process in which the information may well not be forthcoming in time to assist in therapy. When available, the poison container with residual contents should be brought to the emergency room with the patient; otherwise, the assistance of the police should be enlisted so it may be obtained. The prescribing druggist, regional poison-control center, or manufacturer can identify the contents, or the ingredients may be listed on the label. At times more than one toxic substance is contained in commercial products, particularly in insecticides.

Knowledge of the relative incidence of the different types of poisonings is of some assistance in symptomatic therapy. For example, in children about 50 percent of ingested poisons are from the medicine cabinet and consist of aspirin, laxatives, cough medicine, sedatives, and tranquilizers. Another 25 percent are from bleaches, lyes, furniture polish, silver polish, and cleaning agents found beneath the kitchen sink in most homes. Kerosene and gasoline account for from 10 to 30 percent of the remaining, depending upon geographical and socioeconomic factors. Kerosene ingestion and accidental carbon monoxide inhalation frequently relate to the use of kerosene stoves for heating and are most prevalent in slum or rural areas. The burning of battery casings as fuel by slum dwellers may produce lead poisoning.

The National Clearinghouse for Poison Control Centers has provided from the 105,178 reports of poisoning sent to them the following list of the thirty most frequently named trade items, which appear below in decreasing order of total reports received in 1968. In parentheses after the product name is the order in which that product would be placed if the list were in numerical order for the under-5 age group. To complete the list of the top thirty products ingested by children under 5 years of age, add "D-Con Rat Poison"

(4); "Lomotil" (19); "Ajax Cleanser" (20); "Contac" (21); "Head and Shoulders Shampoo" (22); "Mellaril" (27); Holly berries (30).

This list can be shown to the family members to assist in the recalling of products within the home to which the child might have had access.

30 Most Frequently Named Items

Name	Under 5 Years	Name	Under 5 Years
1. "Clorox"	(1)	16. Yew plant	(8)
2. "Librium"	(12)	17. "Pine Sol"	(11)
3. "Valium"	(7)	18. "Tuinal"	
4. Phenobarbital	(10)	19. "Placidyl"	
5. "Ex Lax"	(2)	20. "Darvon"	
6. "Excedrin"	(16)	21. "Noludar"	
7. "Drano"	(5)	22. "No Doz"	(17)
8. "Congespirin"	(3)	23. "Comet"	(13)
9. "Sominex"		24. "Equanil"	
10. "Anacin"	(28)	25. "Ben Gay"	(14)
11. "Doriden"		26. "Purex"	(15)
12. "Nembutal"		27. "Dilantin"	(37)
13. "Lysol"	(9)	28. "Butisol"	
14. "Testor's Cement"	(6)	29. "Harris Famous Roach Tablet"	(15)
15. "Thorazine"	(29)	30. "Stelazine"	

The following list of the toxic constituents of commonly ingested substances will assist in both symptomatic and specific therapy.

Toxic Constituents of Commonly Ingested Household Substances

Medicine Cabinet

Antiseptics: phenol (carbolic acid), boric acid, mercuric chloride, iodine
Aspirin and headache pills: salicylate, acetanilid, or acetophenetidin
Belladonna (atropine)
Cold tablets, seasick pills, over-the-counter "tranquilizers," antihistamines
Cough mixtures: codeine, ethylmorphine, methadone
Hair and dandruff lotions: salicylic acid, kerosene, alcohols, pilocarpine, cantharidin, acetic acid
Heart medicine: digitalis, Diamox, veratrum preparations
Laxatives: phenolphthalein, magnesium sulfate
Nose drops: ephedrine, Neo-Synephrine, steroids
Reducing pills: amphetamines, thyroid hormone
Shampoos: denatured alcohol, sodium hexametaphosphate
Sleeping pills: barbiturates, antihistamines, chloral hydrate
Tonics: iron, strychnine, amphetamine
Tranquilizers: phenothiazines

Kitchen

Bleach: sodium hypochlorite, oxalic acid
Boric acid
Deodorizing tablets: formaldehyde
Detergents: sodium hydroxide, sodium hypochlorite, tetrasodium phosphate, ethylene glycol
Drain flusher: lye, sodium acid sulfate
Dry cleaning fluids: hydrocarbons, acetone, methyl alcohol, trichloroethylene
Inhalation of cooking gas
Lighter fluid: hydrocarbons
Liquor: alcohol
Polish (silver): cyanide, sulfuric acid
Polish (stove): kerosene
Polish (wood): kerosene
Rat, mouse, and ant poisons: strychnine, sodium fluoroacetate, cyanides, phosphorus, nicotine
Rug cleaner: hydrocarbons, usually chlorinated
Shoe paste: kerosene
Soaps: generally nontoxic; a few have sodium hydroxide, tetrasodium phosphate
Window cleaner: ammonia

Garage

Antifreeze: ethylene glycol, alcohols
Antirust compounds: oxalic acid, hydrofluoric acid, hydrocarbons
Car polish: hydrocarbons, kerosene, oxalates
Charcoal lighting fluids: hydrocarbons, methyl alcohol, denatured alcohol
Flower sprays: nicotine sulfate, chlordane and lindane, arsenic, benzene, DDT, tetraethyl pyrophospate, parathion and malathion
Gasoline in soft-drink bottles
Paint: lead, arsenic, hydrocarbons, zinc, chromium, titanium
Paint cleaners and thinners: turpentine, phenols, methyl alcohol, alkalies

Yard

DDT and toxaphene
Fertilizers: phosphates of metal and ammonium
Plants: mushrooms (atropine), thorn apple (atropine), cherry (cyanide), foxglove (digitalis), castor bean (ricin)
Rodenticides: phosphorus, strychnine, cyanides, thallium, sodium fluoroacetate, methyl bromide, arsenic, bishydroxycoumarin
Suntan lotions: methyl salicylate, alcohol

Basements

Black widow spider bite
Bleach soaps, aniline dyes (laundry ink)
Fire extinguishers: carbon tetrachloride, methyl bromide
Fire-starting fluids: petroleum hydrocarbons
Fuel gas, sewer gas

Gasoline: hydrocarbon
Insecticides: benzene hexachloride (see also Garage)
Lacquer: methyl alcohol, ethyl, and amyl acetate
Paint and solvents: lead, arsenic, chromium, zinc, titanium, hydrocarbons
Plastic glues: formaldehyde, ethylene, dichloride
Rat, mouse, and ant poisons: strychnine, sodium fluoroacetate, cyanide
Rug cleaner: chlorinated hydrocarbon
Shellac: methyl alchohol
Wallpaper cleaner: hydrocarbons, kerosene

Attic

Bat and squirrel feces: salmonella, unknown emetic substances
Christmas bulb fluid: methylene chloride
Cleaning agents: carbon tetrachloride
Moth balls or flakes: naphthalene
Smoke inhalation: oil fumes, carbon monoxide, formaldehyde

Bedroom

Allergy pills: antihistamines
Aspirin: salicylates
Birth control pills: female sex hormones
Cold wave: potassium bromate
Contraceptive jellies and foam: phenylmercuric salts
Cuticle remover: caustic alkalies
Deodorants: aluminum chloride
Depilatories: calcium thioglycolate, soluble sulfides
Hair dye: silver salts, anilines, ammonia, metallic dyes, sodium hypochlorite
Moth balls and flakes: naphthalene
Nail preparations: esters, ketones, alcohols
Neutralizers: acetic acid, potassium bromate
Sleeping pills: chloral hydrate, barbiturates

SUMMARY OF EMERGENCY MANAGEMENT

I. Upon receipt of telephone call:
   1. Be calm and reassuring to avert panic.
   2. Obtain name and telephone number.
   3. Ask age and sex.
   4. What was the type of poisoning—for example, oral, eye, skin, and so forth?
   5. Ask name of the product and the amount ingested or missing.
   6. Ask caller to bring container to phone and read label.
      a. Presence of *Poison* label
      b. Inflammable warning (hydrocarbons)
      c. Use and contents if given
      d. Physical state of product and odor

e. Manufacturer or druggist's name and telephone number on label

7. If product or container is not found, inquire what is suspected and ask for clues as to the area of the home, factory, or yard where the poisoning occurred. Any drugs missing? What medicines have been lying around?

II. Decide need for treatment.

1. If substance is innocuous, praise the party calling for his alertness and reassure him that treatment is unnecessary.
2. If the call suggests potential poisoning, advise him to bring the patient to the emergency room quickly.
3. Tell him to bring can or container with the patient.
4. Tell him the lay emergency measures to be given in transit or if some distance from hospital.

III. Emergency measures to be carried out by *layman:*

1. Ingested poison
   a. Hydrocarbons (kerosene, lighter fluid, rug cleaner, turpentine, gasoline): Give milk or quickly prepared flour suspension, 1 to 3 cups.
   b. Corrosives
      (1) Acid: Give milk of magnesia or aluminum hydroxide, 60 ml in 3 cups water. If not available, give milk or flour suspension.
      (2) Alkali: Give dilute vinegar half and half with water or dilute citrus fruit juice. If not available, give diluent demulcent as above.
   c. Other substances: Stimulate vomiting with finger or syrup of ipecac. If unsuccessful or after vomiting, give milk or flour suspension. Bundle patient warmly and transport to hospital.
2. Inhaled toxic substances
   a. Supply fresh air and loosen undergarments and collars.
   b. Give artificial respiration by mouth-to-mouth method if needed.
   c. Bundle the patient warmly and transport to hospital.
3. Eye contamination
   a. Use *no chemical antidotes.*
   b. Wash eye out for at least 5 minutes with running water.
4. Body or skin contamination
   a. Remove clothes immediately while rinsing with running water.

b. Immerse in tub or shower.

c. Use *no chemical antidotes.*

5. Scorpion or snakebites

  a. Keep patient calm and insist upon no bodily movements.

  b. Tourniquet above the site. This should not create a throbbing sensation or complete abolition of pulse. Loosen every 20 minutes.

  c. Pack with ice cubes.

  d. Give antiserum, preferably brought to patient.

  e. If patient is moved, carry him on stretcher and insist on cooperation.

6. Injected allergens, poisons, or overdose of toxic drug

  a. Prone position must be maintained.

  b. Tourniquet above the site of injection. This should not create a throbbing sensation or complete abolition of pulse. Loosen every 20 minutes.

  c. Pack with ice cubes.

GENERAL EMERGENCY MEASURES IN THE HOSPITAL

When the patient is brought to the hospital following poisoning, either internal, inhaled, or the contact type, delays in decision should be avoided. A 20-minute delay may prove fatal. General measures to remove the poisons should be instituted while the specific treatment or antidote is obtained from the card file, texts, and reference material on hand. A call may be required to the area poison-control center or the manufacturer. The product name, constituents, use, physical state, and antidote, if given on the label, should be noted.

Specific treatment must be given. This may consist of physiological agents to counteract the pharmacological effects of poison after assimilation, or agents which render the toxic substance innocuous or unabsorbable. In the majority of cases, if the patient is seen within one hour, the general measures for removing poisons will be sufficient.

The technique of treatment is as follows.

Skin Contamination

Body surfaces and orifices should be washed copiously with water if the poison is of the contact type. All clothing should be removed, with irrigation, and the patient should be immersed in tub or shower if contamination is widespread over the body. Chemical antidotes are not advised because of the heat liberated. Toxic oils can be removed with organic solvents.

Snakebites

Use of a tourniquet above the site of the bite should be continued and ice packs applied locally. Polyvalent antisnakebite serum is given. Study of snake reference books may well identify the snake by description and occasionally by fang marks. *The patient must not be allowed to move for several hours!* Crisscross incision and suction do not remove significant serum and are not advisable.

Eye Contamination

See Chapter 16.

Ingested Poisons

Stomach lavage is definitely indicated within 3 hours after ingestion of poison. If milk or flour mixture has been used at home, the time can be extended. This will apply to enteric coated tablets as well.

Stomach lavage is *contraindicated* if there has been ingestion of strong alkali or acid, kerosene, and oils. Convulsions may result if the patient has taken strychnine. Aspiration pneumonia may result if the patient has lost the cough reflex, as in coma.

In all instances of significant poisoning, after initial emergency measures have been completed the patient should be admitted to the hospital or observation unit for continued care or observation.

TECHNIQUE OF GASTRIC LAVAGE

The ideal tube to use for gastric lavage is the Moss* double-lumen tube, which permits constant infusion and suction. Other gastric tubes can be used, the larger the better. Occasionally light anesthesia is necessary when the patient is uncooperative and cannot be restrained. Most children can be "mummified" in a sheet and

* U.S. Catheter and Instrument Co., Glens Falls, N.Y.

placed on their left side with the head hanging over the edge of the table and with the face down. The foot of the table should be raised. This minimizes aspiration. The tube is passed by mouth, gently and without force, and the patient is encouraged to swallow to avoid gagging and choking. One must be certain that the tube is not in the trachea by listening or noting bubbling when, after passage, the end is immersed in water. Isotonic saline solution should be used for lavage. With a single-lumen tube only small amounts of fluid (150 to 200 ml) should be injected at a time to avoid forcing the poison into the duodenum. Repeat lavaging 15 to 20 times or until returns are clean. With the Moss double-lumen tube only about 10 minutes is required to empty the stomach satisfactorily.

Specific antidotes may be added to the saline solution. For example, potassium permanganate (1:5000) can be used as an oxidizing agent to neutralize strychnine or nicotine. Ordinary evaporated milk serves as a good demulcent. Sodium bicarbonate (5% solution) is recommended for iron poisoning. Calcium salts are helpful in fluoride and oxalate poisonings. Starch is used specifically for iodine. A weak iodine solution, 15 to 20 drops of the tincture of iodine in a cup of water, will precipitate mercury, lead, and strychnine.

GENERAL REFERENCES

Boys, F., and Smith, H. M. *Poisonous Amphibians and Reptiles, Recognition and Bite Treatment.* Springfield, Ill.: Thomas, 1959.

* Dreisbach, R. H. *Handbook of Poisoning.* Los Altos, Calif.: Lange Medical Publications, 1963.

* Gleason, M. R., Gosselin, R. E., and Hodge, H. C. *Clinical Toxicology of Commercial Products* (3d ed.). Baltimore: Williams & Wilkins, 1969.

Halstead, Bruce W. *Poisonous and Venomous Marine Animals of the World.* Washington, D.C.: U.S. Government Printing Office, 1965.

* Hayes, W. J. *Clinical Handbook on Economic Poisons.* U.S. Department of Health, Education, and Welfare, Public Health Service, Communicable Disease Center, Atlanta, Georgia, 1963.

Hughes, W. T., Jr. *Pediatric Procedures.* Philadelphia: Saunders, 1964.

Kingsbury, J. M. *Poisonous Plants of the United States and Canada.* Englewood Cliffs, N. J.: Prentice-Hall, 1964.

Moeschlin, S. *Poisoning, Diagnosis and Treatment.* New York: Grune & Stratton, 1965.

* National Clearinghouse for Poison Control Centers, Card Index Files. Periodic additions and information bulletins. U.S. Department of Health, Education, and Welfare, Public Health Service, Washington, D.C.

* References for poison treatment cabinet.

New and Nonofficial Drugs. Philadelphia: Lippincott. Annual publication.
* *Physicians' Desk Reference.* Oradell, N.J.: Medical Economics, Inc. Free of charge to physicians. Annual publication.
Segar, W. E. The Critically Ill Child: Salicylate Intoxication. *Pediatrics* 44:440, Sept. 1969.

* References for poison treatment cabinet.

Gastrointestinal Emergencies

JOHN A. BALINT

GASTROINTESTINAL BLEEDING

Overt Hemorrhage

DIAGNOSIS. In emergency-room practice the patient is most likely to present with overt bleeding. The problem basically then is to determine its severity.

1. A history of the amount of blood lost as related by the patient or other witness will help establish the severity of the bleeding. Thirst is a common symptom of dehydration and continuing hemorrhage.

2. The circulatory state of the patient (see Chapter 7) is another clue. Signs of reduced circulating volume include: rapid pulse, sweating or peripheral cyanosis with dry extremities, and low blood pressure, which falls when the patient sits or stands up. Anxiety often accompanies these signs.

3. Blood count and hematocrit reading are of little value in the acute stages because of delay in hemodilution after acute blood loss. Since hemodilution may take 24 to 36 hours to be complete, these determinations are helpful only as a base line, or if bleeding has occurred some 24 or more hours earlier.

SITE. If the patient has vomited blood or has passed melena, bleeding is likely to have occurred in the upper gastrointestinal tract or small intestine (melena only). In the case of bleeding from the large bowel, bright-red blood passed per rectum is the rule. Two notable exceptions must be borne in mind. Massive bleeding from peptic ulcer may lead to passage of red blood per rectum, whereas slower bleeding from the cecum may produce melena.

If bleeding is from the upper gastrointestinal tract, the diagnoses in Table 19-1 must be considered. It is beyond the scope of this work

Table 19-1. Causes of Upper Gastrointestinal Bleeding

Peptic Ulcer Group	Percent of Total
Chronic gastric ulcer	15 to 20
Chronic duodenal ulcer	30 to 40
Acute ulcers	25 to 30
Hiatus hernia	2 to 3
Marginal ulcers	5 to 8
Causes Other Than Peptic Ulcer	
Carcinoma of stomach	2 to 3
Portal hypertension (esophageal varices)	5 to 10
Other causes	5 to 10

After F. A. Jones, and J. W. P. Gummer, *Clinical Gastroenterology.* Oxford: Blackwell, 1960.

to review the differential diagnosis. For this, the reader is referred to the standard texts listed at the end of the chapter. The following pointers are worth bearing in mind: (1) Bleeding peptic ulcer accounts for 75 to 80 percent of the cases. If the patient has epigastric pain relieved with the onset of bleeding, an ulcer is the probable source. (2) A history of alcoholism, together with an enlarged liver, and perhaps splenomegaly and the extrahepatic stigmata of liver disease, especially in a patient who is confused or comatose, suggests bleeding from esophageal varices. It is important to remember, however, that 20 percent of cirrhotic patients may bleed from peptic ulcer or gastritis.

If hemorrhage is from the lower gastrointestinal tract, benign or malignant tumors of the colon, ulcerative colitis, diverticulitis, hemorrhoids, and fissures must be considered. In such patients a rectal examination and sigmoidoscopy are mandatory. It is also important to remember that the majority of these lesions are within reach with a sigmoidoscope.

MANAGEMENT. Patients who present with overt upper gastrointestinal hemorrhage in general will require admission to hospital. They are a joint responsibility of the medical and surgical services, and both should be notified immediately. While awaiting the patient's transfer to the ward, the following should be done:

1. Blood is drawn for typing and cross matching as well as prothrombin time, base line blood count, and platelet count.

2. If the patient shows signs of circulatory embarrassment, intravenous infusion of saline solution is started.

3. For anxiety, and if there is no suspicion of cirrhosis, morphine is given, 8 to 15 mg intramuscularly, depending on the patient's size and pulmonary status.

4. Vasopressor agents, such as norepinephrine, are generally contraindicated in this situation. However, the patient should be kept lying down and, if necessary, the foot of the bed elevated on blocks.

5. A Harris or Ewald tube should be passed into the stomach and the stomach washed out with cold saline solution until clear. Once clots are removed, a Levin tube should be passed, left in place, and attached to a suction pump. Even in patients who have not vomited blood, insertion of a nasogastric tube to ascertain the presence or absence of blood in the gastric content is helpful and indicated. In such patients, if no blood is found in the stomach and vomiting is not a symptom, the tube may be removed once its diagnostic function has been accomplished.

For patients presenting with overt lower gastrointestinal hemorrhage, the procedure outlined above should be followed except for step 5. Instead, as stated, a rectal, proctoscopic, and sigmoidoscopic examination should be performed. The lesions that are likely to be seen include polyps, carcinoma, ulcerative colitis (page 318), hemorrhoids, and fissures. In the last two instances, emergency admission will rarely be necessary; the patient may be referred to the appropriate clinic or service as an outpatient.

Occult Bleeding

All the conditions considered above may cause occult bleeding, in which case the patient will present with fatigue, weakness, even dyspnea or heart failure secondary to anemia. In addition he will usually have symptoms of the underlying disease, e.g., peptic ulcer, regional enteritis, hiatus hernia, and so forth. In such patients emergency-room studies should include the following:

1. A full history is taken and a physical examination is made. It is worth looking for the rarer causes of bleeding, such as hereditary telangiectasia shown by mucosal hemangiomas, tigroid streaking of the retina and Morocco leather skin in pseudoxanthoma elasticum, and purpura as a sign of hematological disorder. It is important also to inquire for a history of drug ingestion, e.g., salicylates, reserpine, or anticoagulants.

2. A rectal examination should be made.

3. The stool is examined for occult blood using stool obtained by the examining finger. Suitable tests include the benzidine or guaiac procedures or the hematest tablets.

4. A complete blood count is taken, including erythrocyte count, hematocrit reading, hemoglobin value, leukocyte count, and differential cell and platelet counts.

5. Sigmoidoscopy is done.

Management will depend on the severity of anemia and the secondary manifestations, as well as the patient's age and the presence of associated disease. In general, if anemia is severe (Hgb<8 gm) and the patient over 50, admission to a hospital will be indicated, especially if the patient is having cardiac or pulmonary difficulties. The less seriously ill may be evaluated on an outpatient basis with barium enema, upper gastrointestinal and small-bowel series, and liver studies if indicated.

ULCERATIVE COLITIS

Ulcerative colitis is a nonspecific chronic inflammatory disease affecting the large bowel only. Depending on the location, extent, and severity of the disease, it may present in various ways.

Acute or Fulminant Disease

Although most commonly seen in young adults, acute ulcerative colitis may effect patients at all ages. The symptoms are fever, abdominal cramps, severe diarrhea with blood, mucus, and pus in stools, and tenesmus. There may be associated anemia, dehydration, and more rarely extracolonic manifestations such as arthritis, uveitis, or erythema nodosum. Physical examination is otherwise unremarkable in most cases. The presence of abdominal distension, especially when accompanied by diminished or absent bowel sounds, should raise suspicion of actual or impending perforation, even in the absence of severe pain.

The differential diagnosis must be made from acute bacterial enteritis, e.g., *Salmonella* or *Shigella* infections, and regional enteritis (see Regional Enteritis, below). The diagnosis is made by proctoscopic or limited sigmoidoscopic examination, performed without preparation of the bowel and without air insufflation. Adequate suction is necessary. In patients with ulcerative colitis the rectal mucosa is edematous, reddened, freely bleeding, and friable. In some instances actual ulceration may be seen. The disease affects the entire mucosa, so that no normal mucous membrane is evident. Such an appearance is diagnostic of the disease. By contrast, in patients with amebic dysentery, discrete reddish ulcers are seen with normal intervening mucosa. In bacillary dysentery, the rectal mucosa may show some granularity or edema but is not friable.

If abdominal distension is present, roentgenograms should be taken to rule out toxic megacolon (massive colonic distension, either generalized or localized) or perforation with free air in the abdominal cavity.

The patient presenting with acute ulcerative colitis requires immediate admission to a hospital. While he awaits admission, both medical and surgical services should be notified. In addition blood should be drawn for (1) typing and cross matching; (2) base line complete blood count; (3) serum electrolyte determination including sodium, potassium, chlorides, carbon dioxide content, calcium, and phosphorus; and stool should be collected and sent for culture. If the patient shows signs of dehydration, an intravenous infusion of 0.85% saline solution or Ringer's lactate solution should be started while the results of the blood studies are awaited.

Chronic or Subacute Disease

Patients of any age may be affected. The presenting attack may be the first the patient has had or a relapse. The patient will complain of bloody diarrhea, and often cramps and tenesmus. There is usually some fever, often nausea, and even vomiting. The patient has usually lost weight. In this instance also the extracolonic manifestations of the disease may be present. Physical examination will usually reveal anemia, but otherwise nothing of note beyond the findings listed above. However, rectal and sigmoidoscopic examination will reveal findings similar to those seen in the acute state but usually with a lesser degree of active bleeding.

The differential diagnosis includes regional enteritis, rectal neoplasm, or dysentery. Again, the endoscopic appearance is diagnostic.

Management depends on the assessment of the patient's overall state. Unless his general condition is good and the disease clearly of long standing, admission to a hospital for complete evaluation and treatment is indicated. Milder cases, especially those without significant systemic symptoms—fever, weight loss, and so forth—may be evaluated on an outpatient basis. However, at least a hemoglobin level, hematocrit reading, and leukocyte count should be obtained before the patient is considered for outpatient care. If there is any doubt, the patient should be admitted.

Mild cases may be treated with a high-protein, low-roughage diet and psyllium hydrophilic mucilloid (Metamucil) to help add bulk to the stool. Morphine and its analogues are best avoided. Salicylazosulfapyridine (Azulfidine), 1 to 1.5 gm four times daily, may be helpful in more symptomatic cases. Barium enema should be delayed if possible until the disease is under control. In such patients with mild disease, whether treatment as outlined is instituted or not, arrangements must be made for careful follow-up by a physician at frequent and regular intervals.

REGIONAL ENTERITIS

Regional enteritis or Crohn's disease is a chronic granulomatous inflammatory disease usually involving the ileum, but it can also affect the colon, rectum, perianal region, jejunum, or stomach.

Modes of Presentation

1. There may be acute abdominal pain strongly suggesting acute appendicitis. The pain is often colicky; it is periumbilical or in the right lower quadrant, with tenderness and guarding and even rebound tenderness. Low-grade fever and leukocytosis are common. There may be constipation or diarrhea. In such instances differentiation from appendicitis is usually impossible except at abdominal exploration. There may be no previous history of abdominal complaints.

2. Regional enteritis may present as intestinal obstruction. The patient complains of cramping abdominal pain with or without vomiting, and constipation. Complete obstruction is unusual. In this instance there will usually be a preceding history of abdominal pain over a period of months or years associated with diarrhea and weight loss. The patient will often have fever and anemia.

3. About 16 percent of patients with this disease will present with overt gastrointestinal hemorrhage (see Gastrointestinal Bleeding, above), though this is rarely massive.

4. The patient may seek attention because of fever of several days' or weeks' duration. Associated symptoms usually include diarrhea and abdominal cramps as well as weight loss. Anemia is often present, and abdominal examination may reveal a mass usually in one or other lower quadrant or in the pelvis.

5. Regional enteritis may look like ulcerative colitis, accompanied by severe diarrhea with blood and mucus in the stools, fever, and cramps.

6. Chronic nonspecific diarrhea may be the presenting symptom associated with weight loss. Other symptoms cited above may be present but are not prominent in such patients.

7. The development of a fistula may bring the patient to the hospital. Fistulas may be mucocutaneous, e.g., fistula in ano or rectal fistula, or ileocutaneous; or they may occur from bowel to bladder leading to foul-smelling urine and pneumaturia and urinary tract infection, or from bowel to bowel causing severe diarrhea and weight loss.

8. More rarely the patient presents with steatorrhea, with foul, bulky, pale stools which often appear greasy. This is usually preceded by a long history of abdominal pain for which an appendectomy may have been performed in the past without benefit. This complication is likely to result either from very extensive disease involving the jejunum or from fistula formation.

9. Sometimes the patient presents with erythema nodosum or, less commonly, skin ulceration. If this is associated with abdominal cramps, diarrhea, and fever, the possibility of regional enteritis should be considered.

Diagnosis

Although diagnosis is often difficult, the following findings in patients presenting with any of the above-mentioned complaints should raise the suspicion of Crohn's disease.

1. Tender abdominal or pelvic mass.
2. Fever.
3. Perianal fistulas or other sinuses or perianal ulceration.
4. Erythema nodosum or pyoderma.
5. Clubbing of the fingers.

Sigmoidoscopy often reveals normal mucosa and thus helps to rule out ulcerative colitis. More rarely the rectal mucosa is thickened and has a somewhat cobblestone appearance. This finding is very suggestive of regional enteritis.

Laboratory data of value are a low serum albumin, iron-deficiency anemia with leukocytosis, and positive stool test for blood.

Management

In general, once the diagnosis is suspected, the patient should be admitted to a hospital for full evaluation and treatment, particularly if he presents the picture of an acute abdominal emergency (see Regional Enteritis, Modes of Presentation, items 1–3, above). Anyone presenting with perianal or rectal fistula must be carefully evaluated by means of rectal examination, proctosigmoidoscopy, and, where indicated, barium enema. Milder cases may be treated symptomatically on an outpatient basis with a high-protein, low-residue diet, antispasmodics, and iron replacement. Such patients, unless recently evaluated, will need full gastrointestinal radiologic evaluation.

JAUNDICE

Above all, the correct treatment of the jaundiced patient depends on correct diagnosis. *It is primarily a clinical diagnosis.*

Types and Diagnoses

History and the physical findings, including examination of urine and stool, are the primary means of determining type and diagnosis.

In *hemolytic disease* jaundice is present *in the presence of normal-colored urine*. There may be a family history. Splenomegaly and leg ulcers often occur.

In *viral hepatitis* there is often a history of contact with another case or of transfusions or injections within the preceding 1 to 6 months. The patient usually has a prodromic influenza-like illness with fever which subsides with the onset of jaundice. Anorexia is almost always present. The patient is jaundiced, the liver is usually moderately enlarged, and the spleen is palpable in about 10 percent of patients. The urine contains bile, as shown by the color and yellow froth on shaking. Urobilinogen is also present on appropriate testing of the urine. The stools are usually pale.

Another form of viral hepatitis seen with increasing frequency is homologous serum jaundice of drug addicts who have been "mainlining" their narcotics. The presence of needle marks over the veins is telltale evidence of this source of infection.

Cirrhosis of the liver is suggested by a history of excessive alcohol intake with poor nutrition. The patient is often wasted and may have ascites. Spider angiomas are present on the arms and trunk and palmar erythema is usually evident. The liver is likely to be markedly enlarged, and the spleen may be palpable. Fever may also be present. The urine contains bile and urobilinogen, and the stool is usually pale or actually acholic.

Weil's disease is now rarely seen. The diagnosis should be considered if the patient gives a history of exposure to rats and presents with fever, conjunctivitis, headache, and jaundice. The presence of not only bile but large amounts of protein in the urine should strongly suggest the diagnosis.

Drug-induced jaundice is suggested if the patient gives a history of ingestion of phenothiazines, anabolic steroids, or mono-amine oxidase inhibitors. Other hepatotoxins must also be considered, such as carbon tetrachloride, phosphorus, or arsenic. When this last group is involved, alcoholism or a suicidal tendency may be complicating features. Many hepatotoxins affect the kidneys also, and evidence of renal damage such as albuminuria may be present. The urine contains bile and urobilinogen, and stools may be pale.

Extrahepatic obstructive jaundice is generally due to common duct stone or carcinoma of the pancreas, ampulla of Vater, or bile ducts. In the former case, jaundice is usually associated with biliary colic, often with fever and shaking chills. In patients with calculus disease the liver is usually not significantly enlarged and the gallbladder is not palpable. By contrast, in patients with malignant obstruction, pain is less likely, the liver is often greatly enlarged, and the gallbladder may be both visible by inspection in a good light and palpable. In either case the urine contains bile, but commonly little or no urobilinogen, and the stools are acholic. *The combination of jaundice, fever, shaking chills, and pain suggests ascending cho-*

langitis with obstruction of the bile ducts and indicates the need for urgent surgical consultation.

Familial jaundice usually is seen in the neonatal period or is mild and seldom presents in the emergency room. Conditions falling in this category include Crigler-Najjar syndrome, Gilbert's syndrome, Dubin-Johnson syndrome, and so forth.

Recurrent jaundice of pregnancy occurs in patients in the third trimester of pregnancy and commonly presents an obstructive pattern. This is not usually accompanied by constitutional symptoms other than itching. The urine contains bile, and the stools are pale.

Metastatic liver disease with jaundice should be suspected in patients with weight loss, anorexia, and jaundice who have a very large, hard, irregular liver. Ascites is rare in this situation. The urine contains bile and urobilinogen, and stools may be pale.

The patient with *liver abscess* usually presents with right upper quadrant pain, septic fever, and marked weight loss. Hepatomegaly with tenderness of the liver and sometimes a friction rub is present. Ascites and peripheral edema are common. Most patients are jaundiced, with bile and urobilinogen in the urine.

Management

With the exception of patients presenting with Charcot's triad (pain, shaking chills, and jaundice), jaundice is *not* an emergency. Nonetheless, the appearance of jaundice may be an indication of either hepatic decompensation, as in cirrhosis, or biliary obstruction, both of which are best evaluated and treated in a hospital. Patients with viral hepatitis may be managed at home if the domestic situation permits. Most other patients should be admitted.

Useful Tests

1. Alkaline phosphatase. This is usually more than double the normal value in extrahepatic obstruction. Lesser elevations are often seen in hepatocellular disease.
2. Transaminase. Marked elevation (over 400) is rarely seen in conditions other than viral hepatitis or after ingestion of hepatotoxins.
3. Complete blood count.
4. Prothrombin time and response to parenteral vitamin K. Good response indicates extrahepatic obstructive jaundice.

5. Urobilinogen in urine.
6. Total serum bilirubin.

Do not do Bromsulphalein test.

HEPATIC DECOMPENSATION

Hepatic decompensation is caused by progressive hepatocellular disease due to viral hepatitis, alcoholic cirrhosis, or hepatotoxins.

Presentation

1. The patient may be brought in because of inappropriate or odd behavior or because of progressive drowsiness, stupor, and confusion. (For differential diagnosis, see Chapter 6.)

2. There may be jaundice (see preceding section).

3. Ascites is usually due to increased portal pressure associated with lowered plasma oncotic pressure. It may also be due to carcinomatosis or cardiac failure. Looking for extrahepatic stigmata of liver disease and a history of alcoholism or other hepatotoxins will help with diagnosis. Ascites due to heart failure is usually accompanied by dyspnea, and ankle-swelling precedes the appearance of ascites. It is well to look for evidence of heart disease.

4. Gastrointestinal bleeding (see above) or generalized bleeding tendency may be present, due to failure of the clotting mechanism secondary to liver failure.

Most commonly several of these phenomena are found in the same patient, making diagnosis easier.

Precipitating Factors

Precipitating factors must be investigated by careful history from the patient (or relatives or others), for treatment is based almost entirely on their elimination or correction. The following are the most common:

1. Hemorrhage into the gastrointestinal tract leading to hepatic coma or precoma due to absorption of breakdown products (see Gastrointestinal Bleeding, above).

2. Dietary indiscretion, e.g., excessive protein intake causing coma, or excessive salt intake causing ascites.
3. Alcoholic excess.
4. Intercurrent infection, usually pulmonary or of the urinary tract.
5. Ingestion of drugs, e.g., marsalid or morphine, or of poisons, e.g., phosphorus.
6. Hypokalemia due to excessive diuretic therapy, or hypomagnesemia.

It must be remembered that alcoholics often fall and may sustain a head injury. Therefore, subdural hematoma must be borne in mind.

Diagnosis

The following physical findings are most helpful:

1. Fetor hepaticus—a sweet, musty odor.
2. Flapping tremor of the hands (asterixis).
3. Apraxia.
4. Extrahepatic stigmata of liver disease, e.g., spider angioma, palmar erythema.
5. Signs of liver disease, e.g., hepatomegaly, jaundice, ascites, splenomegaly.
6. Neurological signs—variable. Reflexes may be increased or decreased; plantar responses may be extensor.

Laboratory Tests

Tests to reveal elevated blood ammonia, prolonged prothrombin time, low serum albumin, and elevated serum bilirubin should be done.

Management

Patients with evidence of hepatic failure should be admitted to the hospital for treatment. Depending on precipitating factors present in the patient, therapy should be instituted in the emergency room as outlined in the appropriate sections above.

GENERAL REFERENCES

Gastrointestinal Bleeding

Chirr, A. B., Littell, A. S., Badger, G. F., and Beams, A. J. Acute hemorrhage from peptic ulcer. *New Eng. J. Med.* 255:973, 1956.

Jones, F. A. Hematemesis and melena. *Gastroenterology* 30:166, 1956.

Jones, F. A., and Gummer, J. W. P. *Clinical Gastroenterology.* Oxford: Blackwell, 1960. Pp. 393–429.

White, R. L., Healy, W. V., and Habif, D. V. Diagnostic aids in localizing the site of upper gastrointestinal hemorrhage. *Surg. Clin. N. Amer.* 42:1091, 1962.

Ulcerative Colitis

Brooke, B. N. *Ulcerative Colitis and Its Surgical Treatment.* London: E. S. Livingstone, 1954.

Edwards, F. C., and Truelove, S. C. The course and prognosis of ulcerative colitis (Parts 1 & 2). *Gut* 4:229, 1963.

Edwards, F. C., and Truelove, S. C. The course and prognosis of ulcerative colitis (Parts 3 & 4). *Gut* 5:1, 1964.

Kirsner, J. B. (Ed.). New frontiers in ulcerative colitis. *Gastroenterology* 40:286, 1961.

Regional Ileitis

Cornes, J. S., and Stecher, M. Primary Crohn's disease of the colon and rectum. *Gut* 2:189, 1961.

Lockhart-Mummery, M. E., and Morson, B. C. Crohn's disease of the large intestine. *Gut* 5:493, 1964.

Pollack, A. V. Crohn's disease. *Brit. J. Surg.* 46:193, 1958.

Van Patter, W. N., Barger, J. A., Dockerty, M. B., Feldman, W. H., Mayo, C. W., and Waugh, J. M. Regional enteritis. *Gastroenterology* 26:347, 1954.

Jaundice

Hanger, F. M. Diagnostic problems in jaundice. *Arch. Intern. Med.* (Chicago) 86:169, 1950.

Schenker, S., Balint, J. A., and Schiff, L. Differential diagnosis of jaundice; report of a prospective study of 61 proved cases. *Amer. J. Digest. Dis.* 7:449, 1962.

Hepatic Decompensation

Adams, R. D., and Foley, J. M. *The Neurological Disorders Associated with Liver Diseases in Metabolic and Toxic Diseases of the Nervous System.* Baltimore: Williams & Wilkins, 1953.

Davidson, C. S. Hepatic Coma. In L. Schiff (Ed.), *Diseases of the Liver* (3d ed.). Philadelphia: Lippincott, 1969.

Sherlock, S.   *Diseases of the Liver and Biliary System*. Oxford: Blackwell, 1958.

Sherlock, S., Summerskill, W. H. J., White, L. P., and Phear, E. A.   Portal-systemic encephalopathy, neurological complications of liver disease. *Lancet* 2:453, 1954.

Infectious Disease 20

HARVEY R. BERNARD
DUMONT F. ELMENDORF, JR.

Although the diagnosis and treatment of infectious disease in the emergency room depend more on clinical impression derived from history and physical examination than upon laboratory procedures, accurate identification of the causative organism or organisms and a knowledge of their sensitivities to the more frequently used antimicrobial agents are essential to good medical practice. Accurate microbiological identification depends upon the transmission of an adequate, representative, and viable sample of the material to be tested to a laboratory which has been informed of the clinical problem. This liaison permits the laboratory to select media and techniques appropriate to the organisms most likely to be important and encourages the laboratory to report expeditiously to the clinician both presumptive and final identifications.

Many patients with infectious disease who are brought to the emergency room do not have life-threatening illness; in fact, their complaints really do not constitute true emergencies. Frequently, however, the illness is viewed as such by the patient, and thus appropriate preliminary management is most important. It is often most difficult to distinguish between patients whose illness requires immediate hospitalization and those who can be managed safely without hospitalization.

In addition to a determination of the seriousness of the illness, the danger of its transmission to other patients and the staff must be assessed. A coughing patient may present little dramatic appeal in comparison with a major accident case, but if the cougher has tuberculosis the drama may unfold weeks or months later to those individuals who were inadvertently exposed! An enclosed room should be provided in the emergency room for examination of patients with suspected infectious disease in order to reduce the risk of general contamination. All patients with fever, skin rash, sores, prostration, cough, coryza, or diarrhea should be kept from contact with others until the necessity for formal isolation is determined. For such seriously ill patients, early hospitalization and isolation are indicated. Further diagnostic and therapeutic measures should be pursued thereafter by those who will be responsible for definitive care.

However, concern over the possibility of cross infection must be rational. The protective measures should be appropriate to the disease under consideration. For example, isolation of a patient suspected of suffering from smallpox requires attention to infinite detail regarding all possible avenues of spread, while the prevention of cross infection from a patient suffering from a perforated colonic diverticulum is essentially the same as that used for the case of the patient with a colostomy, i.e., effective disposal of the infectious material and dressings and protection of the attendants through careful gloving and handwashing. Isolation precautions should never constitute an impediment to the therapy of the individual.

HISTORY

The history should include information concerning known or possible exposure to contagious disease while at work, in the home, while traveling, or during recreation. A knowledge of the seasonal incidence and prevalence of infection within the community is helpful. Since adequate quarantine is now impractical owing to the speed of air travel, it is important to know the disease problems not only within the home community but in cities the world over. Exposure to animals and insects should be noted. Malaria, for example, is endemic in many resort areas in subtropical countries frequented by our population. The local health agencies are the best source of current information of this nature.

All previous immunizations and the approximate dates thereof should be ascertained. Since some immunization procedures are extremely effective, while others provide merely a partial degree of protection, it is generally useful to make distinctions along these lines. Usually, the more severe and acute the infectious process, the more effective are the immunization procedures currently available or likely to become available for protection. For example, poliomyelitis immunization provides long-term protection for years, while typhoid immunization confers only partial protection, inasmuch as cases of this disease occasionally occur in patients who have been properly immunized. Immunization procedures for truly chronic disease such as tuberculosis continue to provide a ground for dispute as to their relative effectiveness.

Past history of infections and predisposing factors such as diabetes and other metabolic endocrinological and congenital abnormalities is important. The physician should also know of allergies to previously used antimicrobials and serums, including the species from which the serums are prepared, before prescribing for the patient.

The standard review of systems often discloses information the patient thinks irrelevant to the present illness, or he views them as related to a separate illness. For example, a patient may demonstrate urinary tract symptoms and neglect to disclose a history of an antecedent sore throat, or the finding of a past heart murmur.

PHYSICAL EXAMINATION

The physical examination should be thorough. Much time will be saved by disrobing the patient fully. The entire surface of the skin and mucous membranes may be viewed efficiently, disclosing rashes, rose spots, petechiae, purpura, and other diagnostically helpful lesions, frequently unnoticed by the patient.

The general state of the patient and the degree of preoccupation with his illness constitute most valuable information in determining the seriousness of a given illness. A seriously ill person is usually introspective and depressed and relates with difficulty to the physician or others. Lack of cooperation or frank hostility, particularly in children, may be a more important indicator of disease than fever or generalized lymphadenopathy.

DIAGNOSIS

After the history and physical examination have been recorded, a formulation of the problem should be made and documentation and exclusion begun by means of (1) complete blood count, (2) urinalysis, (3) chest roentgenograms, (4) rapid diagnostic microbiological procedures, and (5) appropriate cultures.

Complete blood counts disclose a wide variety of unexpected findings. Urinalysis, performed with a well-maintained modern microscope, can detect many unexpected findings, including bacilluria. Methylene blue, 1% aqueous, will help as a stain of wet preparations and is useful in distinguishing cocci from amorphous material. If a fresh, well-mixed, uncentrifuged sample is used, all elements visible under high-power magnification ($\times$45) will have concentrations of over 100,000 per milliliter.

Chest films, especially the lateral view, often disclose patches of early pneumonitis in noncoughing patients.

Among the rapid diagnostic bacteriological procedures, Gram's stain applied to appropriate secretions will be most helpful. The modification using 1% basic fuchsin in place of the customary safranin demonstrates *Haemophilus influenzae* and other usually poorly staining slender gram-negative organisms.

The acid-fast stain, when applied to sputum, may save time and needless exposure for the prompt diagnosis of many cases of tuberculosis.

Newer, rapid methods of diagnosis detect antigen in either localized or diffuse forms but for many reasons these methods may not be practical in a variety of infections. Fluorescent antibody identification and particle agglutination techniques, when available, may be of distinct aid in effecting at least a tentative bacteriological diagnosis, which may be confirmed at leisure by cultural methods under continuing revision, and they differ widely for the different types of organisms sought.

It is helpful if cultures are obtained before antimicrobial drugs are used. However, a history of antimicrobial administration does not preclude the detection of the offending microorganism since some microorganisms are much more readily masked than others. Under these circumstances cultures should be taken and the laboratory informed of the drug in use, so that measures may be taken to neutralize it, a standard practice in the processing of blood cultures obtained during the course of penicillin treatment of endocarditis, for example.

CLASSES OF INFECTION

General classes of infection likely to be encountered in the emergency room are as follows:

1. Pyodermas and abscesses
   a. *Streptococcus pyogenes*

    b. *Staphylococcus aureus*
    c. *Candida* (*Monilia*) and dermatophytes
    d. *Treponema pallidum*
2. Burns
    a. *Streptococcus pyogenes*
    b. *Staphylococcus aureus*
    c. *Pseudomonas aeruginosa*
    d. Proteus sp.
3. Wounds (traumatic as well as surgical)
    a. *Staphylococcus aureus*
    b. *Streptococcus pyogenes*
    c. Enterobacteriaceae
    d. Anaerobic and microaerophilic streptococci
    e. Clostridium sp.
    f. Bacteroides sp.
4. Eyes: Cornea and conjunctiva
    a. Viruses—adenoidal, pharyngeal, conjunctival, inclusion, trachoma, lymphogranuloma venereum
    b. *Staphylococcus aureus*
    c. *Diplococcus pneumoniae*
    d. *Haemophilus influenzae*
    e. *Diplococcus gonorrhoeae*
    f. Enterobacteriaceae
    g. Koch-Weeks bacillus
5. Respiratory: Ear, nose, and throat
    a. *Streptococcus pyogenes*
    b. Viruses—APC, adenoviruses, herpes
    c. *Diplococcus pneumoniae*
    d. *Staphylococcus aureus*
    e. *Haemophilus influenzae*
    f. *Neisseria meningitidis*
    g. *Pseudomonas aeruginosa*
    h. *Candida albicans*
    i. *Listeria monocytogenes*
    j. *Klebsiella aerobacter*
    k. Infectious mononucleosis agent
    l. *Mycoplasma*
    m. Vincent's infection
    n. *Corynebacterium diphtheriae*
6. Trachea and bronchi
    a. *Diplococcus pneumoniae*
    b. *Haemophilus influenzae*

    c. *Staphylococcus aureus*
    d. *Mycoplasma*
    e. Viruses—influenza, adenoviruses
    f. *Pseudomonas aeruginosa*
    g. *Klebsiella aerobacter*
    h. Proteus sp.
    i. *Mycobacterium tuberculosis*
    j. Rickettsia
    k. *Streptococcus pyogenes*

7. Intestinal tract
    a. Viruses
    b. Enteropathogens, *Escherichia coli*
    c. *Staphylococcus aureus*
    d. *Staphylococcus aureus* enterotoxin
    e. Salmonella sp. (includes typhoid)
    f. Shigella
    g. *Pseudomonas aeruginosa*

8. Penis, urethra, cervix, and prostate
    a. Trichomonas
    b. *Candida albicans*
    c. *Mycoplasma*
    d. Herellea-Mimea
    e. *Neisseria gonorrhoeae*
    f. *Treponema pallidum*
    g. *Lymphogranuloma venereum*
    h. *Diplococcus pneumoniae*
    i. *Streptococcus pyogenes:* group A, B, C, or E

9. Kidney, urinary tract, and bladder
    a. *Escherichia coli*
    b. *Pseudomonas aeruginosa,* Proteus sp.
    c. *Staphylococcus aureus*
    d. Anaerobic and microaerophilic streptococci
    e. *Streptococcus pyogenes,* group A
    f. *Klebsiella aerobacter*
    g. Proteus sp.

THERAPY

The treatment of infection varies. Most medical and many minor surgical infections constitute the primary illness and are caused by a single organism. In these instances effective therapy must be directed at the offending organism. However, many infections, especially surgical infections are secondary to other conditions. In many instances treatment of the primary condition will also result in cure of the infection and in most instances treatment of the primary disease must be effected before cure of the secondary infection is effective or permanent. Determination of appropriate chemotherapy is more difficult in these instances because a mixed bacterial flora is usually involved.

As all surgical wounds are contaminated by bacteria to some degree, surgical illnesses, especially acute traumatic ones, afford a unique opportunity to prevent infection through appropriate wound care. These details have been discussed previously in Chapter 11. Since the timing of the onset of the illness or injury may be accurately assessed in many instances, chemoprophylaxis may be utilized effectively in surgical diseases when it is much more difficult in medical ones. The basic ingredient of successful chemoprophylaxis is the provision of adequate serum and tissue levels of an effective antimicrobial when the bacterial inoculum is the smallest. In practical terms, antimicrobials are most effective when present at the time of bacteria inoculation and less effective as time passes until they become ineffective at preventing infections after 3 to 4 hours. Drugs given preventively should be administered for a short period (8 to 24 hours) to help the host defense cope with bacteria introduced with the onset of surgical disease. Antimicrobial drugs when used against established infections are most effective in limiting the spread of localized infection through local tissues and in minimizing danger of the dissemination of bacteria through the bloodstream; they are less effective against bacteria within a localized infection. These must be dealt with by the host defenses aided appropriately by incision and drainage or débridement by the surgeon. Antimicrobials may be used to prevent primary lodgement of an infection in otherwise normal tissue during surgical operations to cure deeply seated infections (e.g., appendiceal abscess).

It is important to realize that many virus infections are complicated by secondary bacterial infection. *Streptococcus pyogenes,* group A, for instance, frequently exists in a subclinical or carrier state that is often raised to the clinical level by an intercurrent respiratory virus infection. A history of recurrent respiratory infections or ear infections can be a clue to underlying chronic bacterial disease of this variety. In addition, true virus influenza is often a diphasic illness also, in which a bacterial component characteristically becomes significant and may be fatal if unrecognized.

The seriousness of the clinical illness determines how much risk is justified in the decision of whether to use drugs at all, and if so, whether a more effective but potentially more toxic agent is warranted. Judgment is always required. For example, there is little doubt that coryza should not be treated with an antimicrobial agent under most circumstances and there is no doubt that chloramphenicol is worth its risk in *Haemophilus influenzae* meningitis.

A list of infectious agents together with recommendations for the antibacterial agent of choice follows.

Microorganism	*Drugs of Choice*
Bacteroides sp.	Tetracycline, chloramphenicol
Candida albicans	Amphotericin B, nystatin locally
Clostridium sp.	Penicillin, cephalothin
Staphylococcus aureus	Penicillin, methicillin, oxacillin, cephalothin
Corynebacterium diphtheriae	Antitoxin, penicillin, erythromycin
Dermatophytes	Amphotericin B locally
Escherichia coli	Variable, sulfonamides, etc.
Haemophilus influenzae	Chloramphenicol, sulfonamides, ampicillin, etc.
Klebsiella aerobacter	Variable
Koch-Weeks bacillus	Chloramphenicol, sulfonamides
Listeria monocytogenes	Variable, tetracyclines
Lymphogranuloma venereum (LGV)	Tetracyclines
Monilia—*Candida albicans*	Amphotericin B, nystatin locally
Mycobacterium tuberculosis	Isoniazid, streptomycin para-amino-salicylic acid (PAS)
Mycoplasma	Erythromycin, tetracyclines
Neisseria gonorrhoeae	Penicillin
Neisseria meningitidis	Sulfonamides, penicillin
Diplococcus pneumoniae	Penicillin, erythromycin
Proteus sp.	Variable, high-dose penicillin
Pseudomonas aeruginosa	Variable, colistin, polymyxin, gentamycin
Rickettsia	Chloramphenicol, tetracyclines
Salmonella sp. (includes typhoid)	Chloramphenicol, ampicillin
Shigella	Sulfonamides
Streptococci, anaerobic and microaerophilic	Penicillin
Streptococcus pyogenes, group A	Penicillin, erythromycin
Treponema pallidum	Penicillin
Trichomonas vaginalis	Metronidazole
Vincent's infection	Penicillin

Neurological Emergencies 21

WALTER J. FRIEDLANDER

Patients with a multitude of neurological problems are seen in the emergency room, but only a few require immediate recognition and treatment. Some of these cases are dealt with elsewhere in this volume and will not be further considered. To be discussed here are problems of (1) sudden onset of weakness as exemplified by myasthenia gravis and (2) seizures.

MYASTHENIA GRAVIS

Release of acetylcholine from the presynaptic nerve ending at the myoneural junction causes a muscle to contract. The acetylcholine must then be destroyed by the action of acetylcholinesterase in order for the muscle to be "reset" so that it can again contract when it is once more subjected to acetylcholine release. Therefore, weakness in patients with myasthenia gravis may be due to either (1) the disease itself, which is probably the result of an insufficient but not totally absent acetylcholine effect, or (2) the administration by the physician of too large a dose of anticholinesterase drug (e.g., neostigmine) so that acetylcholine is not destroyed at the myoneural junction and hence the muscle cannot be "reset" for another contraction. The latter condition is referred to as a *cholinergic crisis*.

337

Diagnosis

Myasthenia gravis usually has a gradual onset but occasionally it begins suddenly, so that the patient may present in the emergency room with a history of a sudden onset of weakness. The weakness may involve only one set of muscles or may be generalized. The cases that begin suddenly usually do not have such profound weakness that emergency treatment is required; immediate therapy is more likely to be necessary in the patient with a previously established diagnosis who now suffers a sudden exacerbation of his weakness, constituting a myasthenic crisis. There are a number of key points in establishing the diagnosis.

1. It is observed that with increasing activity of the muscle(s) about which the patient complains there is increasing weakness. This can be tested by asking the patient to contract the supposedly involved muscle rapidly for 10 to 20 seconds (for example, blink if the levator palpebrae is weak, open and close the grip if the fingers are weak) and then making as objective a comparison of strength before and after exercise as is possible (for example, measurement of the palpebral fissures in millimeters, dynometric measurement of grip).

2. The acute illness is unassociated with fever, objective sensory findings, or impairment of consciousness. Exceptions to each of these exist: The patient with myasthenia may have a complicating infection with resultant fever, and not infrequently an infection will cause an exacerbation of the myasthenia; the patient may complain of paresthesias but will not have demonstrable sensory disturbances; finally, profound weakness of the respiratory muscles may cause anoxia, which in turn may impair consciousness.

3. If extraocular muscles are involved, the pupillary reactions to accommodation or light are *not* affected.

4. Deep muscle reflexes are normal unless there is extremely profound weakness.

5. There is a positive response to the parenteral administration of an anticholinesterase drug such as edrophonium (Tensilon). Edrophonium test: 2 mg of edrophonium is rapidly given intravenously and if no effect is seen within 30 seconds, an additional 8 mg is given; the optimum effect is seen almost immediately or cer-

tainly within a few minutes. A positive response should be a *definite,* not just an equivocal improvement in strength. Failure to effect a definite improvement may mean: (1) the patient does not have myasthenia gravis; (2) the myasthenia gravis is so severe that even larger doses of medication are needed; or (3) the patient is in a cholinergic crisis and is weak because he has already received excessive anticholinesterase.

DIFFERENTIAL DIAGNOSIS. Myasthenia gravis is characterized by a local or a generalized weakness. Local myasthenia implies a major involvement of only a limited number of muscles (not necessarily symmetrical in distribution). The weakness of extraocular muscles or other limited muscle groups due to localized myasthenia gravis must be differentiated from other disorders manifested by *local weakness* (see Table 21-1); the diffuse weakness of generalized myasthenia gravis must be differentiated from other disorders manifested by *generalized weakness* (see Table 21-2).

Treatment

Emergency-room treatment of a mild case of myasthenia gravis (which means most cases of local myasthenia) probably is not indicated once a diagnosis has been established. Therapy is a long-term process often requiring frequent changes in dosage of medicine in order to "titrate" the patient; it should be undertaken by the physician who will assume responsibility for the patient.

In cases of severe weakness in which cholinergic crisis has been ruled out as the cause, neostigmine (Prostigmin) may be given intramuscularly in doses of 1 to 2 mg every 1 to 3 hours. In great emergencies, 1 mg can be given intravenously. In order to decrease the undesirable parasympathetic side effects, 0.2 to 0.6 mg of atropine every 3 to 6 hours can be given intramuscularly.

If respirations are embarrassed, an endotracheal tube or tracheostomy with use of a mechanical respirator is indicated.

In cases of *cholinergic crisis,* all anticholinesterase drugs should be withheld. In addition, if the patient shows evidence of respiratory embarrassment, assisted breathing through an endotracheal tube or cuffed tracheostomy tube will be necessary. The least that should be done in all cases is to have a respirator immediately available.

Sudden death is not unknown either in myasthenic or in cholin-

Table 21-1. Differential Diagnosis of Local Myasthenia Gravis from Other Causes of Acute Focal Weakness

Disorder	Aids in Differential Diagnosis	Emergency Measures
Neurasthenia, hysteria	Ptosis and difficulty in swallowing respond only equivocally to edrophonium test or respond as well to a placebo History of previous psychiatric difficulties Episode precipitated by emotional situation	None
Cerebrovascular insufficiency	History of previous transient ischemia attacks Presence of "neighborhood" signs such as crossed hemiparesis Ipsilateral paresis of facial muscles associated with lateral rectus palsy Horner's syndrome may accompany difficulty in swallowing Presence of upper motor neuron signs Slight elevation of cerebrospinal fluid protein Other evidences of cardiovascular disease	None
Unruptured intracranial aneurysm	Presence of headache or retro-orbital pain ipsilateral to extraocular muscle palsy When oculomotor nerve is involved, loss of pupillary reflex is common	None
Multiple sclerosis	History or presence of patchy central nervous system involvement Cerebrospinal fluid may show mild pleocytosis, slight elevation of protein, and abnormal colloidal gold curve	None
Postinfectious encephalomyelitis	History of recent illness (particularly an exanthem) or history of an infection Recent history of antitoxin administration Patchy neurological signs Cerebrospinal fluid may show slight elevation of protein and slight pleocytosis	None
Diabetic neuritis	Presence of diabetes If oculomotor nerve is involved, pupillary reflex is usually present	None

Condition	Findings	Treatment
	Signs of peripheral polyneuritis Cerebrospinal fluid protein may be elevated	
Wernicke's encephalopathy	History of nutritional deficiency or acute alcoholism Usually some impairment of consciousness Nystagmus often present with extraocular palsy May have signs of cerebellar dysfunction May have polyneuritis	100 mg of thiamine chloride with added B complex in 5% glucose in water given as intravenous drip
Acute poliomyelitis	Fever, myalgia, stiff neck Weakness may be patchy and progressive over period of several days Urinary retention may be present Cerebrospinal fluid pleocytosis	None usually required, but when muscles of respiration are involved, a respirator may be lifesaving
Botulism	History of recent ingestion of rancid food Pupillary reflexes lost Deep muscle reflexes decreased or absent	Antitoxin
Diphtheria	History of sore throat 2 to 3 weeks previously Pupillary reflexes lost Deep muscle reflexes decreased or absent Cerebrospinal fluid protein may be elevated	Antitoxin
Guillain-Barré syndrome	May present with oculomotor or facial paresis Ascending weakness over hours or days Deep-muscle reflexes decreased or absent May have sensory findings Cerebrospinal fluid protein elevated with few if any cells	None usually required, but tracheostomy and a respirator may be lifesaving
Todd's paralysis	History of a seizure beginning in or limited to the now paretic limb Contralateral electroencephalographic focus	None

Table 21-2. Differential Diagnosis of Generalized Myasthenia Gravis from Other Acute Generalized Weaknesses

Disorder	Aids in Differential Diagnosis	Emergency Measures
Neurasthenia and hysteria	Table 21-1	
Poliomyelitis	Table 21-1	
Botulism	Table 21-1	
Diphtheria	Table 21-1	
Guillain-Barré syndrome	Table 21-1	
Familial periodic paralysis	Often familial History of previous attacks usually present Frequently occurs after heavy carbohydrate intake followed by rest Deep muscle reflexes decreased or absent Cranial nerves not commonly involved Serum hypokalemia	None
Hyperkalemic periodic paralysis	Often familial History of previous attacks usually present Frequently occurs after period of exercise followed by rest Deep muscle reflexes decreased or absent Cranial nerves not commonly involved May have myotonic response to percussion of muscle Serum hyperkalemia Made worse by administration of potassium	None
Sodium-responsive periodic paralysis	Familial history Precipitated by rest after exercise	None

Condition	Features	Treatment
	Deep muscle reflexes decreased or absent Cranial nerves above the glossopharyngeal not involved Made worse by potassium administration Serum potassium normal	None
Hypokalemic weakness	History of excessive potassium loss, e.g., chronic administration of mercurial diuretics, overpurging, or use of corticosteroids Deep muscle reflexes decreased or absent Greatest weakness in proximal muscles Electrocardiographic changes (depressed ST, prolonged QT, small T fused with U) Serum hypokalemia	
Hyperkalemic weakness	Oliguria with renal failure Electrocardiographic changes (symmetrical peaking of T, later prolonged PR and QRS) Serum hyperkalemia	None
Hypoglycemia	Sweating Hypotension Sometimes Babinski's reflex is present Hypoglycemia Reduced cerebrospinal fluid glucose levels	Glucose (after blood is drawn for determination of plasma glucose level)
Tick paralysis	Ascending paralysis Deep muscle reflexes decreased or absent Late cranial nerve involvement Tick present, frequently in hair	Remove entire tick
Cholinergic crisis	History of taking anticholinesterase drugs May have signs of parasympathetic stimulation such as miotic pupils, abdominal cramps, or diarrhea Edrophonium test makes condition worse	See text

ergic crisis. Since death may be caused by cardiac arrest, continuous electrocardiographic monitoring is desirable in all seriously ill patients.

If a cholinergic crisis cannot be differentiated from a myasthenic crisis, the best emergency procedure is to stop all drugs and have a respirator at hand. The patient must be watched very carefully!

The immediate goal of treatment in either myasthenic or cholinergic crisis is some definite improvement in the patient's condition rather than quick restoration to complete normality.

SEIZURES

A seizure is the clinical manifestation of a "discharge" from an abnormally "irritable" area of the central nervous system. Although the basic neurophysiological mechanism of all seizures is probably the same, there are many different etiologies for the abnormal "irritability" (see Table 21-3). The clinical characteristics of a particular seizure depend on the specific area of the central nervous system that is involved. For example, if the entire brain is involved, there is a generalized convulsion; if the frontal, adverse area is involved, there is contralateral turning of the eyes, then head, and perhaps the whole body; if the temporal lobe is involved, there may be automatic activity or emotional disorders such as fear or depression, and so forth.

Diagnosis

As thorough a search as possible for the etiology of the seizure should be made so that specific treatment can be instituted (see Table 21-3).

A history from relatives or acquaintances of the patient or witnesses to the seizure is helpful. Seizures seen in the emergency room should be described in as much detail as possible, since this information may be of inestimable value later in the definitive diagnostic work-up and care of the patient. Diagnostic terms such as *grand mal, petit mal, Jacksonian,* and so forth, should be avoided, but *all* details should be reported such as: was there a focal onset to the generalized convulsion? which side of the body was first involved? was there impairment of consciousness? was there urinary incontinence? did the patient bite his tongue (not just cheek)? A detailed neuro-

Table 21-3. Etiology of Seizures

Etiology	Aids in Differential Diagnosis
I. Primary in central nervous system	
A. Idiopathic	Onset usually in the first two decades of life, but seldom during first year. Nothing in history to account for seizures. Nothing focal either in the seizure or on neurological examination. Electroencephalogram is without lateralizing focus and often shows bilateral, synchronous "discharge."
B. Symptomatic	Onset at any age. Frequently there is something in history to account for brain damage.
1. Trauma	Often seizure has a focal onset even though it may become generalized. Neurological examination may show focal abnormalities. Electroencephalogram may show focal abnormality.
2. Cerebrovascular accident	
3. Infection	
4. Tumor	
5. Cortical degenerative disease	
C. Febrile convulsions of infancy	Previous history of seizures with febrile illness may exist. Rare after 6 years of age. No evidence of focal neurological abnormality in either the seizure, neurological examination, or electroencephalogram. The nonspecific effect of fever must be differentiated with care from actual infection of the central nervous system accompanied by fever.
II. Drugs	
A. While on medication	
1. Atropine	Associated delirium. Signs of parasympathetic block including mydriasis, dry mouth, etc.
2. Phenothiazines	Usually on large dosage. Often history of previous seizures.

(*Continued on page 346*)

Table 21-3. (*Continued*)

Etiology	Aids in Differential Diagnosis
3. Hydrazides, e.g., Isoniazid, Iproniazid	Receiving antituberculosis therapy if isoniazid, or antidepressive therapy if iproniazid. Deep muscle reflexes may be increased. When other evidence of polyneuritis is present, deep muscle reflexes may be decreased. Improvement with pyridoxine 50 to 100 mg intramuscularly.
4. Cycloserine	Receiving antituberculosis therapy. Improvement with pyridoxine as above.
5. Cocaine	May have received topical, local anesthetic. Evidence of narcotic addiction including nausea, sweating, mydriasis, and fever.
6. Meperidine (Demerol)	Seizures are dose-related although patient need not otherwise be toxic.
7. Imipramine, e.g., Tofranil or Elavil	History of receiving psychopharmacological drugs for depression.
8. Ethyl alcohol	No history of withdrawal. It is important to search for related disorders such as epilepsy secondary to old head trauma, recent trauma with a subdural hematoma and so forth. Focal seizures imply focal brain pathology that may or may not be complicated by vitamin B_6 deficiency, hypoglycemia, or withdrawal (see below); *withdrawal per se produces generalized convulsions.*
B. Withdrawal from medication	
1. Ethyl alcohol	This diagnosis should be made with care, for not all patients who drink are alcoholics. Withdrawal seizures are generalized and occur hours to several days after stopping or greatly reducing alcohol consumption.
2. Sedatives	History of chronic intake and sudden withdrawal of barbiturates, bromides, meprobromate (Miltown, Equanil), glutethimide (Doriden), or benzodiazopines (Librium, Valium). Before making diagnosis, consider underlying problem for which the sedative was given.

III. Toxins — History of exposure to convulsive toxins.

IV. Infections — Primary infections of the central nervous system.

V. Cardiovascular disorders

A. Cardiac arrhythmia — May have converted to normal rhythm at time of examination.

B. Vasculitis — Evidence of other organ systems being involved in addition to central nervous system.

C. Hypertension — Hypertension per se does not cause seizures but may lead to cerebral vascular accidents which may result in seizures.

D. Hypotension — Produces seizures only if significant cerebral anoxia results or if complicated by thrombosis of intracranial artery. If there is no obvious syncope or other explanation, consider an acute myocardial infarct.

VI. Metabolic disorders — In infancy, pyridoxine dependency is a possible etiological factor. In all age groups the following metabolic abnormalities may lead to convulsions: hypoglycemia, nonketotic hyperglycemia, hypocalcemia, hypomagnesemia, hyponatremia, hypernatremia, water intoxication.

VII. Toxemia of pregnancy — This diagnosis should be made with care to exclude all other possibilities, particularly in a woman not at term (see Chapter 10).

VIII. Other organic disorders — Azotemia, sickle cell anemia, porphyria, metastatic carcinoma, etc.

IX. Psychiatric causes — In general, functional seizures are bizarre, long-lasting, and performed to accomplish a psychic need. However, organic seizures can be precipitated by emotional situations and can be bizarre particularly if of temporal lobe origin. A normal electroencephalogram obtained *during* a generalized seizure is highly suggestive of that particular seizure being nonorganic. Neurological findings during a seizure that disappear after the seizure is ended greatly favor a seizure being organic in origin. Such findings include dilated or fixed pupils, Babinski's sign, tongue-biting, and urinary incontinence. The diagnosis of a functional seizure demands great care!

logical examination will also aid in localizing the area of the brain which is "discharging."

The *minimal* laboratory studies that should be obtained when the cause is not known should include the following:

1. Blood count and tests for blood sugar, blood urea nitrogen, and serum calcium.
2. Tests for urinary albumin and sugar.
3. Lumbar puncture with recording of pressure and examination of cerebrospinal fluid for cell count, smear for bacteria, total protein, glucose, serology, and culture.

Other laboratory tests which may be very helpful on an emergency basis are these:

1. Tests for blood magnesium and sodium, and culture for bacteria and febrile agglutinations.
2. Electrocardiogram.
3. Electroencephalogram.
4. Skull roentgenogram.

Treatment

Treatment of a single generalized convulsion or perhaps up to three or four repeated convulsions usually requires *no* medicinal therapy. In fact, in a known epileptic patient, a large dose of anticonvulsant drug given during the convulsion when added to the usual maintenance therapy may at least temporarily complicate further management. Exceptions to this rule are (1) patients with a recent myocardial infarction, surgical incision, and so forth, in whom even one convulsion may have deleterious effects, and (2) a prolonged (20 minutes or more) convulsion even if it is only a single one, particularly in an infant or a young child.

Nonmedicinal treatment of a *single, generalized convulsion* should consist of precautions against self-inflicted injury. A padded tongue blade should be used to prevent tongue-biting, but the tongue blade should not be forced into the mouth against clenched teeth, for the teeth can be broken. The patient should not be allowed to fall from the bed or examining table but at the same time must not be forcibly restrained lest a fracture result. During or immediately after a generalized convulsion the patient should be turned on his side so that he will not aspirate; the airway must be clear in the new position.

Minor seizures need no emergency treatment except, again, to see that the patient does not harm himself. If the patient is wandering about because of automatic activity, he can be appropriately guided, but if forcibly restrained he may become agitated.

Febrile seizures in small children should be treated by an attempt to reduce fever by tepid baths or alcohol sponges. If medication is required because of prolonged or multiple seizures, the same doses of medicine as suggested for treatment of status epilepticus should be given.

Status epilepticus is the occurrence of one seizure after another without return of a good degree of consciousness between seizures, whereas in *frequent* seizures* there is return of consciousness after each seizure. The principal aim of drug therapy in status epilepticus is to stop the seizures without oversedating the patient, for it is desirable to evaluate the postictal state. The decision as to how large the dose of drug is to be must be weighed between the desire to not anesthetize the patient totally and the need to give a dose large enough to control a potentially dangerous situation.

The drug of choice in most cases is diazepam intravenously. Diazepam, 10 mg I.V., given over a period of 2 to 3 minutes is the usual dose for patients 10 years of age or older. The dose is reduced for younger children, e.g., 2 mg under the age of 1 year, and 5 mg for children 1 to 7 years old. If seizures continue, the dose may be repeated two to three times with a waiting period of 20 minutes between injections. Rarely this causes respiratory embarrassment or severe drops in blood pressure.

Another useful drug is sodium phenobarbital given parenterally in a solution of distilled water or saline. It is safer and hence pref-

---

* The term *status* usually refers to repeated generalized convulsions, but there is also a condition of *petit mal status*. Since petit mal status may present only as obtundation with or without twitching, particularly of the eyelids at a rate of three per second, or minor automatic activity, it is a difficult diagnosis to make on purely clinical grounds. However, it can easily be established by electroencephalography. A disorder which can be likened to status is occasionally seen in patients who have a history of seizures and now appear obtunded without unusual motor activity. The EEG shows more-or-less continuing "seizure" activity. In these cases, the treatment of an unconscious or obtunded patient with what, on the surface, appears to be a paradox, i.e., parenteral diazepam (Valium) or phenobarbital (anticonvulsants) may result in the patient's "awakening." Obviously such treatment of an unconscious or obtunded patient is dependent on a correct diagnosis, which can be made only by an EEG.

erable to give the medication intramuscularly, but if the status is severe, the drug may be given intravenously with the important caution that in this case it be administered very slowly over a matter of at least several minutes. An appropriate *initial* dose of sodium phenobarbital in an aqueous solution is:

Children up to 1 year of age	60 mg
Children 2 to 5 years old	120 to 200 mg
Older children	200 to 240 mg
Adults	240 mg

A repeat dose, similar to the initial dose, may be given in 30 minutes if the initial dose does not decrease the frequency or severity of the attacks. An appropriate decrease in dose is advisable if the seizures are continuing but are definitely decreasing in frequency or severity. At least four doses should be given before anesthesia is seriously considered.

Pediatric Emergencies 22

WILLIAM A. PETERSEN

No attempt is made here to include all emergencies of childhood. Emphasis has been placed on those that are most commonly encountered and on suggested outlines for their expeditious management. To deal effectively with sick children in an emergency-room setting the physician must have an organized approach in terms of evaluation, therapy, and disposition. The following is offered as a guide:

1. Establish a *working diagnosis* on the basis of history and physical examination.
2. Institute *supportive measures*—intravenous fluids, lowering of body temperature, etc.—as the case may require.
3. Obtain *preliminary studies* when indicated.
4. Initiate *specific therapy* when possible.
5. Obtain appropriate *consultation* when indicated.
6. Admit to a hospital or arrange for treatment at home.

FEVER

One of the most common complaints in pediatric practice is fever. The degree of temperature elevation, regardless of its cause, usually forms the basis of the parents' concern. The cause of fever should always be investigated, but appropriate antipyretic measures may be instituted before establishment of a diagnosis.

351

Common Causes of Fever

The common causes of fever include acute tonsillitis and pharyngitis, otitis media, acute gastroenteritis, acute nonspecific upper respiratory infections, lower respiratory infections, the numerous exanthemas, and urinary tract infections. Most of these conditions may be diagnosed by history, physical examination, and the use of minimum laboratory study.

Effective Antipyretic Measures

1. Unneeded clothing is removed to allow radiation of heat.
2. The patient may be sponged with tepid water. The effectiveness of the sponging is dependent upon conduction of heat to the water and its subsequent evaporation. Cold water or cold wet towels should *not* be used, for they produce peripheral vasoconstriction with conservation of body heat. They may likewise cause shivering, resulting in heat production.
3. Acetylsalicylic acid (aspirin) is universally available and is the most effective agent for decreasing body temperature. The usual dose is 60 mg for every year of age up to 5 years, given every 4 hours. For the 5- to 10-year-old child, 300 mg suffices, and 600 mg for the older child. If vomiting occurs, double the dose may be given rectally. Acetaminophen (Tempra) in dropper dosage form, 60 mg in 0.6 ml, is convenient during the first several years of life.

Less Common, More Serious Causes of Fever

In most instances children with the following serious infections present with fever. Children with septicemia, bacterial meningitis, or encephalitis are obviously acutely ill at the time they arrive in the emergency room and warrant immediate hospitalization in addition to vigorous antibiotic and other lifesaving supportive therapy. Because they are most often admitted through the emergency room, it is imperative that a concise outline be readily available as a guide to diagnosis and treatment.

SEPTICEMIA. The infant or child who is acutely ill with sepsis will require specific antibotic therapy long before culture results are reported. It is, however, inexcusable to begin antibiotics before certain cultures have been obtained.

1. If the patient is in shock, intravenous fluids by arm vein or scalp vein should be begun while cutdown is being performed. A 0.85% saline solution or a 2.5% glucose-0.45% saline solution may be utilized at a rate of 2500 to 3000 ml per square meter of body surface area per 24 hours. The rate may be doubled in the first hour.

2. Blood, nasopharyngeal, and throat cultures are obtained in addition to a culture of any obvious focus of infection such as a draining ear, a petechial lesion, or an infected umbilical cord.

3. Lumbar puncture is done with simultaneous collection of blood for sugar determination. Specimens are obtained for culture, sugar, protein, and cell count. As soon as feasible, a smear of this fluid should be gram-stained and organisms searched for.

4. An attempt is made to obtain urine for quantitative culture.

5. An appropriate initial dose of antibiotics should be given before the patient is transferred to the ward if cultures have been obtained. Infants under 6 months of age should receive aqueous crystalline penicillin, 500,000 units intravenously, slowly, and kanamycin, 7.5 mg per kilogram of body weight intramuscularly. Infants over 6 months of age should receive aqueous crystalline penicillin 1,000,000 to 2,000,000 units intravenously, slowly, and ampicillin 50 mg per kilogram of body weight intravenously, slowly, after proper dilution.

6. Blood is drawn for complete blood count, typing, and cross matching.

7. Blood should be sent for electrolyte determinations (sodium, potassium, chloride, carbon dioxide content, and blood urea nitrogen).

MENINGITIS. The infant or child suspected of having meningitis should be handled very much like the child suspected of having sepsis. Supportive measures should be instituted immediately but antibiotics withheld until cultures are obtained.

1. Intravenous fluids are administered as outlined under Septicemia (preceding section). These should be given by needle and appropriate vein until cutdown is performed.

2. Blood, nasopharyngeal, throat, and other cultures are obtained as expeditiously as possible.

3. Lumbar puncture is done with simultaneous collection of venous blood for sugar determination.

4. Blood is drawn for electrolyte determination, complete blood count, and blood urea nitrogen determination.

5. Initial doses of antibiotics are given before transfer to the ward if all cultures have been obtained. These drugs, as detailed under Septicemia, should be given immediately by the appropriate route.

6. Sedation with phenobarbital may be required if seizures have occurred.

WATERHOUSE-FRIDERICHSEN SYNDROME. The Waterhouse-Friderichsen syndrome is an acute state of shock seen in fulminating meningococcemia. Children with this condition are desperately ill and usually demonstrate numerous petechial and ecchymotic skin lesions. Considerable controversy has arisen surrounding certain aspects of treatment, but the following measures should be utilized in addition to the antibiotic coverage listed under Septicemia and Meningitis (preceding sections), depending on the age of the patient.

1. Hydrocortisone 5 to 7.5 mg per kilogram of body weight is given every 24 hours.

2. Intravenous fluids are started, 0.85% saline solution or 2.5% glucose in 0.45% saline at 2500 ml per square meter of body surface area per 24 hours.

3. A single fresh blood transfusion of 6 to 8 ml per kilogram body weight is administered if available.

ENCEPHALITIS. Encephalitis or encephalomyelitis may be caused by any one of a group of neurotropic viruses but may likewise be induced by viruses that are not specifically neurotropic in action. It may also occur as a postinfectious complication of mumps, measles, chickenpox, and other viral illnesses as well as after smallpox vaccination. In the emergency ward the most important purpose of evaluating a child suspected of having encephalitis is to be certain that the symptoms are not due to acute bacterial meningitis. Lumbar puncture should be performed if funduscopic examination has ruled out increased intracranial pressure. Following this, cultures of nose, throat, and blood should be obtained and the patient admitted for supportive care.

Coexisting symptoms which may need emergency care prior to admission are (1) hyperpyrexia, (2) airway insufficiency, (3) convulsion, and (4) dehydration with fluid and electrolyte imbalance.

RESPIRATORY DISTRESS

Acute Laryngotracheobronchitis (Croup)

Most children seen in the emergency room with croup are between the ages of 2 and 5. They have usually been put to bed with a history of being perfectly well except perhaps for a mild cold. In many cases of croup there is an element of inflammatory edema of the vocal cords as well as laryngospasm; therefore, symptoms may vary from time to time and may diminish following spontaneous vomiting of swallowed mucus. Hoarseness, inspiratory stridor, cough, dyspnea, and sternal or subcostal retraction are present to varying degrees. The presence or absence and severity of each will help dictate the need for hospitalization. Most children may be successfully treated with (1) humidified air, (2) an expectorant cough mixture, (3) adequate fluid intake, and (4) broad-spectrum antibiotics (frequently prescribed but probably of little help in shortening the duration of symptoms because of the predominant viral etiology of this condition).

The child under 2 years of age who demonstrates retraction at rest is best treated in the hospital. Although less than 1 percent of children with this disorder will require tracheostomy, evidence of restlessness, agitation, or decreasing air exchange must be closely watched for. Consultation with specialists trained in doing tracheostomy should be obtained if there is doubt.

If a child is to be hospitalized and is in severe distress in the emergency room, no attempt should be made at that time to visualize the throat. It is far better that he be placed in a steam room and that appropriate emergency equipment be made available before such an examination.

Acute Epiglottitis

Acute epiglottitis is a syndrome of acute respiratory obstruction caused by *Haemophilus influenzae*. The children are obviously acutely ill when first seen and are usually between 3 and 8 years of age. The illness is characterized by an abrupt onset of respiratory obstruction due to edema of the epiglottis and a fulminating course. It is frequently a surgical emergency as well, for approximately 50 percent of afflicted children will require tracheostomy. Although the symptoms are similar to croup symptoms, they are more severe and progress more rapidly.

Treatment consists of the following measures: (1) immediate admission, (2) immediate consultation with a specialist qualified to perform tracheostomy, (3) throat and blood cultures after airway is secure, (4) ampicillin, 50 mg per kilogram of body weight intravenously, *immediately*, and (5) ampicillin, 150 to 200 mg per kilogram of body weight per day intravenously, in divided doses during the first 24 hours, changing to the intramuscular route as the child improves.

Foreign Body

The parents of any child presenting with cough, stridor, or dyspnea should be diligently questioned regarding possible aspiration of vomitus, food particles, buttons, toys, and the like. Plain films of the chest may demonstrate radiopaque objects, but films obtained during deep inspiration and forced expiration, as well as fluoroscopy, may be required to demonstrate partial obstruction with a nonradiopaque object. If the likelihood of this diagnosis is great, the services of a specialist trained in bronchoscopy should be immediately sought and treatment by removal carried out as soon as possible.

Acute Bronchitis

Acute bronchitis or tracheobronchitis may occur secondary to a purulent upper respiratory infection or be caused by any one of a number of viral agents. The most prominent symptom is cough, though there is usually a low-grade fever and occasionally some wheezing. Treatment is satisfactorily carried out at home in most instances with the same regimen as is utilized for croup. There is growing evidence that most cases are viral in origin; antibiotic treatment is therefore probably unnecessary.

Acute Bronchiolitis

Acute bronchiolitis is a clinical syndrome, probably of varying etiology, most commonly seen in infants under 6 months of age and rarely seen after 2 years. The presenting signs and symptoms are primarily the result of obstruction of terminal bronchioles by inflammatory edema, tenacious secretions, and bronchiolar spasm with production of dyspnea, increased respiratory rate, retraction, and an audible expiratory wheeze. Unlike the child with croup, these infants have no disturbance of phonation and no inspiratory stridor.

Since many of these infants are only mildly ill, the prime decision to be made is whether or not admission to the hospital is necessary. Mild cases may be treated at home with (1) elevation of the head of the crib; (2) humidification of the room air with a vaporizer; (3) frequent suctioning of the nose and mouth with a soft rubber bulb syringe; (4) phenylephrine nose drops as needed; (5) syrup of ipecac, 5 drops every 4 to 6 hours for infants less than 1 year old, and 10 drops for infants 1 to 2 years of age; and (6) tetracycline syrup, 20 mg per pound per day given in four divided doses by mouth, each dose followed by adequate fluids. Although many cases are of viral etiology, articles continue to appear indicating that *Haemophilus influenzae* may be the cause.

Many infants are brought to the hospital in severe distress and may be moribund on initial evaluation. In selected instances immediate bronchoscopy has been lifesaving by removing tenacious secretions and giving the physician time to utilize other therapeutic measures. Infants who are cyanotic or severely tachypneic, or who are becoming fatigued, should be promptly hospitalized and vigorously treated. A number will develop congestive heart failure, a complication which must always be watched for.

Acute Asthma Attack

The emergency treatment of an acute asthma attack will depend in great measure on what drugs have been given before the patient's arrival. The fewer the drugs previously used, the easier the plan of attack.

1. Epinephrine solution 1:1000 in doses of 0.15 ml subcutaneously for small children, 0.25 ml for larger children, is usually the first drug utilized. This may be repeated in 15 minutes.

2. If a good response is obtained with the first dose, a dose of an aqueous suspension of epinephrine in concentration of 1:200 is given (Sus-Phrine). The dose is 0.1 to 0.3 ml, depending on the weight of the patient. Relief for 8 to 12 hours is usually provided.

3. Simultaneously with the above, an oral theophylline or theophylline-ephedrine mixture should be prescribed for home use. We prefer a theophylline glyceryl guaiacolate mixture (Elixir Quibron),

one-half teaspoonful for each 10 pounds of body weight given every 8 hours.

4. Humidification of air at home is essential.

If the above measures fail to alleviate the attack, the child is probably best hospitalized so that appropriate intravenous fluids may be given and environmental factors eliminated.

Pneumonia

Although many children with pneumonia present with classic symptoms and physical findings, a large number are detected in the emergency room only after a chest film has been ordered as part of the evaluation of a febrile patient. Many are only mildly ill and may be treated adequately at home if proper follow-up is available. Some are obvious candidates for immediate admission, among them the child with pleural effusion, the child with cyanosis or severe respiratory distress, and the child with secondary cardiac failure.

The most common bacterial pneumonia in children is pneumococcal in origin and will respond to adequate penicillin therapy. For the average child this consists of 600,000 units of procaine penicillin intramuscularly in the emergency room with prescription of a dose of 200,000 to 400,000 units of phenoxymethyl penicillin by mouth every 6 hours, depending on size and age, to be taken at home for 7 to 10 days.

The child who is to be admitted should receive only supportive therapy in the emergency room pending completion of appropriate bacteriological studies. Antibiotics based on the assumed pathogenic organism may be ordered following admission.

Pneumothorax

See Chapter 3.

Other Upper Respiratory Illnesses

OTITIS MEDIA. The typical clinical findings in acute otitis media have been outlined in Chapter 17, as has the technique of myringotomy. Since many children are seen with lesser degrees of involvement, the following treatment plan is offered as a guide:

CHILDREN OVER AGE 3. Most bacterial middle ear infections in this age group are due to beta hemolytic streptococcus or pneumococcus.

For that reason, penicillin is the drug of choice. It should be given in an oral dosage of 200,000 to 400,000 units four times daily, depending on age, for 8 to 10 days. If vomiting is present, the initial dose should be 600,000 units of procaine penicillin by the intramuscular route.

Other ancillary measures include (1) aspirin for fever and pain, (2) phenylephrine nose drops every 4 hours, and (3) Auralgan solution, warmed and instilled in the affected ear every 2 hours for pain if *no* drainage is present.

CHILDREN UNDER AGE 3. Since *Haemophilus influenzae* may be etiologically responsible for as many as 20 percent of the bacterial ear infections in this age group, drug treatment must include an agent effective against it. It is therefore recommended that either of the following schedules be utilized: (1) ampicillin oral suspension, 100 mg per kilogram per day in divided doses every 6 to 8 hours for 7 to 10 days, or (2) phenoxymethyl penicillin or penicillin G, 200,000 to 400,000 units every 6 hours, in conjunction with a triple sulfa suspension in doses of 150 mg per kilogram per day in divided doses. Other ancillary measures outlined above may likewise be taken.

TONSILLITIS.   See Chapter 17.

PHARYNGITIS.   See Chapter 17.

PERITONSILLAR ABSCESS.   See Chapter 17.

Aspirin Poisoning

Any child with rapid respirations unexplained by history and physical examination should have appropriate urine and blood tests performed to detect aspirin overdosage. Blood may be sent directly for salicylate level measurement and urine may be tested with ferric chloride, which will give a burgundy color that remains after boiling. Outpatient treatment or admission will depend on salicylate level, state of hydration, and coexisting illness.

ALLERGIC EMERGENCIES

The acute asthma attack has already been discussed. Other common allergic emergencies are:

Reactions to Stinging Insects

Allergic reactions to insects vary from limited swelling at the site of the sting to a delayed type of reaction consisting of localized swelling, generalized urticaria, and angioneurotic edema. Most children who react to stings, however, will present with an immediate systemic response consisting of generalized flushing, itching, urticaria, and angioneurotic edema of the eyes, lips, hands, and feet. Severe anaphylactic reactions are infrequently seen in the pediatric age group.

Children with localized reactions may be effectively treated by removal of the stinger, if present, and application of ice packs or cold compresses to the swollen area. Children with generalized reactions should be given: (1) an injection of epinephrine hydrochloride 1:1000 subcutaneously in a dose of 0.2 to 0.5 ml depending on the size of the child; (2) an intravenous or intramuscular injection of diphenhydramine hydrochloride (Benadryl) 25 to 50 mg.

Parents should be apprised of the dangers of subsequent reactions and referred to a competent allergist for possible hyposensitization and instructions in emergency measures to be utilized at home.

Urticaria

Many children will present in the emergency ward during the warmer months of the year with urticaria of varying degrees of severity. Often the etiology is impossible to ascertain and most can be adequately treated at home as follows: (1) diphenhydramine (Benadryl Elixir), 40 to 120 mg daily, in divided doses, depending on age; (2) if considerable itching or angioneurotic edema is present, an injection of epinephrine hydrochloride 1:1000, 0.2 to 0.5 ml subcutaneously, may bring prompt relief.

CARDIAC EMERGENCIES

Congestive Heart Failure

Congestive heart failure in infancy and childhood gives predominant symptoms of acute right-sided failure, for the underlying cause is usually an acute pulmonary infection or a congenital heart defect, which places a greater strain on the right side of the heart. Examples are acute bronchiolitis, pulmonary stenosis, and left-to-right intracardiac shunts. Regardless of etiology, the emergency care is quite similar.

Classic symptoms in order of decreasing frequency are dyspnea (tachypnea), cardiomegaly, hepatomegaly, and rales. Peripheral edema is seen in only 25 percent of cases. Emergency measures include the following:

1. The patient is placed in semi-Fowler's position.
2. Oxygen is given by funnel or face mask.
3. Digitalization with lanatoside C (Cedilanid) or digoxin is started in dosage outlined below.
4. Morphine sulfate is occasionally helpful in a dosage of 1 mg per 10 pounds of body weight.
5. Diuretics may be given after admission.
6. Appropriate measures are taken to treat infection if present.

Paroxysmal Supraventricular Tachycardia

Paroxysmal supraventricular tachycardia is usually seen in the first 4 to 6 months of life. Presenting symptoms are the sudden onset of pallor or cyanosis in association with rapid respirations. Other findings are cardiac enlargement, hepatomegaly, pulmonary congestion, and a cardiac rate between 200 and 300 per minute. An electrocardiogram will confirm the cardiac rate and should demonstrate normal QRS configuration.

Treatment consists of attempts to induce vagal stimulation by the use of unilateral carotid sinus pressure or bilateral eyeball pressure. If these fail, digitalization should be carried out according to one of the schedules listed below. The route and speed of digitalization will depend upon the severity of the symptoms.

DIGITALIZATION DOSE. For rapid digitalization either lanatoside C or digoxin may be used by the intravenous or intramuscular route. The total digitalizing dose varies with age and is as follows: 0.02 to 0.03 mg per pound for infants less than 2 years; 0.01 to 0.02 mg per pound for infants over 2 years.

DIGITALIZATION SCHEDULES. Schedules for giving the drugs vary, but I have found the following two plans useful depending on the severity of the clinical situation.

Plan A 1. One-half total digitalizing dose of lanatoside C intravenously immediately.

        2. One-half total digitalizing dose of digoxin intramuscularly immediately, with direction to continue digitalization with digoxin by the intramuscular route on arrival on the ward.

Plan B 1. One-half total digitalizing dose of digoxin intramuscularly immediately.

        2. One-quarter total digitalizing dose of digoxin intramuscularly in 6 to 12 hours.

        3. One-quarter total digitalizing dose of digoxin intramuscularly in 18 to 24 hours.

Maintenance doses may be found in any standard pediatric text.

VOMITING AND DIARRHEA

Vomiting

Vomiting is an extremely common complaint during infancy and childhood. It may occur as an isolated phenomenon or be associated with any number of childhood illnesses. An adequate history, with emphasis on feeding habits and exposure to illnesses, as well as the performance of a complete physical examination, will aid in detecting underlying predisposing factors.

Acute nonspecific gastroenteritis is one of the most usual causes of vomiting in children, and to a slightly lesser degree in small infants. It is characterized by an abrupt onset and a benign course in most instances. Although the condition is self-limited, there are a number of measures which may be instituted to aid the family in coping with it.

1. Give nothing by mouth for 1 to 1½ hours.

2. Begin teaspoonful quantities of a clear liquid such as carbonated beverage every 15 minutes for 1 to 2 hours. If vomiting does not recur, the quantity may be increased to 1 to 2 tablespoonsful every 30 minutes and eventually to 1 to 2 ounces every hour.

3. Totally avoid milk and solid food for 12 to 24 hours.

4. Antiemetic drugs in suppository form are occasionally required for the child who fails to respond to the above regimen. One-half of a trimethobenzamide (Tigan) or promethazine (Phenergan)

suppository inserted rectally may be utilized prior to institution of the above regimen.

Diarrhea

Diarrhea, which usually accompanies or follows the vomiting, is a frequent cause for visits to the emergency room. The more severe and specific types of diarrhea should always be remembered, but the vast majority of young children will be found to have nonspecific diarrhea. Treatment measures may be taken after the vomiting has subsided.

1. Give clear liquids, 4 to 8 ounces every 4 hours depending on the age of the child.
2. Gradually add half-strength boiled skimmed milk, especially in small infants.
3. Maintain a bland, low-fat diet for several days afterward.
4. Selective use of antidiarrheal agents containing kaolin and related compounds is indicated in certain instances. The dose should be calculated according to the manufacturer's directions.
5. Infrequently, an antidiarrheal agent containing an antispasmodic is required for relief of crampy abdominal pain. We prefer a mixture of kaolin, pectin, and atropine (Donnagel-PG) in a dose of one-half teaspoonful for each 10 pounds of body weight every 4 hours for the first day, every 6 hours for the next day or two. Although most children with vomiting and diarrhea may be treated at home, the physician evaluating such a child must separate out those who are obviously dehydrated and in need of admission for parenteral fluid therapy.

Minor Feeding Problems

Many infants are brought to the emergency room each year because of excessive crying, excessive gas, "spitting," "colic," and the like. Since these do not, except to the parents, represent true emergencies, the physician's job is to rule out organic illness for which specific therapy is indicated.

Often infants who are otherwise healthy will regurgitate small quantities of formula or food during the first 6 months of life. In many instances reassurance to the parents that the infant is well is all that is required. Improper feeding techniques or excessive quantities of formula are other causes for discomfort and "spitting." The infant who is constipated may frequently be helped by the addition of 1 teaspoonful of Karo syrup to each bottle of formula.

DEHYDRATION—SHOCK

At the risk of oversimplification, the management of the dehydrated child will be divided. We will discuss (1) those who are in shock and are desperately ill, and (2) those who demonstrate evidence of mild to moderate dehydration.

Severe Dehydration with Shock

The general principles in management are similar to those described in Chapter 2.

1. A cutdown should be performed, with insertion of a plastic catheter into a suitable vein so that replacement therapy can be expeditiously carried out.

2. In our experience a very satisfactory fluid for starting therapy has been a 0.45% solution of sodium chloride, to which may be added additional lactate in the form of $\frac{1}{6}$ molar sodium lactate solution. Lactate should be added only when the CO_2 content of serum is below 12 mEq per liter. To raise the CO_2 content 1 mEq per liter will require 4.2 ml of $\frac{1}{6}$ molar sodium lactate per kilogram of body weight.

3. When fluid replacement therapy is started, blood should be drawn for complete blood count and blood urea nitrogen, sodium, potassium, chloride, and CO_2 content.

Mild to Moderate Dehydration

After appropriate blood studies have been obtained, children only mildly to moderately dehydrated are best handled by being given nothing by mouth and admitted to the hospital for replacement therapy.

Adrenal Insufficiency

CONGENITAL ADRENAL HYPERPLASIA. One of the common forms of adrenal insufficiency seen in pediatrics is that associated with the salt-losing variety of congenital adrenal hyperplasia. Infants with this condition present during the first 2 weeks of life with vomiting, dehydration, and rapid collapse. Survival depends on vigorous treatment on suspicion of this entity. The enzymatic defect may be confirmed at a later date in order to substantiate the diagnosis.

Females will be promptly diagnosed because of the obvious masculinization of the external genitalia present at birth. Infant males usually have normal-appearing genitalia, for the minimal increase in phallus size and pigmentation of scrotum is easily missed. This condition should be considered in any infant male presenting with severe dehydration or with a clinical picture compatible with pyloric stenosis. Treatment is as follows:

1. Intravenous fluids consisting of 0.85% saline or 10% glucose in normal saline solution.
2. Plasma, 5 ml per kilogram of body weight.
3. Hydrocortisone, 1.5 mg per kilogram intravenously, immediately.
4. Deoxycorticosterone in oil, 2 mg per kilogram intramuscularly, immediately.
5. Admission to a hospital as soon as the above have been carried out.

WATERHOUSE-FRIDERICHSEN SYNDROME. See Fever, page 354.

ABDOMINAL PAIN

Most parents who bring a child with abdominal pain to the emergency room do so suspecting acute appendicitis. In the great majority of cases this diagnosis will not be substantiated, but any one of a large number of extra-abdominal conditions amenable to nonsurgical therapy will be implicated. Acute gastroenteritis, otitis media, tonsillitis, and pneumonia are frequently accompanied by abdominal pain and may be readily diagnosed by thorough examination and minimal laboratory study. Urinary tract infections are common in pediatrics, and no emergency-room evaluation of a child with abdominal pain or fever is complete without a urinalysis.

In the neonatal period, milk intolerance or improper feeding technique is frequently blamed. Intussusception must always be remembered, especially in the 3- to 12-month age group. In many instances an emergency barium enema will be indicated to establish or rule out this diagnosis.

On occasion the parent's suspicion will be confirmed; however, acute rheumatic fever must not be overlooked as it is most prevalent in the same age group in which appendicitis occurs. Only on direct questioning will the fleeting complaints of arthralgia be mentioned and the cardiac murmur take on significance.

COMA

This section will serve primarily to point out differences in etiology, evaluation, and treatment of coma in the pediatric age group. Emphasis will be placed on common causes and on initial supportive therapy.

Common Causes of Coma

Only with an appreciation of the common causes of coma in this age group can one proceed with a logical investigation. Many standard supportive measures are applicable to all cases, but suspected etiology will markedly influence the choice of diagnostic studies in most instances.

TRAUMA. Head injury is one of the most frequent causes of loss of consciousness in children. Careful examination will generally enable detection of the site of injury, following which a brief evaluation to determine the severity must be made. Management is expectant except in the child with a penetrating skull fracture or in whom there is evidence of a progressing lesion such as an epidural or subdural hematoma.

CONVULSIVE OR POSTCONVULSIVE STATES. Inasmuch as 5 to 6 percent of all children will experience at least one seizure during the first decade of life, this condition must always be considered. Initial examination may reveal a transient localized paralysis of muscle groups, but pupillary reaction is usually normal. Appropriate studies to determine the underlying cause must be carried out.

INTOXICATION. Accidental ingestion of drugs and various toxic agents available in any household continues to account for an appreciable number of children presenting in the emergency room in an unconscious state. Substances which may produce convulsions and/or coma are barbiturates, phenothiazines, salicylate, antihistamines, alcohol, central nervous system stimulants, parathion and other organic phosphate insecticides, hydrocarbons, and a host of others. Specifics concerning diagnosis and treatment are outlined in Chapter 18.

LEAD ENCEPHALOPATHY. Lead intoxication is mentioned separately because convulsions and coma occur only after a prolonged period of chronic lead ingestion. This condition should always be considered in the 1- to 4-year age group, especially in children residing in the older section of a city. Lead encephalopathy is encountered more frequently in the spring and summer when exposure to increased sunlight results in greater gastrointestinal absorption of lead.

INFECTION. Severe infections, either generalized or limited to the central nervous system, are seen with reasonable frequency in any busy emergency room. Meningitis, encephalitis, and overwhelming sepsis have been discussed previously. The possibility of a brain abscess must be seriously considered in any child with cyanotic congenital heart disease who presents with an unexplained convulsion or with coma.

METABOLIC DISORDER. Of the various metabolic disorders resulting in coma, severe fluid and electrolyte imbalance, diabetes mellitus, and hypoglycemia warrant consideration and appropriate studies to rule them in or out.

Supportive Measures

Before a definitive diagnosis is established, a number of supportive measures will be required and should include the following:

1. Establishment and maintenance of an adequate airway and adequate air exchange.
2. Provision of oxygen by face mask or catheter.
3. Control of any frank blood loss.
4. Maintenance of normal body temperature.
5. Gastric lavage.
6. Appropriate intravenous fluids to correct shock and dehydration.
7. Appropriate selection, on the basis of preliminary examination,

of those tests most likely to aid in establishing a definite diagnosis.

Emergency Laboratory Evaluation

Because of the life-threatening nature of most conditions resulting in coma, preliminary investigation must be carried out as rapidly as possible once the supportive measures have been instituted. The laboratory procedures required in a given case will depend to a great extent on history and the impression gained from preliminary examination. Tests to be considered include the following:

1. Blood, for sugar, electrolytes, blood urea nitrogen, calcium, and phosphorus content.
2. Blood, for complete blood count and platelet count and for screening for basophilic stippling.
3. Blood, for typing, cross matching, and culture.
4. Blood, for salicylate, barbiturate, or lead level when these conditions are likely.
5. Urine, for sugar, albumin, and acetone content and microscopic examination.
6. Urine, for testing with ferric chloride to detect the presence of salicylates or phenothiazine derivatives.
7. Urine, for detecting coproporphyrins when lead poisoning is suspected.
8. Analysis of gastric aspirate when intoxication is suspected.
9. Lumbar puncture, in absence of papilledema, when meningitis, encephalitis, or lead poisoning is suspected. Lumbar puncture may be safely performed in a child with lead encephalopathy after initial neurosurgical evaluation.
10. Neurological and neurosurgical consultation.
11. Films of the wrists and knees for lead line if lead poisoning is suspected.

Definitive Treatment

The definitive treatment of a number of the entities producing coma have been previously discussed in this or a preceding chapter. A few comments will be made concerning therapy in children, which differs greatly from therapy in an adult.

DIABETIC ACIDOSIS. After appropriate studies have confirmed the presence of diabetic acidosis, the following measures are suggested:

1. Intravenous 0.85% saline solution at a rate of 350 ml per square meter of body surface area per hour for the first 24 hours.
2. Initial dose of crystalline insulin in a total of 2 units per kilogram of body weight, one-half intravenously and one-half subcutaneously.
3. Admission to ward for continued treatment.

POISONING. Before the child with lead encephalopathy is transferred to the ward, a 30% solution of urea in a dose of 1 gm per kilogram of body weight should be started and continued at a rate of 150 to 200 ml per hour. Sedation may be required if seizures are a problem.

CONVULSIONS

Febrile Convulsions

Febrile convulsions are the most common form of seizure in children seen in the average emergency room. They usually occur between 6 months and 4 years of age in association with an acute febrile illness. Certain criteria have been established to define simple febrile convulsions, and these should be adhered to. The seizures should be of brief duration in a previously healthy child in the above-mentioned age group. There are usually no postictal phenomena, and an electroencephalogram after the illness has subsided should be normal.

Treatment usually consists of appropriate antipyretic measures in addition to treatment of the underlying infectious process. The seizure will be over by the time the child arrives, but phenobarbital, 15 mg every 6 hours, should be prescribed for the remainder of the febrile illness. Most infants seen following their first febrile convulsion should have a lumbar puncture to rule out acute bacterial meningitis.

Nonfebrile Convulsions

Since there are a great many causes for nonfebrile seizures in infancy and childhood, the concern of the emergency-room physician will be primarily to arrest the seizure and to make the necessary arrangements for admission and diagnostic evaluation. The following is a rough outline for initial care:

1. An adequate airway must be maintained.
2. Sodium phenobarbital is given intramuscularly in a dose of 60 mg per year of age up to 3 years, 200 mg for a 4-year-old, and 240 mg for the child over 5 years of age. Half this dose may be repeated in 30 minutes if seizures persist. The most common cause of failure to control seizures is the use of an *inadequate initial dose.*
3. An alternative form of therapy that is very effective is intramuscular paraldehyde 1.5 ml per 10 pounds of body weight with a repeat of half this dose in 30 minutes. Paraldehyde must be given by deep intramuscular injection to avoid a slough.
4. Oxygen by funnel or face mask may be needed.
5. Suctioning of secretions is done as needed.
6. Intravenous fluids are administered.
7. Any underlying predisposing condition, such as drug ingestion, lead intoxication, fluid and electrolyte imbalance, and so forth, is treated.

Psychiatric Emergencies

23

JULES S. GOLDEN

A. M. MARCHIONNE

The vast majority of people function within social, familial, psychological, and physiological systems. For practically all individuals there is some disorder, either within these various biological and social fields, or at their interfaces. Such turbulence may be of diverse quality and severity, but generally the feelings, thinking, and behavior of the population are not deemed so remarkable that professional appraisal is requested or professionals see it as their role to intervene.

In appraising a patient in the emergency room, be alert to current situational problems or deficits. What are the circumstances or events that have led an individual to seek help, or to identify himself or be identified by others as suffering a psychiatric disorder? What apparent social, familial, behavioral, or physiological change or culmination of changes has emerged that an individual now presents with a loss of psychological equilibrium?

Conversely, it may be equally important to identify various strengths or assets. What have been the patient's adaptive patterns and relations with others that have permitted him to function in and with the community thus far?

Finally, what in the overall situation suggests intervention? In the balance, how desirable, imperative, and extensive need it be? Reassurance about how well things seem to be going, despite problems, may be the patient's and the family's need. In emergency

371

rooms as elsewhere, health professionals increasingly deal with re-inforcing health and well-being rather than single-mindedly stamp-ing out disease.

This chapter attempts to define as brief a psychiatric evaluation and therapeutic engagement as the nature of the presenting dis-order and good practice permits.

RAPID APPRAISAL OF PSYCHIATRIC DISORDER

General Objectives

Effectiveness in caring for disturbed patients is well served if initial efforts are directed to answering certain key questions:

1. What are the vital signs and the gross neurological status?
2. Can the patient himself give minimal identifying data, define what is troubling him, and say to what he attributes his troubles?
3. Is the patient a danger to himself or others?
4. With whom else is it necessary or desirable to communicate about the patient and the apparent disturbance?
5. Can the emergency-room personnel influence members of the family, friends, or authorities, in order to alleviate or lessen stress on the patient?
6. What therapy, observation, or confinement, if any, is desirable or imperative? Does it appear feasible to avoid hospitalization, yet avert more severe disorder subsequent to the emergency-room visit?

Answers to the first five questions may directly affect the sixth.

Technique of Examination

Psychiatric evaluation depends upon effective communication with the patient or those who accompany him.

The initial questions to the patient, which may be specific and direct, establish the level of alertness and crucial identifying data: "What is your full name?" "How old are you?" "Your marital sta-tus?" "What work do you do?" "Where and with whom are you living at the present time?"

Then, paradoxically, the history and mental status are most often quickly and easily obtained through "open-ended" questions that begin with words like *what* and *how:* "How is it that you are here?" "What about thoughts or attempts to injure yourself?" Questions such as "Do you wish to commit suicide?" "You don't wish to kill yourself, do you?" are likely to inhibit communication of the patient's feelings by evoking monosyllabic responses. The direct question that begs a yes or a no answer may heighten fears of the consequences of revealing thoughts or put dangerously misleading responses into the patient's mouth. This applies in questioning others about the patient, as well.

Chief Complaints and Present Illness

Many psychiatric patients seen in the emergency room suffer an exacerbation or culmination of a long-standing disorder. If the patient's symptoms are a distinct departure from the premorbid personality, even if vital signs are essentially normal, the mental aberrations may well be the presenting signs of a primarily medical rather than psychiatric emergency—e.g., meningitis, aortic endocarditis, porphyria, brain tumor or abscess, head injury, and so forth —that may require direct questioning, neurological examination, blood-level measurements and cultures, urine analyses, spinal tap, and so forth. Interruption of the psychiatric examination per se may be imperative. Inordinate rage reactions or threats of violence require comprehensive neurological and psychiatric evaluation before the patient is released.

For patients able to communicate, initial questions concerning identification are followed by "What problems bring you to the emergency room?" Almost as routinely the next remark by the physician may be "Tell me more about . . ." or "What about . . ." the problems enumerated. In relation to the present illness the physician asks, "What are things like at home?" "What are things like at work?"

Only now does he ask, *"For how long* have you had these problems?" *"What* has happened recently, in any way, that things are worse for you?"

Past History

Begin with "How many times have you been in hospitals for problems before this?" Also, "What other troubled times have you had?" If there are positive answers, "What happened in the past when you had these problems?" and "What kinds of treatment did you have in the past; where; and for how long?" "With what results?"

For a brief survey of other significant illnesses, ask "What sicknesses or accidents have you had in the past that required treatment or hospitalization?" "What recent illnesses or accidents have you suffered?" Always: "What medicine have you been taking recently or in the last months?"

Questions on drug use are imperative to ask of the under-thirty age group: *"What drugs* have you taken today and in the last month?" *"When have you last* used marijuana ('grass'), LSD ('acid'), amphetamines or pep pills ('speed'), or any other drugs?" If responded to positively, "How often and how much?"

Since there are many preparations and combinations of drugs in use, and many present bizarre mental and neurological pictures, regardless of the reported preparation, ask "When you have (or he has) had such a reaction or a bad trip, what usually is effective in bringing you (or him) down?" (See Treatment of Drug-Induced Aberrations, later in this chapter.)

Some Options

(See also other headings in this chapter as noted below.)

On the basis of findings thus far, the patient or the history may give indications of the following:

ACUTE MEDICAL, SURGICAL, OR NEUROLOGICAL DISORDER. Do requisite physical and laboratory examinations and procedures first, and then if the mental status and behavior of the patient remain a problem refer to this chapter. (In most medical disorders phenothiazines are not contraindicated. See Drug Therapy, also When to Hospitalize.)

PRIMARILY A DRUG REACTION OR BAD TRIP. Defer rest of examination temporarily, and see Treatment of Drug-Induced Aberrations. For ingestion of poisons and overdoses see Chapter 18.

PRIMARILY A PSYCHIATRIC DISORDER. For the patient apparently suffering a psychiatric disorder or emotional crisis, continue to Mental Status and Target Symptoms.

COMMON PROBLEMS IN LIVING. For a patient who is not unduly distressed over a definable common problem in living, e.g., marital disorder, work problems, and so forth, consider the approach under Emergency Room Supportive Psychotherapy, or continue with examination for Mental Status and Target Symptoms.

NEED FOR REFERRAL. For the patient who clearly has appeared because he is unaware of another more appropriate therapy resource, and also perhaps is testing whether he is accepted by others despite his problems before seeking help elsewhere, see Referring Patients.

Mental Status and Target Symptoms

The examination of the patient thus far generally reveals (1) general appearance and orderliness of attire; (2) rate of speech (retardation or pressure of speech), distractability, and any inappropriateness of behavior; (3) adequacy of memory, level of alertness, and ability to communicate coherently; (4) general level of intellectual functioning; and (5) willingness and ability to relate and cooperate.

Asking the patient several proverbs, "What does this saying mean to you?" e.g., "You can't tell a book by its cover?" and also *"What if* you saw a letter on the ground that was addressed, sealed, and had an uncanceled stamp?" may reveal unsuspected concreteness of thinking (organicity, psychotic trends) or antisocial attitudes.

The remainder of the examination may now be directed at considering the following signs or symptoms and assessing just how prominent, disabling, or dangerous those that are present may actually be.

DEPRESSION. Regardless of the presenting problems, a careful appraisal of depressive trends and suicidal risk is essential for *every* patient. Ask "With the troubles you have told me about, just how down in the dumps, blue, or depressed have you been or are you now?" (If the question is posed, "You don't get depressed, do you?" many patients will say, "No, I don't" even though they may be suicidal.) Then, "Everybody has ups and downs in moods or feelings. What is it like when you are at your worst?" An easy approach to suicide is, "Practically everyone at some time has feelings he would be better off dead or has thoughts of suicide. What about yours?" If the answer is, "I think about it but I wouldn't do it because (1) I am too much of a coward, (2) it is against my religion, (3) I couldn't do it to my family," in the absence of previous suicidal attempts it is a reasonable assumption that the patient is not currently a significant suicidal risk.

If the patient has suicidal ideation, inquire, "What plans have you made?" and "What alternatives do you see to ending it all?" If the patient (1) has specific plans, (2) sees no alternative to suicide, (3) has made previous attempts, or (4) has a family history of suicide, he must be considered a danger to himself. In particular, if the patient (1) contemplates or has used firearms or hanging as a method, (2) reveals recent writing of or change of a will, (3) has bought a burial plot, (4) has written a note indicating disposition of his remains and effects, prospects for suicide are ominous (and hospitalization probably imperative). There is a greater risk, statistically, if the patient is separated or divorced, has remained single, or lives alone [3]. (Phone calls from or about patients threatening suicide should be evaluated in the same light. Many patients make last-minute efforts to communicate their intentions. Police or hospital ambulances *immediately directed to the scene* save lives. Meanwhile, if possible, keep the patient on the phone to delay an attempt.)

RETARDATION. Retardation is generally obvious, as manifested by a crouched position, unhappy expression, slow bodily movement, slow speech, and paucity of thoughts.

CATATONIA. The catatonic patient often presents himself as immobile. His limbs can be moved, but he will not move voluntarily. He may say nothing, although he is aware of what is going on about him.

PARANOIA. Some patients readily reveal paranoid ideation. Ask all others, "With the troubles you have, to what extent are things in life stacked up against you?" "How much do people notice you or talk about you?" "To what extent are people out to get you?"

DELUSIONS. The acutely delusional or psychotic patient is more likely to be brought by others than to seek help himself. Unless obviously delusional, ask all patients, "What is the strangest thing that has happened to you recently?" "To what extent do parts of your body feel different, detached, or do things seem different to you?" "Many people in a storm hear their names called when no one is there. What experiences like this have you had?" "Some people believe that others control their thoughts or actions. How about you?"

CONFUSION, DELIRIUM, OR AMNESIA. Confusion or delirium may be due to toxicity, drugs, brain damage, temporal lobe seizures, acute psychoses, and so forth. Etiology may not be obvious, but the preceding questioning should make the degree of confusion or presence of delirium evident. Amnesia due to fugue states and the like requires psychiatric and perhaps police consultation.

ANXIETY AND AGITATION. Patients can suffer severe anxiety, yet not convey it in their demeanor or expression. There may or may not be gross physiological reactions; the pulse may, for example, be normal. A patient can appear anxious and show physiological alterations and not seem fully aware of his distress.

The patient of particular concern, however, is frankly agitated. He cannot sit still, complains of unbearable tension, and often cannot relate these feelings to environmental pressures.

HYPOMANIA. The hypomanic patient expresses a sense of well-being, sees no reason for being in the emergency room, usually talks incessantly, changes the subject frequently, and does not sit still. Hypomania need not be obvious, but heed the family's report.

HOSTILITY, AND HOMICIDAL TENDENCIES. The hostile patient is most often brought by others. By questioning others, the physician must ascertain "Just how threatening has he been?" "What has he actually done?" Dangerous patients generally are somewhat paranoid, have a chip-on-the-shoulder attitude, or have frank delusions of persecution. (Many persons who have committed premeditated murder, however, are meek and docile.) Patients under the influence of alcohol, even small amounts, can be dangerously assaultive.

Ask all patients, "With the troubles you have, what about feelings of harming someone else?" A positive answer requires asking "What are the feelings, against whom, and why?" and "What about wishes to kill someone?"

Impulsive aggression is inferred from history, recent scrapes with the law, fights, or other ill-considered behavior. If it seems indicated, ask, "How much trouble have you had with the police?"

Many patients express fear of injuring others, but without a history of actual violence such action is unlikely. (The woman who has an obsession that she will injure her child should be reassured, but also referred for further help.)

SOCIOPATHIC BEHAVIOR. Sociopathic patients may be brought by family or authorities for various transgressions but act cooperatively, suavely, or with frank hostility. From their own story alone it may be difficult to detect sociopathic trends. Be wary of the patient who comes for drug prescriptions or other secondary gain. (Sociopathic behavior does not exclude suicidal risk.)

HYPOCHONDRIASIS. History of repeated negative examinations for numerous or persistent physical complaints is characteristic. Peculiar complaints—odd responses to "To what extent do parts of your body feel different?"—with agitation suggest onset of acute psychosis.

INSOMNIA OR ANOREXIA. Ask each patient, "How much sleep have you been getting?" "How about frightening dreams?" "What about recent gain or loss of weight?" Diminished sleep, frequent nightmares, or rapid changes of weight often are prodromes of acute psychosis.

INSIGHT. If the patient's awareness that he is disturbed appears lacking, ask "With all the problems you have told me about, just how disturbed or mixed-up do you feel you really are?"

IMPRESSIONS AND TREATMENT

With the exception of the diagnosing of an organic or drug reaction that may require specific and immediate treatment, the primary concern in the emergency room is *not the specification of an etiology but the evaluation of the general degree of disturbance, psychologically and socially*. Can the patient return after the emergency-room visit to his environment, and under what circumstances? The presence or absence of certain symptoms, however, indicates urgent care. The presence or absence of others suggests minimal involvement by emergency-room staff. Certain guide lines are here presented, but ultimately disposition must rest on the judgment of the concerned staff. Also, the consultative and special services available in the particular hospital or the community may be a factor.

When to Hospitalize

DEPRESSION AND SUICIDAL BEHAVIOR. If the patient is severely depressed, reveals previous suicide attempts, or shows more than casual suicidal ideation, immediate hospitalization with constant observation is generally imperative.

Depression may be related to difficult life situations, be without apparent provocation, or be a side effect or sequela of various medications and drugs, e.g., rauwolfia compounds, amphetamines, corticoids, contraceptive medications, and LSD. Of primary importance is not the presumed etiology but the depth of the depression and suicidal drive.

The emergency room is a dangerous place for the depressed person. Scalpels and other potentially lethal implements are everywhere in abundance. The patient must be kept physically separated from what may not appear to be obvious danger. A person may regard coming to the emergency room as a psychiatric patient a uniquely disgraceful or humiliating experience and hence be prompted to make an attempt on his own life.

Psychiatric patients requiring emergency-room surgery must have their limbs firmly bound and immobilized to prevent their seizing a scalpel and committing suicide. A gentle but firm approach, telling the patient what is being done and why, is always indicated. Also, an attendant must be watching the patient without interruption. Emotionally disturbed persons can show a totally unexpected and phenomenal strength at a moment's notice. It is well to be particularly wary of the apparently semiconscious patient who has made a recent suicidal effort.

DELUSIONS AND CONFUSION. The patient who is acutely delusional or confused generally requires immediate hospitalization, particularly if his delusion shows a persecutory or paranoid content. (Paranoid delusions are frequent sequelae of amphetamines.)

AGITATION, RETARDATION, CATATONIA, DELIRIUM, AND HYPOMANIA. The patient who is clearly retarded, agitated, delirious, or catatonic needs hospitalization. For the hypomanic patient, although he may try to talk his way out of it, hospitalization is usually essential. If the hypomanic patient is told to return at a later time, it is unlikely that he will, and *in a short time he may do untold damage to himself or others.*

WEIGHT LOSS AND INSOMNIA. Patients who indicate a rapid weight loss or increasing lack of sleep with even minimal signs of mental aberration, such as looseness of association or paranoid trends, should be considered for hospitalization, in order that they may be studied and an onset of a more frank psychosis prevented. Users of amphetamines, "STP," and "DMT" may show insomnia and weight loss, and be euphoric and unmindful of it.

ANXIETY, HYPOCHONDRIASIS, PARANOIA, AND HOSTILITY. Hospitalization is likely only to aggravate the disturbance of patients who show themselves as somewhat anxious, hypochondriacal, suspicious, paranoid, or hostile, but not delusional or homicidal.

HISTRIONIC, MANIPULATIVE, OR SOCIOPATHIC BEHAVIOR, OR NARCOTICS ADDICTION. Unless the organic condition or serious depression makes hospital care necessary, such patients should not be admitted to other than special-treatment units.

How to Hospitalize

The physician will be most effective if his approach is kindly but firm. He should not equivocate.

VOLUNTARY ADMISSION. The patient with insight may be asked, "How do you feel about coming into the hospital?" If he objects, then, "I feel it is of the *utmost importance that you enter the hospital now.*" The suicidal, agitated, or acutely delusional patient is told, "It is *necessary* that you come into the hospital *now.*" If he is willing, he himself should *at this time* sign any forms required by state law or the hospital for *voluntary admission and treatment* of a mental disorder. When electroshock treatment is utilized (the treatment of choice for the severely depressed, suicidal, and often the acutely psychotic and hypomanic), forms granting permission for electroshock therapy should also be signed. All forms should be duly witnessed by a hospital employee.

INVOLUNTARY ADMISSION. Nearest of kin, if present, should be informed immediately of the physician's intention; if not present, he should be contacted by phone. Depending on a particular state's laws and the hospital's policy, the relatives should sign various forms, duly witnessed, indicating permission or request for hospitalization and treatment. Again, signing for electroshock is best accomplished at this time.

The frankly suicidal, homicidal, or acutely psychotic patient, depending on a particular state's laws, can be involuntarily confined for limited periods of time. Sometimes enlisting the aid of county health officers and the police is necessary to effect such confinement. It may be legal to admit, sedate, and seclude mentally deranged patients against their will, but treatment may be possible only after a court-directed hearing. (With others, if hospitalization is declined but not deemed essential, there should be secured from the patient or next of kin a signed statement that release is against medical advice.)

TYPE OF HOSPITALIZATION. Hospitalization may be possible on the hospital psychiatric ward or, lacking such facility, on a non-psychiatric service, preferably in a private or semiprivate room with constant observation by an experienced nurse or, if this is not feasible, by attendants or family members; otherwise immediate transfer to a hospital with psychiatric facilities may be necessary.

THE PROCRASTINATING PATIENT. Many patients say, "I will enter the hospital, but let me go after my things or make arrangements for my family." Such arrangements are tasks for the family, social service, or community agencies. A hemorrhaging patient would not be permitted to go home for his toothbrush; it may be just as catastrophic to let a psychiatric patient leave the emergency room if the physician concludes that hospitalization is urgent.

THE RESISTIVE PATIENT. If there is the slightest suspicion that the patient will flee or physically resist necessary confinement, *at least* three or four able-bodied staff or other personnel should stand by when it is explained to the patient that he is ill and is to be hospitalized. Some patients will become assaultive if only one or two staff members are present, but sufficient personnel, just by their presence, enhance cooperation. The staff should not leave if at first the patient cooperates until the patient is heavily sedated, because the few remaining may then be dangerously assaulted.

For the patient who threatens to be or actually becomes assaultive, intravenous amobarbital sodium (Sodium Amytal), 0.5 gm (7½ grains) well diluted (20 ml), is the drug of choice, provided there is no indication that the patient has already imbibed a potentiating or respiratory-depressant drug. The intravenous injection should be already prepared when a potentially resistive patient is informed he will be confined. Injection should be administered as slowly as feasible (several minutes) and the minimum amount that sufficiently quiets the patient given. When it is deemed necessary, a larger dose should be used with caution. Chlorpromazine, 50 mg or 100 mg intramuscularly, may be an alternative, but is slower to act.

Despite frank psychotic behavior, patients are generally more cooperative immediately and subsequently if they are told what is intended; otherwise they may distrust the staff because they feel they have been "tricked" into admission.

THE PATIENT WHO FLEES. If a psychotic or suicidal patient runs from the emergency room, it is necessary to recruit any help available while following him. Then, his arms and legs are firmly grasped, unneeded bystanders are dismissed, and the patient is carried back for confinement or sedation. At such times, by giving sharp, explicit orders to anyone who hesitates in doing his bidding, the physician can usually avert a potentially dangerous situation.

THE CRIMINAL OFFENDER. If the patient has reportedly committed a serious offense, or if he threatens to do so, state law or the safety of others may make it imperative that police authorities be immediately advised of the situation regardless of the decision concerning the need for hospital care.

If the police bring a patient who allegedly has committed an offense, it may be necessary to allow an officer to stand guard, but routine emergency-room procedures should not be altered. *Any* information about the patient should not be made available to the authorities without the approval of the hospital administration. The patient should not be interrogated by the police in the emergency room. Relatives can be informed of the patient's physical and mental condition.

TRANSFERRING AND TRANSPORTING PATIENTS

Transfer to Another Hospital from the Emergency Room

If appropriate facilities are not locally available, take the following measures: (1) *Phone the other hospital* to describe the patient and make certain that he will be accepted on arrival. (2) Inform the patient (unless violence is a threat) and family of reasons for transfer. (3) Be certain necessary forms are properly prepared that must accompany the patient (commitment papers, and so forth) and a copy of emergency-room findings and reasons for transfer. (4) *Sedate patient.* If there is a history of violent behavior or threat of violent behavior, for a trip of up to 1 hour intramuscular or intravenous sodium amytal, from 0.25 to 1 gm, may suffice. For longer journeys, chlorpromazine, 50 to 100 mg intramuscularly, may suffice; but in very resistive and excited patients, combining the two medications may be necessary. (5) Transfer in an ambulance if the patient is not fully cooperative. More than one attendant may be necessary if the patient has been violent and effective restraints are not available. (6) A staff woman (nurse) or family member should accompany women patients. (7) Travel at an hour when it is unlikely traffic will cause undue delays.

How to Bring Acutely Disturbed Patients to the Emergency Room

The emergency room may receive queries about such situations. (1) For a patient who has ingested a drug with suicidal intent, or a disturbed but cooperative patient, use the most readily available vehicle, e.g., a taxi. (2) For an aggressive or potentially dangerous patient, use the police, or, if necessary, the rescue squad or voluntary firemen, to diminish likelihood of injuries. (3) The hospital may have its own ambulance service available.

DRUG THERAPY

Choice of drug, dosage, and route of administration are largely dependent on the degree of disturbance rather than the type of disorder. With the exception of the phenothiazines—chlorpromazine (Thorazine), thioridazine (Mellaril), trifluoperazine (Stelazine), prochlorperazine (Compazine), and so forth—most other ataractic drugs are potentially habit-forming or addicting, and only sufficient medication for the immediate situation should be prescribed. For the emergency room, without provision for routine follow-up, the suggested drugs are deliberately few and deemed relatively safe.

Control of Severe Disturbance

Amobarbital sodium (Sodium Amytal) 0.25 to 1 gm may be administered, slowly, intravenously, to the *severely depressed* or *agitated* patient, the patient deemed *suicidal,* the *acutely psychotic* patient, and the *hypomanic* or *manic* patient to expedite hospitalization (as discussed under How to Hospitalize, above) or transfer in an ambulance to another facility. Attendants and proper restraints may be essential for transporting patients for any distance in a vehicle, but, as shown below, phenothiazines by mouth or intramuscularly may effectively tranquilize for several hours.

Moderately Severe Disorder

For the moderately *anxious, agitated, panicky* patient and the *delusional, paranoid,* and *hypomanic* patient, current drugs of choice are the phenothiazine tranquilizers. Chlorpromazine or thioridazine, 25 mg by mouth is the usual dosage, but as high as 50 mg can be given to adult patients without undue concern, and prescriptions can be given for sufficient tablets (25 mg up to 100 mg four times a day) until psychiatric consultation can be arranged. If such tranquilizers have been prescribed previously with good result, but the patient has failed to take medication, give the dose reported effective previously immediately and *insist on resumption of medication at previous levels* [4].

For the more disturbed, 100 mg of chlorpromazine—or, when the response to the drug is already well known, 200 mg—can be given by mouth if the patient can be observed for several hours in a reclining position, or if he can return home and be given the medication and remain in bed under observation for 5 or 6 hours. (Chlorpromazine may also be used to expedite transportation.)

Patients who complain of drowsiness on receiving chlorpromazine and do not appear overactive can be given trifluoperazine, 2 mg to 5 mg by mouth during daytime hours, and a prescription for additional tablets to be taken, one on awakening in the morning and a second in the early afternoon. (The dose of chlorpromazine should be reduced 25 mg for every 2 mg of trifluoperazine.)

Patients should be warned against (1) driving until they have become accustomed to these drugs and (2) any prolonged exposure to the sun. They should be routinely told to phone the emergency room should there be untoward effects.

Acute Anxiety, Agitation, Excitement

When hospitalization is not necessary or feasible, the *acutely anxious, agitated,* or *excited patient,* and the patient who shows these signs or *aggressiveness as a reaction to alcohol,* should be given chlorpromazine 50 to 100 mg intramuscularly, *but should be observed for at least one hour* for a precipitate fall in blood pressure or other untoward physical reaction. The excited patient who requires transportation likewise may receive intramuscular chlorpromazine.

Mild to Moderate Depression

The mildly to moderately *depressed* patient should not be given barbiturates, meprobamate, or amphetamines. Administration of "antidepressant drugs," monamine oxidase inhibitors, and so forth, by the nonpsychiatrist in the emergency room is considered by the authors a risky procedure, potentially precipitating a psychotic reaction or dangerous physical side effects. The mildly to moderately depressed patient can be given trifluoperazine safely, 2 mg by mouth immediately and 2 mg morning and early afternoon each day, until a psychiatric consultation can be arranged or the patient can be referred to a physician in the community experienced in the treatment of depression. The intravenous use of drugs for the rapid relief of depression remains the domain of the expert.

Mild to Moderate Anxiety, Hypochondriasis, or Hostility

Chlordiazepoxide (Librium), 10 mg to start with, and then 10 mg four times a day, can be safely given to the *mildly anxious, hostile,* or *hypochondriacal* patient. The moderately anxious, hostile, or hypochondriacal patient can be given 25-mg doses, but he must be warned of slowed responses and directed not to drive a car. (If medication for more than several days is indicated, trifluoperazine, 2 mg morning and early afternoon, should be substituted, to avoid possible drug habituation.)

Insomnia, Weight Change

Chloral hydrate, 100 mg (several capsules only), can be prescribed for *insomnia.* Referral to an outside physician or clinic may be indicated for this or rapid *change in weight,* if it is not so severe as to require hospitalization.

Conversion Reaction

Amobarbital sodium may be utilized to promote a hypnoid state in the emergency room to relieve conversion symptoms or make a differential disgnosis between *hysterical neurosis* and neurological disorder, *but this procedure should be undertaken by a psychiatrist or neurologist.* Inexperienced handling of the amobarbital interview may precipitate an apparently neurotic patient into a frank and dangerous psychosis! The differential diagnosis or relief of symptoms can generally await a specialist's consultation.

Sociopathic, Histrionic, Manipulative

The *sociopathic, histrionic,* or *manipulative* patient is best denied medication. Trifluoperazine, 2 mg twice a day (enough for several days), however, is not contraindicated for relief of tension or depression.

Acutely Psychotic

The excited or acutely *psychotic* patient who requires higher than the above suggested doses of phenothiazines for tranquilization is probably a candidate for immediate hospitalization.

PALLIATIVE EMERGENCY-ROOM CARE AND REFERRALS

The Mildly to Moderately Anxious or Depressed, and the Chronically Delusional

Many patients will appreciably benefit from the opportunity to tell an attentive professional person of their difficulties. Among these are (1) the mildly or moderately depressed patient, (2) the chronically but mildly delusional patient suffering a moderate exacerbation of symptoms, (3) the mildly hysterical patient or one with hysteroid symptoms, (4) the anxious patient, and (5) the hypochondriacal patient who does not have somatic delusions or is not in a panic.

The patient can be told with good effect, "I understand why you have come for help. It seems to me, from (the examination and) what you have told me, that things will work out. There is no need in my opinion for you to be admitted to the hospital. I can give you some medication that is helpful, but I wonder if you feel you really need it?" Generally, do not give medication if the patient states that he can do without it—he may feel much relieved and improved because the doctor believes he is not so disturbed that medication is necessary—unless it appears important in order to avert further and more severe exacerbation of disturbance.

The delusional patient should be asked what medication has helped him in the past, and this or a phenothiazine can be prescribed. He can be encouraged to take it for a time until he is less troubled.

Depending on the facilities available, the patient can be told, "If you feel the need for help later: (1) you can call one of the following mental hygiene or psychiatric clinics; (2) you can call a practicing psychiatrist from the following list; or (3) you can always phone us or come to the emergency room again." Paradoxically, for many patients, assurance that help is available at any time is a major factor in allaying the anxieties or panic that provoke further calls for emergency help; hence, this invitation usually reduces the incidence of return visits.

Referring Patients

Some patients come to emergency rooms seeking acceptance and referral because of problems that require special mental health services, but do not know where else to go. After evaluation, the patient can be informed of available resources, and how to use them. A list of resources in a particular community, approved by the hospital administration, to which patients may be referred, will be of value. It is well to assure the patient that he can call the emergency room should he have difficulty getting other help, or in the interim until he can be seen elsewhere. Giving the patient this assurance is apt to decrease rather than promote unnecessary return visits.

The Recidivist Patient

The patient who repeatedly visits the emergency room should be referred for psychiatric consultation. If visits relate to antisocial behavior, proper disposition may be the realm of civil or police authorities. The manipulative or exploitative patient who does not require emergency care can be told that examination shows that the emergency room is not the appropriate place for his problems, and if he wishes he must seek help elsewhere.

Symptoms Following Trauma

Psychiatric symptoms subsequent to accidents, whether or not physical trauma is sustained (anxiety, phobias, startle reaction, nightmares, persistent inexplicable pains, and so forth), indicate prompt psychiatric referral [5].

EMERGENCY-ROOM SUPPORTIVE PSYCHOTHERAPY

Common Problems in Living

Patients who present with a problem in living—e.g., marital difficulties, problems at work—but do not show signs of appreciable physical or emotional distress, may not require the routine approach already described and, to a greater or lesser extent, it may be abridged. Depending on time and inclination, such patients may be encouraged simply to elaborate on their problems and life circumstances.

Often, acknowledging *the positive* in the past may do well to eliminate *the negative* at present. The interview preferably is conducted in a quiet place. After introducing yourself, begin with, "Tell me more about your problems and yourself." Wait, say little, and listen. Then perhaps, "How have things been in the past?" Later, "It must have been difficult. Anyone would have been frightened, angry (and so forth), in such circumstances. How did you manage then?" From what may be revealed, try commenting on positive aspects of how the patient apparently coped under duress in the past: "From what you have told me, you seemed to have handled difficulties then. I wonder if things are that different now?" By being nonjudgmental and subtly reinforcing self-image and assets, a good listener may facilitate the patient's ability to help himself.

This approach presumes some basic skills in communication or a knack in talking with patients. Several questions regarding suicidal and psychotic trends, however, as delineated earlier under Mental Status and Target Symptoms, should not be omitted.

TREATMENT OF DRUG-INDUCED ABERRATIONS

Drug reactions are increasingly a problem. The drugs used, alone or in combination, and the strengths of preparations vary as do the manifestations.

Often those who accompany the patient know the drug used and, aside from the immediate crisis, may be best able to aid the patient. When the patient is on a bad trip (a "bummer") or morbidly depressed (a "crash"), gaining confidence of the patient and his friends may be essential to discovering the etiological agents and most effective treatment. Ask "What have you (has he) been using?" The initial answer may be "marijuana" ("grass"). If your response to this is in no way judgmental, your next question, "and what else?" may be revealing. Then, "By vein or mouth ('main-line' or 'popping'), and how much?"

Most drugs used may produce, in high doses or with rapid withdrawal, excitement, depression, or psychosis.

Barbiturates and C.N.S. Depressants

Cases seen in emergency rooms show slurred speech, agitation, and so forth, and may require hospitalization to prevent death from overdose, to test for tolerance, and to prevent dangerous convulsions and other withdrawal symptoms. Glutethimide (Doriden) overdose or habituation requires *prompt* medical consultation.

Amphetamines and C.N.S. Stimulants

Speech may be slurred, incessant, and accelerated (rapping); or patients may be morbidly depressed or paranoid and panicky. They may be insomniac and euphoric; but also emaciated. Chlorpromazine per os or intramuscularly is the usual form of tranquilizer; hospitalization is dependent upon severity of symptoms. Methylphenidate (Ritalin) (a nonamphetamine) habituation may be associated with seizures.

Hallucinogens

LSD, mescaline, and so forth, may produce major distortions in perception and gross alterations in behavior. The bad trip, and recurrence (flashbacks) of hallucinatory experience even years after the LSD was imbibed, call for reassurance, verbal attempts to calm the patient, and phenothiazines. If recovery is prompt, the patient may be released to someone else's surveillance. If not, hospitalization may be indicated.

Preparations popularly named STP and DMT may produce manic-like psychosis and destructive behavior. There are reports that phenothiazines are contraindicated. Barbiturates or paraldehyde may be necessary to control behavior, and hospitalization is generally indicated.

Cannabis

Marijuana, hashish, and so forth, of themselves are not usually responsible for emergency-room visits. If such patients do present, treat symptomatically.

Narcotics

For management, consult standard texts and hospital policy.

FAMILY OF THE ACUTELY ILL OR DECEASED

If the family of the seriously ill or of a patient dead on arrival show an untoward or extreme emotional response, it may be desirable to accept them as patients and treat them (perhaps with phenothiazine tranquilizers) in accordance with Impressions and Treatment, above.

RECORDS AND DIAGNOSIS

Emergency-room records, though brief, should include (1) identification, (2) source of referral and who accompanied the patient, (3) chief complaints or reason for visit, and present illness, (4) observed physical or medical abnormalities, (5) pertinent positive findings on mental status, (6) impression, (7) recommendations, (8) treatment given and drugs prescribed (dose, amount, directions), and (9) actual disposition.

At the cost of redundancy, it is essential to begin each paragraph citing chief complaints, history, and mental status with "The patient states . . ." "The husband, police officer, and so forth, states . . ." or the physician may invite legal action against himself and others for recording presumed rather than established facts.

Diagnoses in psychiatry, other than of organic conditions, are essentially descriptive rather than etiological. They are dependent upon extensive observation and study that are not feasible in the emergency room. These diagnoses fall into the following main groups: (1) psychotic, (2) psychophysiologic, (3) neurotic, (4) personality disorders, and (5) transient situational disorders. The diagnostic manual of the American Psychiatric Association (DMS-II) describes them [1]. Of particular interest and help is a category entitled Nondiagnostic Terms for Administrative Use [2].

Since there remains an unwarranted stigma associated with mental disorders, and since many psychiatric diagnoses, once placed on a patient's records, may (1) hurt the patient socially, (2) interfere with present or future job opportunities, or (3) prejudice adversely the patient's own expectations and treatment prognosis, it is recommended that the impression recorded be restricted to *the most general possible category,* e.g., psychotic disorder, neurotic disorder, personality disorder, and so forth. It is always proper, however, to add "manifested by," e.g., depression, delusions of persecution, or whatever the most prominent symptoms may be.

It is always desirable also to state, below Impression, "In my opinion at this time the patient is (or is not) a serious threat to his own (or others') well-being, and immediate confinement is (or is not) now necessary."

Under Recommendations, it is essential to record *what* was recommended and *to whom.*

CONCLUSION

In examining mentally disturbed patients, it must be considered to what extent organic factors contribute, i.e., infection, intoxication or drugs, trauma, metabolic or degenerative diseases, neoplasms, nutritional deficiencies, and exhaustion.

With the above factors ruled out, open-ended questions to the patient and those with him should reveal the degree of danger of the patient to himself or others. Acutely depressed, suicidal, confused, and delusional ideation or behavior strongly suggests hospitalization; histrionic, manipulative, and sociopathic behavior rapid release and perhaps referral elsewhere. But in general, mild disturbance indicates reassurance, moderate disturbance medication (preferably the nonaddicting phenothiazines) and referral, and severe disorder preparation for immediate hospitalization.

If there is no immediate psychiatric consultation available, the physician must rely ultimately on his own judgment for treatment and disposition. The key data and reasoning responsible for his decisions must be recorded.

REFERENCES

1. Committee on Nomenclature and Statistics of the American Psychiatric Association. *Diagnostic and Statistical Manual of Mental Disorders.* Washington: American Psychiatric Association, 1968.
2. *Ibid.,* p. 13.
3. Farberow, N. L., and Shneidman, E. S. (Eds.). *The Cry for Help.* New York: McGraw-Hill, 1961.
4. Gantz, R. S., et al. Phenothiazine reduction as a cause of rehospitalization. *Arch. Gen. Psychiat.* (Chicago) 12:586, 1965.
5. Golden, J. A traumatic syndrome. *Minnesota Med.* 44:24, Jan. 1961.

Drug Abuse

24

JOHN E. GAINOR

In recent years drug addiction, always a problem, has become a much greater one, involving an increasing proportion of the population with a wider variety of agents. The problem among the young is particularly serious. "Young persons today use a farrago of drugs and, less and less frequently, confine their use to a single pharmacologic agent; euphoriants, stimulants, and hallucinogens are mixed in the perpetual search for thrills, alteration of consciousness, and escapism. Because so many drugs are used, the physician treating drug overdose in the emergency room faces an increasingly difficult task." *

HALLUCINOGENS

Names of Agents

Commonly Used

MARIJUANA	female hemp plant *Cannabis sativa*
Slang	pot, tea, weed, Mary Jane, grass, love weed, reefer, joint, hay, hashish, joy smoke, stinkweed, etc.
LSD	lysergic acid diethylamide
Slang	acid, cubes, pearly gates, heavenly blue, royal blue, wedding bells

* Editorial, *J.A.M.A.* 211:36, Jan. 5, 1970.

Less Commonly Used

MMDA	3-methoxy-4-5-methylenedioxy amphetamine is obtained from nutmeg; three times as strong as mescaline
MESCALINE	3, 4, 5, trimethoxy-phenylethylamine is obtained from the peyote cactus; bitter taste, usually ingested with tea, coffee, or milk
MESCAL	obtained from a cactus in Mexico, for many years used in Indian ceremonies; mydriasis is the only constant symptom; buttons may be eaten, or a "tea" may be made; symptoms may be flashing lights and bizarre color configurations
DMT	synthetic derivative of tryptamine
DET	synthetic derivative similar to DMT
PSILOCYBIN	extracted from Mexican mushroom, chemically known as ortho-phosphoryl-4-hydroxy-*N*-dimethyl-tryptamine
PSILOCIN	same source and action as psilocybin
68	similar to banana peel; may be a hoax; FDA reports "68" is nothing more than oil of peppermint
Slang	sex-juice, sexy-68
MORNING GLORY SEEDS	contain lysergic acid amide; this alkaloid derivative is about one-tenth as potent as LSD
STP	4-methyl-2,5-dimethoxy alpha methylphenethylamine; a powerful hallucinogen; chlorpromazine may *intensify* the action of STP
Slang	serenity, tranquility, peace, "dom"

MARIJUANA. Marijuana comes from the female hemp plant *Cannabis sativa,* which develops a resinous material that incorporates the active pharmacological principals. This resin can be extracted from the dried tops of the plant, leaves, or flowers, and may be pulverized and smoked with or without admixture with tobacco. There are several kinds of marijuana. In Persia it is called *hashish*. This form is four to five times as powerful as our native marijuana. In India the liquid form is known as *bhang*. Recently the active ingredient of the cannabis resin has been synthesized. It is tetrahydrocannabinol (THC), and is comparable to LSD in its psychic effects. The actions of cannabis are exerted primarily on the central nervous system, but the mode of action is poorly understood. When smoked, the effects are felt in a few minutes and may persist for as long as 12 hours.

SYMPTOMS. Subjectively, smoking marijuana results in one or more of the following: a feeling of well-being, hilarity, euphoria, distortion of time and space perception, impaired judgment and memory, irritability, and confusion. After repeated administration and high dosage, other effects are noted, such as: hallucinations, illusions and delusions that predispose to antisocial behavior; anxiety and aggressiveness as a possible result of the various intellectual and sensory derangements. Sleep disturbances are frequent. Among the somatic effects are injection of the ciliary vessels, laryngitis, chronic bronchitis, and asthma. These conditions and hypoglycemia, with ensuing bulimia are symptoms of intoxication, not of withdrawal. There is little difficulty in recognizing the intoxication of a person who has smoked a significant amount of marijuana in the preceding few hours. Marijuana smoke has a characteristic acrid odor and dried marijuana can be identified by narcotics control laboratories. No blood test is available.

TREATMENT. Ordinarily, minimal protection during the period of acute intoxication is all that is required. During the initial phase, ambulatory treatment of the person with psychological dependency (as contrasted with the experimenter) is generally not satisfactory because of the tendency to relapse. At least, brief hospitalization is recommended to separate the patient from his supply, establish relations between the patient and the physician, and initiate treatment.

LYSERGIC ACID DIETHYLAMIDE—LSD. LSD is obtained from two sources: (1) ergot, the parasitic fungus found on wheat, rye, and other grasses, and (2) morning glory seed. Because of its potency and general availability on the illicit market, LSD is by far the most important hallucinogen. It is sold either in the form of tablets or as saturated sugar cubes.

SIGNS AND SYMPTOMS. The pupils are widened, the pulse is rapid, there is some degree of motor restlessness with hyperreflexia, and sometimes there is a fine tremor. The blood pressure is labile but generally elevated. Not infrequently the patient will complain of vertigo, headache, and nausea. The body temperature is often slightly elevated.

In LSD intoxication the hallucinations are usually visual, but about 25 percent of patients also report auditory hallucinations. By contrast, in schizophrenia hallucinations are predominately auditory.

A typical and diagnostically important symptom of LSD intoxication is the patient's diminished ability to screen out irrelevant stimuli. Under ordinary circumstances a person maintains a focus of his attention on those aspects of his environment which interest him. Irrelevant sounds, such as a dog barking outside, a clock ticking, voices in the next room, remain unnoticed. The patient on LSD, however, responds indiscriminately to all these stimuli. This makes it impossible for him to maintain the focus of his attention and also makes him a victim of outside stimuli, just as he is a victim of his own thoughts and images.

LSD may cause complete personality changes. Hallucinations, exhilaration, or depression, psychotic manifestations, and suicidal or homicidal tendencies may all occur as acute or chronic manifestations of LSD use.

The most frequent complications of LSD include the following: (1) The hallucinated disorganized state reappears without further ingestion of an hallucinogen. (2) There is frequent panic. Hospitalization may be sought owing to a sense of terror with which the patient cannot cope. (3) An extended period of psychosis is seen, particularly in individuals with a history of a previous psychosis or in prepsychotic persons. (4) Grandiose hallucinations are manifested by stepping in front of trains or trying to fly from roof tops, etc.

TREATMENT. The patient should be hospitalized for a brief period of time or, when available, admitted to a holding unit. If frightened, the patient should be reassured; chlorpromazine, 50 mg intramuscularly, is given every 3 or 4 hours and repeated every 3 or 4 hours as necessary. The blood pressure should be monitored because of the hypotensive effects of chlorpromazine.

The patient may derive considerable gratification from the interest which physicians and nurses show in his toxic state. If he shows a dramatic quality in his behavior, he should be dealt with matter-of-factly and without any display of special interest in his verbal productions. It is best to assure the patient that his symptoms are due to LSD, that these will be rapidly counteracted by the drug being injected, and that he is expected to rest after the injection. Tranquilizers, such as diazepam (Valium) and chlordiazepoxide (Librium), also have been used.

Occasionally there is a paradoxical response to chlorpromazine with resultant augmentation of psychotic manifestations. The cause of this is unclear. In such cases an attempt to influence the patient's condition with other phenothiazines or barbiturates may be made. However, the potentiating effects of phenothiazines and barbiturates should be kept in mind. These patients usually require prolonged psychiatric therapy.

NARCOTICS

Names of Agents Commonly Used

HEROIN	may be taken orally or by inhalation—usually I.V.
Slang	horse, Harry, white stuff
MORPHINE	may be taken orally, I.V., and I.M.
Slang	hard stuff, unkie, Miss Emma
CODEINE	less potent in inducing euphoria
HYCODAN	has lost its popularity
DILAUDID	does not have the "thrill" possessed by heroin
DEMEROL	addiction has been proved
METHADONE	addiction has been proved
PERCODAN	recently changed from class B to A because of addiction
EXEMPT NARCOTIC COUGH MEDICINES	
Slang	A–C
PAREGORIC	not exempt in most states

Exempt narcotics have for years been the target of drug abusers. Although not responsible for hard addiction, their easy availability has made them ideal for thrill-seeking young teen-agers and certain elements of the adult population. Many an addict has admitted his road to addiction began with the exempt narcotic cough preparations or marijuana.

Of the many exempt narcotic preparations available, the most popular are the codeine-containing cough mixtures, and paregoric. The cough preparations contain approximately 1 grain of codeine per fluid ounce and they are usually available in 4-oz containers. Paregoric, when available as an exempt preparation, is packaged in 1- or 2-ounce containers, depending on the state law. The usual 5-ml dose of paregoric contains 2 mg of morphine.

Consuming two or three bottles of elixir of terpin hydrate and codeine or paregoric can supply 8 to 12 grains of codeine or 24 to 36 mg of morphine. With the alcoholic content high, the appeal of these compounds is obvious.

These preparations are usually administered orally, although paregoric addicts have been known to inject the product intravenously; the jugular vein in the neck and the antecubital veins are locations of choice. Ulcerating sores of the neck, arms, and leg may develop from the attempted intravenous injection of paregoric. A common method of preparing paregoric is to boil the product until it takes on a cloudy appearance (precipitation of camphor). The camphor is removed with cotton and the remaining material injected. Amphetamines and barbiturates have been used as additives to increase the effect.

A favorite mixture among users of these preparations is a combination of elixir of terpin hydrate and codeine and tablets of tripelennamine (Pyribenzamine) called "Blue Velvet." The codeine and the high dose of antihistamine have a combined depressant effect desired by some individuals.

The combination of antihistamines with codeine cough preparations has gained in popularity recently. Robitussin A–C (a mixture of codeine, pheniramine maleate, glyceryl guaiacolate) particularly has been in demand. A–C is frequently mentioned as a problem by mothers.

Heroin.   Heroin is from two to ten times as potent as morphine, depending upon the measuring techniques. The intense euphoria produced by the drug has made it one of the most popular as well as one of the most dangerous. Heroin is synthesized from morphine by process of acetylation, using acetic anhydride. The process, carried out with simple and inexpensive equipment, will produce a high-quality product with a good yield. Since heroin is more potent than morphine and the yield is high, it is economically desirable to convert morphine to heroin. Opium grown in Turkey is shipped to Lebanon, where morphine is extracted. The morphine is then sent to France, where it is converted to heroin. From France the heroin is sent to Italy for smuggling to New York.

The popularity of the narcotics with escapists lies in the effect of these drugs on the mind. The feeling of being "high," which is similar to the feeling obtained with amphetamines, is desirable among addicts. In addition, euphoria, tranquility, and somnolence are also desirable features. Another effect is the "thrill," a feeling of warmth and a tingling sensation in the abdomen similar to orgasm. Following the initial effects, the subject "goes to nod," a dreamy state of imperturbability. Sleep comes easily, but the subject can be aroused with little difficulty.

Continued use of narcotics leads to physical dependence, tolerance, habituation, and addiction. Symptoms of withdrawal from narcotics depend on the severity of the addiction and the degree of tolerance achieved. They range from mild symptoms, such as yawning, lacrimation, and perspiration, to moderate ones such as tremors, loss of appetite, and insomnia, and finally, the severe symptoms are diarrhea, vomiting, muscle pain and cramps, and weight loss. Miosis, dark glasses, and long sleeves are concomitant findings.

The intensity of the withdrawal symptoms varies with the degree of physical dependence. This, in turn, is related to the amount of drugs customarily used. Typically, the onset of symptoms occurs about 8 to 12 hours after the last dose; thereafter they increase in intensity, reach a peak between 36 and 72 hours, and then gradually diminish over the next 5 to 10 days. However, weakness, insomnia, nervousness, and muscle aches and pains may persist for several weeks. In extreme cases, death may result.

Withdrawal symptoms may be brought on by withdrawing the drug or by injecting a narcotic antagonist such as nalorphine (Nalline). This has become the basis of the Nalline Test for narcotic addiction which is used in many parts of the country. A small dose of nalorphine will cause a mild withdrawal reaction such as dilatation of the pupils in the eyes of the subject who has taken narcotics recently.

Addicts live with the perpetual threat of overdosage. This may come about in several ways. An individual who has relapsed after a period of withdrawal may miscalculate the size of his new dose. An addict, while under the influence of narcotics, alcohol, or other drugs, may miscalculate his dose; or the drug which is usually cut with an excipient, may be stronger than the "pusher" has represented it to be. *In 1969 over two hundred teen-age heroin addicts died in New York City.* Death from narcotic overdosage is caused by respiratory depression, from selective depression of the respiratory center.

Further Facts About Narcotics

(1) Users live in suburbia as well as in the ghetto. (2) Heroin is adulterated so flagrantly that the withdrawal can often be treated with mild sedation. (3) Heroin is so impotent at times that abusers often add either barbiturates or amphetamines.

Major Medical Complications

Abscesses	Pneumonia
Cellulitis	Septic pulmonary embolism
Endocarditis	Tetanus
Hepatitis	Thrombophlebitis
Overdose	

The endocarditis is usually caused by staphyloccocci, *Candida* (*Monilia*), gram-negative enteric bacteria, or enterococci.

Treatment

For overdose, administer nalorphine hydrochloride, 5 mg, or levallorphan tartrate (Lorfan), 1 mg. These drugs are to be given intravenously one to three times at 15-minute intervals, the number of injections depending on the adequacy of the respiratory response.

Further treatment falls in the province of psychiatry, rehabilitation centers, group therapy, "half-way houses," etc. Methadone is currently used extensively in the treatment of the heroin addict. Syrup of methadone seems to be the preferred product for this form of therapy.

STIMULANTS

Names of Agents Commonly Used

BENZEDRINE	amphetamine
Slang	bennie bennie, benzies, peaches, roses, hearts, cartwheels
DEXEDRINE	dextroamphetamine
Slang	hearts, oranges, dexies, footballs
DESOXYN	methedrine
Slang	speed, bomita (when injected)
DEXAMYL	a combination of Dexedrine and Amytal
COCAINE	taken by inhalation or I.V.
Slang	coke, "C," Corine, Carrie, cholly, happy dust, heaven dust, snow, stardust, girl, Bernice, Burese, bennies, flake, gold dust
WYAMINE	mephentermine
	inhaler; probably off the market now
PRELUDEN	phenmetrazine hydrochloride
	usual dose for adults is 25 mg two or three times daily, orally, an hour before meals

AMPHETAMINES.   The underlying reasons for amphetamine abuse vary from person to person, and the drug may serve different purposes at different times for the same patient. Usually, the amphetamine-dependent patient, consciously or unconsciously, seeks to obtain one or more of the following effects: relief from fatigue, increased mental alertness, a heightened sense of well-being (euphoria), and relief from the emotional tone of depression.

When dosage is kept within the therapeutic range, a tolerance to the amphetamines develops rather slowly. However, progressive increments in dosage will speed up development of tolerance to a point that permits injection of amounts hundreds of times greater than therapeutic limits. Cases involving the routine injection of several thousand milligrams have been reported, and chronic abusers of amphetamines can develop a tolerance to amounts far greater than the ordinary minimum lethal dosage.

An unusual feature of amphetamine tolerance which develops after prolonged use is the rapid development of tolerance of the cardiovascular system such that the heart rate and blood pressure may not be significantly increased despite exceedingly large doses. Similarly, the pupils may no longer show dilatation, and findings at physical examination may be within normal limits in spite of active abuse. Usually, the addict will show signs of social, economic, and emotional deterioration; for instance, down-grading of his job, a rundown physical condition, and an unkempt appearance. Such a person also tends to become unreliable, irritable, and unstable. The recent use of amphetamines can be established by testing the urine, but only a few laboratories are equipped for this procedure. It is to be hoped that within a short time testing facilities will be more available. When signs and symptoms of a more specific nature do occur, they are associated with the effect of the drug on the sympathetic nervous system. In cases involving single, *large* doses in nontolerant persons or a sudden increase in dose above the level of tolerance, the following signs may be present: tachycardia, dilated pupils, elevated blood pressure, anorexia, and hyperreflexia. Other indications of the possible presence of amphetamines are nervousness and jitteriness, unclear or rapid speech, and euphoria. The syndrome often may be confused with other types of intoxication or mistaken for an acute anxiety reaction. The duration of the syndrome is variable, and it is generally thought that this variability is related to an underlying or latent psychiatric disorder.

AMPHETAMINE PSYCHOSIS. In some persons, amphetamines produce an acute paranoid psychosis characterized by a paranoid state with auditory and/or visual hallucinations. Although the condition is clearly drug-induced, it lacks certain features of an organic delirium, since there is no disorientation or true confusion. Amphetamine psychosis has been observed after acute poisoning with a single dose of 50 mg and after a "spree" involving increasing doses over 4 to 5 days. However, it is more common in persons who have been taking large amounts for prolonged periods.

Even without specific therapy, the psychiatric manifestations associated with amphetamine psychosis usually disappear in 3 to 6 days after the drug has been discontinued, but they may last for several weeks. However, without definitive or supportive treatment and after-care, relapse to the abuse of amphetamines is frequent and hospitalization may again be required.

WITHDRAWAL. Although there is no characteristic abstinence syndrome, the abrupt discontinuance of amphetamines is not without complications. Withdrawal can uncover an underlying depression or may precipitate a depressive reaction, often with a suicidal potential. There is also some evidence that in certain persons, amphetamine intoxication can precipitate a schizophrenic episode. However, there is no evidence that persons develop physical dependence to stimulant drugs and abrupt withdrawal will not produce symptoms even after prolonged use. Depending on the amount used, all measurable traces should disappear from the body in from 2 to 7 days.

Frequently when the stimulant intake masks chronic fatigue, withdrawal is followed by a 2- or 3-day period of intense tiredness and sleepiness. In patients who are recovering from amphetamine psychosis or in those who exhibit severe restlessness or anxiety, the administration of a phenothiazine tranquilizer may be indicated, as well as a barbiturate at night.

Because of the frequency of multiple dependence patterns, the physician should make every effort to ascertain the patient's drug history before attempting withdrawal. A routine check should be made for needle marks which may indicate concurrent narcotic dependence. As noted, the amphetamine-dependent patient often is also taking barbiturates. If so, procedures should be instituted to withdraw him from the barbiturates as well as amphetamines.

TREATMENT AND AFTER-CARE. Withdrawal is only the beginning of the treatment process for the stimulant-dependent patient. The therapeutic pattern is not significantly different from that used in cases of barbiturates or narcotic dependence.

The physician should be prepared to maintain contact with the patient and be available for specific psychotherapy, or at least supportive help for a long period. If such support is not forthcoming, then the likelihood of relapse and of renewed drug dependence is great.

COMPLICATIONS. As is the case with other intravenous drug intake which is self-administered, the complications include abscesses, cellulitis, thrombophlebitis, hepatitis, and tetanus.

DEPRESSANTS AND TRANQUILIZERS

Names of Agents Commonly Used

NEMBUTAL	sodium pentobarbital, oral or I.V.
Slang	yellow jackets, yellows, ninbies
AMYTAL	sodium amobarbital, oral or I.V.
Slang	blue devils, blue birds, blue heaven
SECONAL	sodium secobarbital, oral or I.V.
Slang	redbirds, red devils, pinks
PHENOBARBITAL	long-acting barbiturate
TUINAL	Amytal and Seconal
ALCOHOL	increases the desire, dulls the performance
BROMIDES	available without prescription
CHLORAL HYDRATE	gastric irritant
Slang	Mickey Finn, Mickey, Peter
LIBRIUM	chlordiazepoxide hydrochloride; prolonged large doses can cause withdrawal symptoms
MILTOWN, EQUANIL	meprobamate; excessive prolonged dosage can cause withdrawal symptoms
DORIDEN	glutethimide; withdrawal can produce hallucinations and grand mal seizures
PARALDEHYDE	similar to chloral hydrate and alcohol in its hypnotic and sedative properties and its side-effects
ASTHMA CIGARETTES	Asthmador—contains the dried parts of *Datura stramonium* (jimsonweed, Jamestown weed, thorn apple), a relative of the belladonna family; stramonium contains atropine and scopolamine
VAPORS	glue, ether, chloroform, gasoline, lighter fluid, refrigerants, carbon tetrachloride, paint thinner, shellac, kerosene (these possibly should be grouped with hallucinogens)
NUTMEG	contains 5 to 15 percent of myristica oil, a volatile oil responsible for the pharmacological action of the fragrant spice; taken orally, the effects appear about 5 hours after ingestion; symptoms are agitation, apprehension, and a sense of impending doom (this is not a popular "cop out")

BARBITURATES. Barbiturate dependence has one characteristic in common with all other states of drug dependence. It is almost always a chronic relapsing disorder, and cycles of withdrawals and reversion to drug use are likely to occur in most cases. Success or failure, however, cannot be measured by the single criterion of relapse. In all cases, continuing treatment of the dependency state and any underlying emotional disorder is essential, even though there is an intermittent, periodic, or even continuing drug use. There is good reason to believe that the total course of this disorder is influenced by adequate treatment over rather long periods.

TYPES OF ABUSER.   Essentially, there are four types of barbiturate drug abuse, and they overlap only occasionally.

1. In the first group are persons seeking the sedative hypnotic effects of the drug in order to deal with states of emotional distress.

2. In the second group there is a paradoxical reaction of excitation that occurs after tolerance has developed because of prolonged use. The drug now stimulates rather than depresses and is taken to exhilarate and animate the person to so-called increased efficiency.

3. In a third group are persons who take barbiturates to counteract the effects of various stimulant drugs, such as the amphetamines.

4. In the fourth category, barbiturate abuse is found in combination with other types of drug abuse, mainly alcohol and/or opiates. Many alcoholic individuals attempt to counteract the withdrawal effects of alcohol with barbiturates. Frequently, alcohol and barbiturates are combined in an attempt to obtain effects that surpass those of either alone. This practice is especially hazardous, as the cumulative effects can easily result in serious intoxication or death.

INTOXICATION.   Early diagnosis based on definitive clinical evidence is essential. Intoxication with barbiturates resembles intoxication with alcohol. Symptoms and signs include various degrees of clouding of consciousness with impairment of mentation, confusion and poor judgment, euphoria or depression, loss of emotional control, irritability, abnormal behavior, and occasionally convulsions or signs of a toxic psychosis. Patients will also show objective signs of dysarthria, ataxia in gait and station, muscular incoordination, nystagmus, ptosis, pupillary changes, and hyporeflexia or areflexia, either symmetrically or asymmetrically. Coma is unusual, as is inanition. Signs of inanition suggest that large amounts of an amphetamine or alcohol have also been used.

WITHDRAWAL SYNDROME.   Sudden and abrupt withdrawal of barbiturates from a person who is physically dependent results in definite abstinence signs and symptoms. Their intensity varies according to the dose taken, length of time the patient has been physically dependent, and individual factors which remain not completely understood. During the first 8 hours after abrupt withdrawal, signs and symptoms of intoxication decline and the patient appears to improve. As these signs and symptoms recede, increasing anxiety, headache, twitching of various muscle groups, nervousness, tremor, weakness, impaired cardiovascular responses when standing, and vomiting become evident. They become fairly intense after 16 hours of abstinence and are rather severe after 24 hours. Between the thirtieth and forty-eighth hour of withdrawal, convulsions of grand mal type are very likely to occur. Occasionally, convulsive seizures are observed as early as the 16th hour and as late as the eighth day. Frequently, there is a period of postconvulsive confusion lasting for 1 to 2 hours. At times there will be increasing insomnia culminating in a state of delirium, closely resembling delirium tremens and characterized by confusion, marked tremors, disorientation, hallucinations, and delusions. Ordinarily the delirium lasts fewer than 5 days and ends with a prolonged period of sleep. Even though no treatment is given, the entire withdrawal syndrome is usually a self-limited condition. Clinical recovery appears to be complete and no organic sequelae are known to occur. However, patients have died during uncontrolled, untreated barbiturate withdrawal syndromes.

Withdrawal of barbiturates from patients with strong physical dependence may be life-threatening and can only be accomplished satisfactorily, and with reasonable safety, in a drug-free environment where hospital and nursing facilities are available. Withdrawal must be accomplished very slowly and carefully. Manifestations of mild barbiturate absence, such as anxiety, weakness, nausea, and tremor, signal the danger of impending convulsions and/or psychosis. Patients in this condition should be given a short-acting barbiturate at once. Experience has demonstrated that sodium pentobarbital, 200 to 400 mg (3 to 6 grains) orally or parenterally, is extremely effective. If the symptoms are not relieved within 1 hour, the dose should be repeated. Subsequent withdrawal consists of a graduated, four times daily administration of barbiturates, at the dose level which just maintains a mild degree of intoxication. Clinical evidence of sedation is essential. Further reduction can begin after one or two days of observation, but the dosage should not be reduced more than 100 mg daily. If signs or symptoms of abstinence recur, the dosage should be temporarily increased. Close observation is required because of concomitant mental confusion, lethargy, muscular incompetence, apprehension, and possible convulsions. Supportive measures such as restoration of electrolyte balance, proper hydration with I.V. fluids, and vitamins are also in order. The usual nursing care and ward routine applicable to patients with convulsive disorders, confusion, or delirium states should be maintained.

LABORATORY TESTS. Identification of a barbiturate can usually be made on 10 ml of unclotted blood or 2 oz of urine.

GLUE-SNIFFING. When a teen-ager sniffs glue, the first stage of intoxication resembles the hazy joyousness produced by alcohol. The ceremony of sniffing glue is usually performed in groups. The glue is squeezed into a paper bag or plastic bag or on a handkerchief or towel and the vapors inhaled. The effects of sniffing glue are similar to those of drinking alcohol: inebriation, exhilaration, euphoria, and stupor. In addition, there are vivid, colorful hallucinations which accompany the experience. Usually the hallucinations appear only during the period of intoxication but in some cases they persist for as long as 2 hours.

Glue contains toluene, which is reported to be responsible for the semibizarre effects. Toluene is irritating to the mucous membrane and causes inflamed nostrils, lips, and eyes in the glue-sniffers. Additional symptoms include nausea, vomiting, and dizziness. Liver damage has been reported, but may not be permanent.

Glue-sniffing may result in aggressive impulses; for example, in an overly ambitious period one boy attacked four Marines.

PRECAUTIONS. In recent months two important recommendations have been advocated and in some localities have been acted upon. One is the addition of mustard to glue, making its inhalation unpleasant. The second forbids the sale of glue to minors unless a parent is present.

TREATMENT. The only treatment needed for the acute episode is to protect the individual from activities harmful to himself or others. The follow-up therapy is family counseling and psychiatric guidance.

GENERAL REFERENCES

Committee on Alcoholism and Addiction and Council on Mental Health. Dependence on amphetamines and other stimulant drugs. *J.A.M.A.* 197:1023, 1966.

Committee on Alcoholism and Addiction and Council on Mental Health. Dependence on barbiturates and other sedative drugs. *J.A.M.A.* 193:673, 1965.

Council on Mental Health and Committee on Alcoholism and Drug Dependence. Dependence on cannabis (marihuana). *J.A.M.A.* 201:368, 1967.

Fras, I., and Friedman, J. J. Hallucinogenic effects of nutmeg in adolescent. *New York J. Med.* 69:462, 1969.

Louria, D. B. *The Drug Scene.* New York: McGraw-Hill, 1968.

Louria, D. B. Medical complications of pleasure-giving drugs. *Arch. Intern. Med.* (Chicago) 123:82, 1969.

Smith Kline & French Laboratories *Drug Abuse: Escape to Nowhere,* 1967.

Index

Abdominal emergencies, 121–133
  acute abdomen, 126–133, 157–159
  examination, 129
  external hernias, 130–131
  nonpenetrating wounds, 123–126
    abdominal wall and retroperitoneal
      injuries, 126
    intestinal, 125
    liver and spleen, 124
    pancreas, 124–125
    rectal, 126
    safety belt injuries, 125
  observation, 133
  pain, 127–128
  penetrating wounds, 121–123
    gunshot, 121–122
    stab, 122–123
  prévious hospitalization and operations,
    128–129
  trauma, 121–126
  treatment, 132–133
Abdominal pain, 127–128
  in children, 365–366
Abortion, 146–148
  septic, 147
Abrasions, 176
Abruptio placentae, 151, 153
Abscess
  collar-button, 247

  in infectious disease, 332
  liver, 324
Achilles tendon
  examination, 185
  ruptured, 218
Acromioclavicular dislocations, 208
Acute abdomen, 126–133, 157–159
  medical, 158–159
  obstetric, 157–159
  surgical, 157–158
Addiction, drug, 128, 393–407
Addisonian crisis, 103
Adrenal insufficiency, in children, 364–
  365
Agitation, 377, 379, 384
Airway maintenance, 24, 34–48
  in burns, 265
  in maxillofacial injuries, 254, 259–260
  in unconsciousness, 87
Alcoholism
  aggressiveness, 384
  diagnosis and therapy, 102
  withdrawal, 346
Allergic reactions, 172
  in children, 359–360
Ambulatory treatment for orthopedic injuries, 199
Amebic dysentery, 319
Amnesia, 90, 377

Amniotic fluid embolus, 154–155
Amphetamines, 389, 400–402
Aneurysms, 117–118
  abdominal, 117
  aortic, 117–118
  traumatic, 111–112
Angiograms
  in intracranial hematoma, 93–94
  renal, 136
Animal bites, 172, 177
Ankle
  examination, 185
  fractures, 213–215
  sprains, 217
Anorexia, 378
Antibiotic prophylaxis. *See also under*
    specific condition
  fever in children, 353–359
  genitourinary, 137, 138, 139, 140
  in maxillofacial injuries, 260
  for open injuries, 109
  in pulmonary edema, 68
  salpingitis, 158–159
  uterine sepsis, 154, 159
  wounds, 175, 180
Anxiety, 65, 377, 380, 384, 385, 386
Aorta, rupture of, 57, 58
Appendicitis, 127, 128, 130, 320
Appendix testis, 142
Arrhythmias, 105. *See also* Dysrhyth-
    mias
Arteriovenous fistula, 111–112
Asphyxia, traumatic, 55
Aspirin poisoning, in children, 359
Asthma, acute, 357–358
Atrial fibrillation, and embolism, 115
Atrioventricular block, 66
Atrium
  fibrillation, 77–78
  flutter, 77–78
  paroxysmal tachycardia, 74–77
  shifting pacemaker, 77
  tachycardia with atrioventricular block,
    76
Auscultation
  in acute abdomen, 129
  in atrial fibrillation, 77
  in respiratory distress, 26
Automobile accidents, maxillofacial in-
    juries in, 252
Avulsion, 234

Bacillary dysentery, 319

Back
  outpatient care, 200–201
  strain and discogenic pain, 218–219
Barbiturates, 102, 389, 403–406
Bennett's fracture, 241
Bhang, 394
Bites
  animal, 172, 177
  human, 177–178, 230
  insect, 360
Bladder
  infections, 334
  injuries, 137
Blood vessels. *See* Cardiovascular system
Body temperature alterations, differen-
    tial diagnosis, 106
Böhler-Braun frame, 195–196, 212
Bone fractures, maxillofacial clinical pic-
    ture of, 258–259
Bones, in hand injuries, 228
Botulism, 341, 342
Breech presentation, 167
Bronchi
  infections, in children, 356
  in infectious disease, 333–334
  rupture of, 57, 59
Bronchiolitis, 356–357
Bronchoscopy, 36–37
Bryant's traction, 190–191
Buck's traction, 191–192
Bullet wounds. *See* Gunshot wounds
Burns
  antibiotics, 273
  circulation in, 268
  contamination in, 268
  depth of, 267–268, 271
  examination, 267–269
  extent of, 267, 270–271
  fluid therapy, 273
  hand, 230
  history, 265–267
  hospitalization, 270
  in infectious disease, 333
  kidney function, 269, 274
  mental state in, 268
  pain, 273
  prognosis, 270–271
  respiratory tract involvement, 269
  significant symptoms, 267
  tetanus prophylaxis, 273, 276
  treatment, 269–274
Bursae, infection of, 249
Business office, 10

"Butterflies," use of, 174

Calcaneus fractures, 215
Cancer
  and bleeding, 316
  genital, 151
Candidiasis (moniliasis), 164–165
Cannabis, 390
Carbon dioxide narcosis, 104
Carbuncles, 244–245
Cardiac arrest, 26, 71–72
Cardiac asthma, 67
Cardiac compression, relief of, 45–48
Cardiac emergencies. *See* Cardiovascular
  system
Cardiac pacemaker implantation, 82–84
Cardiac shock, 65
Cardiac tamponade, 45–46
Cardiopulmonary resuscitation, 71–72
Cardiovascular system, 63–85. *See also*
  under specific condition
  acute pulmonary edema, 67–68
  cardiac arrest, 71–72
  cardiopulmonary resuscitation, 71–72
  cardioversion, 69–70
  cerebrovascular insufficiency, 340
  childhood emergencies, 361–362
  circulation in burns, 268
  circulation in traction, 199
  differential diagnosis, 105
  fibrillation, 27, 66, 70, 77–78, 81
  flutter, 70, 77–78
  heart block, 81–84
  heart failure, 360–361
  myocardial infarction, 64–67
  occlusion, 115–117
  pacemaker, 82–84
  pericardial tamponade, 57–59
  seizures and, 347
  simple faint, 63
  tachycardia, 66, 70, 74–80
  unconsciousness, 367–368
Cardioversion, 69–70, 75
  in ventricular tachycardia, 80
Carotid sinus stimulation, 72–73, 75
Catatonia, 376, 379
Catheter, 141
Central nervous system
  depressants, 389
  lesions, 106
  seizures and, 345
  stimulants, 389
Cerebral concussion, 91–92

Cerebrovascular insufficiency, 340
Cervical spine fractures, 89, 218
Cervix
  infection, 334
  lacerations, 150
Chancroid, 138
Charcot's triad, 324
Chest wall
  defects, 57, 59–60
  splinting, 39–40
Children
  abdominal pain, 365–366
  allergic emergencies, 359–360
  aspirin poisoning, 359
  asthma, 357
  bronchiolitis, 356–357
  bronchitis, 356
  cardiac emergencies, 360–362
  congestive heart failure, 360–361
  dehydration—shock, 364–365
  diarrhea, 362–364
  encephalitis, 354
  epiglottis, acute, 355–356
  febrile seizures, 345, 349, 369
  fetal emergencies, 166–167
  fever, 351–354
  foreign body, 356
  gynecological problems, 168–169
  laryngotracheobronchitis, 355
  meningitis, 353–354
  minor feeding problems, 363–364
  paroxysmal supraventricular tachycar-
    dia, 361–362
  pneumonia, 358
  poisoning, 303, 305–308
  proptosis, 286–287
  respiratory distress, 355–359
  seizures, 369–370
  septicemia, 352–353
  stings, 360
  unconsciousness, 366–369
  urticaria, 360
  vomiting, 362–364
  Waterhouse-Friderichsen syndrome,
    354
Cholangitis, ascending, 323–324
Cholinergic crisis, 337, 339–344
Circulation. *See* Cardiovascular system
Cirrhosis of the liver, 323
Clavicle
  acromioclavicular dislocations, 208
  fractures, 208–209
  sternoclavicular dislocation, 58, 209

Closed-chest cardiac massage, 27
Coadaption splint, 204–205
Coagulation defect, 151
Cold injuries, 114–115
    frostbite, 114, 224, 230
    immersion foot, 114
    trench foot, 114
Colic, ureteral, 140–141
Colitis, ulcerative, 318–320
Collar-button abscess, 247
Colon. *See* Genitourinary emergencies
Coma. *See* Unconsciousness
Communicable diseases. *See* Infectious
    diseases
Compensation cases, 20
Compression injuries
    hand, 234
    thorax, 55
Concussion, 91–92
Condylar fractures, 211
Confusion, 377, 379
Congenital anomalies, 169
Congestive heart failure, 360–361
Conjunctivitis, 285
Consent, 19
Contamination
    control of, 10
    in infectious disease, 330
Contusions, 50
Conversion reaction, 386
Convulsions. *See* Seizures
Cornea. *See* Ocular emergencies
Coronary thrombosis and embolism, 115
Crohn's disease, 320, 321
Croup, 355
Cyanosis, 113
    in respiratory distress, 24, 28

Dacryocystitis, 287
Débridement
    of fractures, 188
    of lacerations, 174–175
Defibrillation, 27–28
Defloration, 162–163
Dehydration, in children, 364–365
Delayed primary closure of lacerations,
    175
Delays in emergency room, 2
Delirium, 377, 379
Delirium tremens, 102
Delivery, in emergency room, 150
Deltoid ligament tear, 214
Delusions, 376, 379, 384, 386

Depressants and tranquilizers, 403–406
Depression, 375–376, 379, 383, 385, 386
Diabetic acidosis, 103
    in children, 369
Diabetic neuritis, 340
Diaphragm, ruptured, 57, 60–61
Diarrhea, in children, 362–364
Digital nerve, 228
Digitalis
    in atrial tachycardia with atrioventric-
        ular block, 76–77
    in cardioversion, 69–70
    in pulmonary edema, 68
Dilatation, gastric, 54–55, 129–130
Dilatation and curettage, 147, 152–153
Diphtheria, 341, 342
Disaster planning, 21
Dislocations. *See specific dislocation*
Diuretics, 31, 68
Dog bites, 230
Donors, potential, 89
Dorsal and lumbar fractures, 218
Dorsal subaponeurotic space, infection of,
    250
Drug abuse, 393–407
    depressants and tranquilizers, 403–406
    hallucinogens, 393–396
    narcotics, 397–400
    stimulants, 400–402
Drug-induced aberrations, 389
Drug therapy, for psychiatric patients,
    383–386
Drug withdrawal, 399, 402, 404–405
Drugs, 13. *See also under specific drug
    or condition*
    seizures and, 345
Duck embryo rabies vaccine, 181–182
Dunlop's traction, 191–193, 198
Dysfunctional uterine bleeding, 152–153
Dysmenorrhea, 160
Dyspnea, in respiratory distress, 24
Dysrhythmias
    drugs for, 65–66
    in myocardial infarction, 64–66
    tachysystolic, 65–66, 72–73

Ear
    cold injuries, 114–115
    foreign bodies, 291–292
    mastoiditis, 291
    otitis externa, 289
    otitis media, 290
    trauma, 292

Eclampsia, 155–157
Ectopic pregnancy, 148–149, 153
Edema, acute pulmonary, 67–68
Elbow injuries, 204
Electrocardiogram
  in atrial fibrillation, 77–78
  in cardioversion, 70
  in dysrhythmia, 73
  in heart block, 82
  in myocardial infarction, 64–65
  in seizures, 349
  in ventricular tachycardia, 79–80
Electroshock therapy, 380
Embolus, 115–116
  amniotic fluid, 154–155
  pulmonary, 84, 118–119
Emergency room
  areas, 6–11
  contagious disease areas, 10
  in disasters, 21
  equipment, 7, 8, 9, 11–13
  examining areas, 7
  physical plant, 6–11
  planning and operation, 5–21
  poison control center, 10
  psychiatric patients in, 10
  scope of treatment in, 5–6
  staff, 13–18
  surgical suite, 7
  unconsciousness, 99–106
Emetics, 302–303
Emphysema
  cervical, 61
  mediastinal, 53
  subcutaneous, 40, 53
Encephalitis, 354
Encephalomyelitis, 340, 354
Encephalopathy
  hypertensive, 105
  Wernicke's, 341
Endometritis, 159
Endotoxic shock, 139, 154
Endotracheal tube, 24, 36, 38, 339
Enteritis, regional, 320–322
Epididymitis, 142
Epiglottis, acute, 355–356
Epileptic seizures, 348–349
Epinephrine
  for cardiac arrest, 27
  in cardiopulmonary resuscitation, 72
Epistaxis, 292–295
Equipment, emergency room, 7, 8, 9, 11–13

poison control center, 299–302
Erythema nodosum, 321, 322
Esophagus, perforation of, 57, 61
Etiology of seizures, 345–347
Examination. *See* Physical examination
Examining areas, 7
Examining tables, 11–12
Extensor tendon injuries of the hand, 225–226, 237–238
External hernias, 130–131
Extradural hematoma, 92, 93
Extrapleural hematoma, 53–54
Extremities
  cold injuries, 114–115
  orthopedic outpatient care, 200–201
Eye(s)
  bright red, 287
  in infectious disease, 333
  painful, 284–286
  tearing and pain, 287

Face. *See* Maxillofacial injuries
Faints, 63
Falls, 252
Familial periodic paralysis, 342
Family
  and consent, 19
  and potential donors, 89
  in stress situations, 19
Febrile seizures, 345, 349, 369
  nonfebrile, 369–370
Feeding problems, in children, 363–364
Felon, 245–247
Femoral fractures
  neck, 210
  shaft, 210–211
  and vascular injuries, 113–114
Fetal emergencies, 166–167
  prolapsed arm, 167
  prolapsed cord, 166–167
  prolapsed foot, 167
Fever, in children
  antipyretic measures, 352
  causes, 351–354
Fibrillation
  atrial, 70, 77–78
  drugs for, 78
  ventricular, 27, 66, 81
Fibula fractures, 213
Fingers
  avulsion, 234
  compression injuries, 234
  fingertip injuries, 230–231

Fingers—*Continued*
  fractures, 240–244
  guillotine amputation, 233–234
  infections, 244–250
  jammed, 234–235
  joints, 238–240
First-degree burn, 267
Fistula, arteriovenous, 111–112
Flail chest, 39–40, 50–52
Flexor tendon injuries of the hand, 225–226, 236–237
Flutter, atrial, 70, 77–78
Foot
  cold injuries, 114–115
  examination, 185
  fractures, 215–216
Foreign bodies
  in children, 356
  ear, 291–292
  eye, 280, 281
  hand injuries, 224, 229
  intrathoracic, 57, 61–62
  nose, 295–296
  pharynx and larynx, 297
Fractures. *See also specific fracture*
  areas for, 8
  multiple, 187–188
  open, 188
  and vascular injuries, 112–113
Frostbite, 114–115, 224, 230
Furuncles, 244

Gangrene
  from cold, 114
  from embolism, 115–116
  gas, 180
  streptococcal, 247–248
Gas gangrene, 180
Gastric dilatation, 54–55, 129–130
Gastric lavage, 311–312
Gastroenteritis, acute, 362
Gastrointestinal emergencies, 315–328. *See also under specific condition*
  hemorrhage
    occult, 317–318
    overt, 315–317
  hepatic decompensation, 325–326
  jaundice, 322–325
  regional enteritis, 320–322
  ulcerative colitis, 318–320
Genital cancer, 151
Genitalia. *See also under specific organ*
  infections, 164–166

injuries, 161–164
phimosis and paraphimosis, 143
ulcerated lesions, 138–139
Genitourinary emergencies
  acute scrotal pain and swelling, 141–142
  acute urinary retention, 141
  hematuria, 142
  infections, 137–140, 334
  injuries, 135–137
  phimosis and paraphimosis, 143
  ureteral colic, 140–141
Genitourinary infections, 137–140
  septicemia, 139–140
  ulcerated lesions of the genitalia, 138–139
  urethritis, 137–138
  urinary, 139
Glaucoma, 284–285
Glue-sniffing, 406
Gonorrhea, 137–138, 158
  of lower genital tract, 166
Granuloma inguinale, 139
Grease gun injury of the hand, 235
Guillain-Barré syndrome, 341, 342
Gunshot wounds, 56, 121–122, 252

Hallucinogens, 390, 393–396
  LSD, 393, 395–396
  marijuana, 393–395
Hand injuries, 221–250
  bones, 228
  closed-reduction technique, 240
  cold, 114–115
  compression, 234
  dislocations, 239–240
  examination, 223–228
  fractures, 240–244
  history, 221–223
  infections, 244–250
  joints, 238–240
  lacerations, 230–232
  nerves, 226–228, 235–236
  skin, 223–224
  sprains, 238–239
  tendons, 224–225, 237–238
  treatment
    general, 228–229
    local, 229–250
  wrist, 112
Hashish, 390, 394

Head injuries
  cerebral concussion, 91–92
  intracranial hematoma, 93–94
  lumbar puncture, 94–95
  skull fractures, 92–93
Heart. *See* Cardiovascular system
Heart block, 81–84
Heart failure, congestive, 360–361
Hematomas
  cervical, 58
  extradural, 92, 93
  extrapleural, 53–54
  intracranial, 93–94
  spleen, 135
  subdural, 93–94
  vulvar and perineal, 162
Hematuria, 142
Hemorrhage
  eye, 287
  gastrointestinal
    occult, 317–318
    overt, 315–317
  in maxillofacial injuries, 253–254, 259
  nose, 292–295
  pectechial, 55
  ruptured spleen, 60
  in shock, 30
  thoracic, indication for surgery, 54, 57–58
  in thoracic injuries, 41–42
  vaginal, 145–153
  in vascular emergencies, 108
  in wounds, 172
Hemothorax, 49, 54
  traumatic, 43–45
Hepatic coma, 103
Hepatic decompensation, 325–326
Hepatitis, 322–323, 324
Hernias
  external, 130–131
  strangulated, 142
Heroin, 397, 398–400
  intoxication with, 102
Herpes simplex, 285
Herpes zoster, 285–286
Hip
  dislocations, 209–210
  fractures, 210
History
  in acute abdomen, 127
  in burns, 265–267
  in hand injuries, 221–223
  in infectious disease, 330–331

  in maxillofacial injuries, 251–253
  in psychiatric emergencies, 372–378
  in unconsciousness, 87–88
  in wound management, 172
Homicidal tendencies, 377
Hospital admission
  for concussion, 92–93
  for orthopedic injuries, 199
  of psychiatric patients, 379–382
  for unconsciousness, 101
Hostility, 377, 380, 385
Human bites, 177–178, 230
Humerus
  fractures, and vascular injuries, 113–114
  injuries, 204–206
Hydatiform mole, 149
Hydrocarbons, ingestion of, 303
Hydrocele, 142
Hymen, imperforate, 169
Hyperkalemia, 84–85
Hyperkalemic weakness, 343
Hyperplasia, congenital adrenal, 364–365
Hypertensive encephalopathy, 105
Hyperthermia, 106
Hyphema, 279–280
Hypochondria, 378, 380, 385
Hypofibrinogenemia, 151
Hypoglycemia, 103, 343
Hypokalemic weakness, 343
Hypomania, 377, 379, 384
Hypotension, 105
Hysteria, 340, 342

Iliofemoral vein thrombosis, 119
Immersion foot (trench foot), 114
Immunization, 330–331
Imperforate hymen, 169
Infarction, myocardial, 64–67
Infection
  in children, 367
  classes of, 332–334
  ear, 289–291
  genitourinary, 137–140
    in children, 168–169
  of hand, 244–250
  lower genital tract, 164–166
  nose, 295
  pharynx and larynx, 297–298
  prophylaxis, 31–32
  seizures and, 346
  severe systemic, 104
  therapy, 334–336

Infectious diseases, 329–336
  area for, 10
  classes of infection, 332–334
  diagnosis, 331–332
  examination, 331
  history, 330–331
  infectious agents and drugs, 336
  therapy, 334–336
Insight, 378
Insomnia, 378, 380, 385
Interphalangeal dislocation, 240
Intertrochanteric and subtrochanteric
    fractures, 210
Intestines
  in infectious disease, 334
  obstruction, 129
  ulcerative colitis, 318–320
Intoxication
  barbiturates, 403–406
  in children, 366–367
  cough medicines, 397–398
  differential diagnosis, 102
  heroin, 102, 397, 398–399
  LSD, 395–396
  marijuana, 394–395
Intracranial aneurysm, unruptured, 340
Intracranial hematoma, 93–94
Intracranial pressure, increased, 88, 95–
    96
Intrapartum hemorrhage, 150
Intra-uterine device, 161
Intravenous therapy, in cardiopulmonary
    resuscitation, 72
Intussusception, 365
Inversion of uterus, 155
Irrigation
  ear, 291–292
  eye, 277–278

Jammed finger, 234–235
Jaundice, 322–325
Jaw movement, 255
Joint injuries of the hand, 238–240

Kidney, 135–136
  function
    in burns, 269, 274
    in shock, 29–30
  infection, 334
  renal failure, 31–32
Kirschner wire, 193–194
Knee
  dislocations, 211–212

  examination, 184–185
  fractures, 211
  injuries, 217

Labor, 149–151, 155
Laboratory, 9
Laboratory tests
  in acute abdomen, 131–132
  barbiturates, 406
  in genitourinary injuries, 135, 136,
    140
  in infectious disease, 331–332
  in pregnancy, 146
  for seizures, 348
Lacerations, 174–178
  hand, 230–232
  vulvar and vaginal, 161
Lacrimal system, lacerations of, 257
Language problems, 2, 16
Large intestine. *See* Intestines
Laryngoscopy, 35
Laryngotracheobronchitis, 355
Larynx, 297–298
  rupture of, 57, 59
Lavage, gastric, 311–312
Laxatives, in poisoning, 302–303
Lead encephalopathy, in children, 367
Level of consciousness, 89–90
Library, 10–11
  poison control center, 300
Ligament injuries, 184–185, 214
Liver
  cirrhosis, 323
  hepatic coma, 103
  hepatic decompensation, 325–326
  injuries, 135–136
  jaundice, 322–325
Lower genital tract infections, 164–166
  bacterial, 165–166
  candidiasis (moniliasis), 164–165
  nonspecific vaginitis, 165
  trichomoniasia, 164
LSD, 390, 393, 395–396
Lumbar
  fractures, 218
  puncture, 94–95
Lysergic acid diethylamide. *See* LSD

Mace injury to eye, 278
Major fascial spaces, infection of, 249–
    250
Malaria, 330

Malleolus fractures, 213–215
Mandible fractures, 261–262, 263–264
Marijuana, 390, 393–395
Mastoiditis, acute, 291
Maxilla fractures, 261–262
Maxillofacial injuries, 251–264
 bones, 261
 examination, 253–259
 fractures, 251, 261–264
 history, 251–253
 soft-tissue injuries, 260–261
 treatment, 259–264
Meatal stricture, 141
Mechanical injuries
 arteriovenous fistula, 111–112
 blunt trauma, 110–111
 penetrating wounds, 110
 traumatic aneurysm, 111–112
Median nerve, 226–227
Mediastinal
 emphysema, 53
 shift, 25
Medicolegal problems, 13, 17, 18–20
 psychiatric hospital admission and,
  380–381
Megacolon, 319
Meningitis, 353–354
 diagnosis and therapy, 106
Meningococcemia, fulminating, 354
Meniscus injuries, 217
Meperidine, intoxication with, 102
Mescaline, 390
Metabolic disorders
 in children, 367
 diagnosis and therapy, 103
 seizures and, 347
Metacarpals, fracture of, 242
Metatarsal fractures, 216
Middle palmar space, infection of, 249
Mitral stenosis, 78, 115
Mittelschmerz, 160–161
Moniliasis (candidiasis), 164–165
Morphine
 in acute pulmonary edema, 68
 intoxication with, 102
 in myocardial infarction, 65
 in paroxysmal atrial tachycardia, 75
Mortality
 from accidental poisoning, 299
 from burns, 265
 from multiple injuries, 23–32
Motion evaluation
 in hand injuries, 224–226

 in maxillofacial injuries, 255, 257
Mouth-to-mouth insufflation, 71
Multiple injuries, 187–188
Multiple sclerosis, 141, 340
Musculoskeletal injuries. *See* Orthopedic
  injuries
Myasthenia gravis, 337–344
Myocardial infarction, 64–67
Myoma
 degeneration of, 159
 submucous, 152
Myringotomy incision, 290

Narcotics, 390, 397–400
 addiction, 380
 heroin, 397, 398–400
 intoxication, 102
Nasogastric tube, 317
 in gastric dilatation, 55
Nasotracheal intubation, 35
Navicular fracture, 239
Neck
 injuries, 89
 outpatient care, 200–201
Negligence, 19
Neoplasms, 139, 142
Nerve palsy, 199
Nerves
 in hand injuries, 226–228, 235–236
 in maxillofacial injuries, 256–257
Neurasthenia, 340, 342
Neuritis, diabetic, 340
Neurosurgical emergencies, 87–97, 337–
  350
 cerebral concussion, 91–92
 cervical fractures, 89
 history, 87–88, 90–91
 increased intracranial pressure, 95–96
 intracranial hematoma, 93–94
 level of consciousness, 89–90
 lumbar puncture, 94–95
 myasthenia gravis, 337–344
 seizures, 344–350
 skull fractures, 92–93
 spinal cord compression, 96–97
 vital signs, 88–89
Nonpenetrating wounds, 123–126
Nose
 cold injuries, 114–115
 epistaxis, 292–295
 foreign bodies, 295–296
 fractures, 262–263
 infection, 295

Nurses, 17

Observation area, 9
Obstetrical and gynecological emergencies, 145–169
  acute abdomen, 157–159
  amniotic fluid embolus, 154–155
  fetal emergencies, 166–167
  genital injuries, 161–164
  lower genital tract infection, 164–166
  pediatric emergencies, 168–169
  pelvic pain, 160–161
  preeclampsia and eclampsia, 155–157
  puerperal inversion of the uterus, 155
  vaginal hemorrhage, 145–154
Occlusion
  acute arterial, 115
    initial management, 116–117
  acute superior mesenteric, 120
Ocular emergencies, 277–287
  abrasions, 280, 281
  bright red eye, 287
  conjunctivitis, 285
  detached retina, 283
  foreign bodies, 280, 281
  glaucoma, 284–285
  herpes zoster, 285–286
  hyphema, 279–280
  irrigation, 277–278
  occlusion, 282, 283
  painful eye(s), 284–286
  proptosis, 286–287
  radiation burns, 281–282
  tearing and pain, 287
  trauma, 277–282
  vision, loss of, 282–283
Olecranon fractures, 204
Open cardiac massage, 27
Oral tracheal intubation, 35, 37
Orthopedic injuries, 183–219
  hospital admission vs. ambulatory treatment, 199
  multiple injuries and multiple fractures, 187–188
  open fractures, 188
  physical examination, 183–185
  precautions with outpatient care, 200–201
  roentgenograms, 185–187
  specific injuries, 201–219
  splinting for transportation, 188–189
  traction, 190–199
Otitis externa, acute, 289

Otitis media, 290
  in children, 358–359
Otorhinolaryngological emergencies, 289–298
  ear, 289–292
  nose, 292–296
  pharynx and larynx, 296–298
Outpatient care, orthopedic, precautions with, 200–201
Ovary
  ruptured cyst, 157
  torsion of cyst, 157
  tubo-ovarian abscess, 158, 159
Oxygen
  in acute pulmonary edema, 68
  in cardioversion, 70
  in life-or-death situations, 23

Pacemaker, cardiac, 82–84
Pain. *See also specific condition*
  abdominal, in children, 365–366
  in burns, 273
  in myocardial infarction, 65
Palpation
  of abdomen, 129
  of maxillofacial injuries, 255
Pancreatic injury, 124–125
Paracentesis
  acute abdomen, 132
  in liver and spleen injuries, 124
Paralysis
  differential diagnosis, 342–343
  Todd's, 341
Paranoia, 376, 380, 384
Paraphimosis, 143
Paronychia, 245
Paroxysmal atrial tachycardia, 74–77
Paroxysmal nodal tachycardia, 76
Paroxysmal supraventricular tachycardia, 361–362
Patella
  dislocations, 211–212
  fractures, 211
Pearson attachment, 194, 197
Pediatric emergencies, 168–169, 351–370. *See also* Children
  bleeding, 168
  congenital anomalies, 169
  infection, 168
  trauma, 168
Pelvic fractures, 209
Pelvic pain, 160–161
  dysmenorrhea, 160

intra-uterine device, 161
Mittelschmerz, 160–161
Penetrating wounds, 55, 110
    abdominal, 121–123
Penis, infection of, 334
Percussion, in acute abdomen, 129–130
Perforation, esophageal, 57, 61
Perfusion, 28–30
Pericardial tamponade, 57, 58–59
Pericardicentesis, 59
Periodic paralysis, 343
Peritoneum, wound penetration, 123
Petechial hemorrhages, 55
Phalanges, 216–217. *See also* Fingers
Pharynx and larynx
    foreign bodies, 297
    infection, 297–298
    trauma, 296
Phimosis, 143
Phlebotomy, in pulmonary edema, 68
Phlegmasia cerulea dolens, 119
Physical examination
    acute abdomen, 129–130
    for orthopedic injuries, 183–185
    in wounds, 172–173
Physical plant, emergency room, 6–11
Placenta abruptio, 151, 153
Placenta praevia, 149
Pneumonia, in children, 358
Pneumothorax, 25, 54
    sealing of open, 40
    tension, 48–49, 54
    traumatic, 43–45
Poison control center, 10, 11, 299–300
Poisoning, 299–312
    aspirin, in children, 359
    in children, 303, 305–308, 369
    equipment for emergency treatment,
        300–301
    gastric lavage, 311–312
    general considerations, 302–304
    general emergency measures in hospi-
        tal, 310–311
    identification of poisons, 305
    ingested, 311
    medication, 301–302
    most common poisons, 305–308
    reference library, 300
    skin contamination, 310–311
    snakebites, 310–311
    summary of emergency treatment, 308–
        310
    treatment (unknown sources), 304–305

vomiting induction, 303
Poisons, common, 305–308
Policy committee, 13–16, 17
Poliomyelitis, 141, 341, 342
Positive-pressure breathing, 68
Postconvulsive state, 105
Postinfectious encephalomyelitis, 340
Postpartum hemorrhage, 150–151
Potassium permanganate, as abortifacient,
    148
Preeclampsia and eclampsia, 155–157
Pregnancy, 146–151
    abortion, 146–148
    antepartum, 146–150
    ectopic, 148–149
    hypofibrinogenemia, 151
    incoagulable blood, 151
    intrapartum, 150
    postpartum, 150–151
    recurrent jaundice of, 324
    toxemia, seizures and, 347
Pressure necrosis, 199
Primary closure of lacerations, 174
Proptosis, 286–287
Prostate infection, 334
Prostatitis, 138
Psychiatric emergencies, 371–392
    appraisal, 372–378
    area for, 10
    diagnosis, 390–391
    drug-induced aberrations, treatment of,
        389–390
    drug therapy, 383–386
    family of acutely ill or deceased, 390
    hospitalization, 379–382
    impressions and treatment, 378–382
    palliative care and referrals, 386–388
    records, 390–391
    seizures and, 347
    supportive psychotherapy, 388
    transferring and transporting patients,
        382–383
Public relations, 1–2, 6, 9
Puerperal inversion of the uterus, 155
Puerperal sepsis, 159
Pulmonary compression, relief of, 40–45
Pulmonary edema, 67–68
Pulmonary embolus, 77, 118–119
Pulverized chest, 51
Puncture wounds, 177
Pyoderma, 332

Queckenstedt's test, 95, 97

Rabies prophylaxis, 180–181
Radial nerve, 227–228
Radiology unit, in emergency room, 8–9
Radius and ulna injuries, 201–204
Rape, 130, 163–164
Records, 13, 14–15, 109, 128
Rectum examination, in acute abdomen, 130
Regional enteritis, 320–322
Renal failure, 31–32
Respiratory distress, 24–28
 in burns, 269
 cardiopulmonary resuscitation, 71–72
 in children, 355–359
 control of, 34–48
 in head injuries, 88–89
 in infectious disease, 333
 in maxillofacial injuries, 254
 in myasthenia gravis, 339–344
 in thoracic emergencies, 34–48
 in vascular emergencies, 108–109
Resuscitation
 cardiopulmonary, 71–72
 in vascular emergencies, 108–109
Resuscitube, 35
Retardation, 376, 379
Retina, detached, 283
Retroperitoneal injuries, 126
Rib fractures
 compound, 57, 59
 multiple, 50–52
 simple, 50
Roentgenograms
 in acute abdomen, 131
 "bad," 49
 in emergency room, 8–9
 hand injuries, 239
 in maxillofacial injuries, 257–258
 in myocardial infarction, 64
 for orthopedic injuries, 185–187
 in thoracic injuries, 48–49
"Rule of nines" in burns, 267–268, 271
Russell's traction, 191–192

Salpingitis, acute, 158–159
Scapular fractures, 207–208
Schiøtz tonometer, 284–285
Scrotal pain and swelling, 141–142
Second-degree burn, 267
Sedatives
 for epilepsy, 349
 intoxication with, 102
 for psychiatric patients, 383–386

seizures and, 345
Seizures, 344–350
 in children, 366, 369–370
 diagnosis, 344–348
 and drug addiction, 345, 404–405
 in eclampsia, 156–157
 etiology, 345–347
 treatment, 348–350
Sensation
 in hand nerve injuries, 227
 in maxillofacial injuries, 256
Septic abortion, 147, 154
Septic shock, 154
Septicemia, 139–140, 352–353
Severe injuries, 23–32
Shingles, 285–286
Shock, 28–30
 in burns, 269
 cardiogenic, 65
 dehydration with, in children, 364
 diagnosis and therapy, 105
 drugs for, 65
 endotoxic, 139, 154
 in maxillofacial injuries, 253–254
 septic, 154
Shoulder
 dislocation, 206–207
 fracture dislocation, 206
Shoulder presentation, 167
Sinus tachycardia, 74
Skeletal traction, 192–199
 methods, 193–195
 precautions, 197–199
 uses, 195–197
Skin
 contamination by poisons, 310–311
 grafts, hand, 231–233
 lacerations of the hand, 230–232
 traction, 190–192
Skull fractures, 92
Small intestine. *See* Intestines
Snakebite, 310, 311
Sociopathic behavior, 378, 380, 386
Sodium-responsive periodic paralysis, 342
Spermatic cord, torsion of, 142
Spinal cord
 compression, 96–97
 lumbar puncture, 94–95
Spinal fractures, 218
Spleen injuries, 135
Splinting
 chest wall, 39–40
 for transportation, 188–189

Sprains, hand and wrist, 238–239
Stab wounds, 122–123
  and cardiorrhaphy, 59
  thorax, 55–56
Staff, 13–18
  house, 16–17
  nonprofessional, 18
Status epilepticus, 349
Steatorrhea, 321
Steinmann pin, 193–194
Stenosis, mitral, 78, 115
Stent pressure dressing, 233
Sterile supplies, 12–13
Sternoclavicular dislocation, 58, 209
Stimulants, 400–402
Stings, in children, 360
Stove-in (flail) chest, 50–52
Strangulated hernia, 142
Streptococcal gangrene, 247–248
Stretchers, 11–12
Subarachnoid block, 97
Subcutaneous emphysema, 40, 53
Subdural hematoma, 93–94
Submucous myoma, 152
Suicidal behavior, 375–376, 378–379, 384
Suicide, 112
Suppurative tenosynovitis, 248
Supracondylar and condylar fractures, 211
Supraventricular tachycardia, 65
Surgery
  area for, 7
  equipment, 7–8
Syphilis, 138

Tachycardia
  atrial, with atrioventricular block, 76, 78
  drugs for, 76–77, 80
  nodal, 70
  paroxysmal atrial, 74–77
  sinus, 74
  ventricular, 66, 70, 78–79, 80
Tachysystolic dysrhythmias, 65–66, 72–73
Talus fractures, 215
Tamponade
  cardiac, 26–27
  pericardial, 57, 58–59
Tarsometatarsal dislocations and fracture dislocations, 216
Tarsus fractures, 215
Tear gas injury to eye, 278
Tendons, hand, 224–225, 236–238

Tenosynovitis, suppurative, 248
Tetanus prophylaxis, 109, 175, 179–180
  in burns, 276
  in hand injuries, 229
  in maxillofacial injuries, 260
Thenar space, infection of, 250
Third-degree burn, 267
Thomas splint, 194, 197
Thoracentesis, 41–42
Thoracic emergencies, 33–62. *See also specific conditions*
  emergency measures, 34–48
  emergency thoracotomy, 57–62
  roentgenography in, 48–49
  wounds, 50–57
Thoracic injuries
  cardiac compression, relief of, 45–48
  pulmonary compression, relief of, 40–45
  restoration of respiration, 34–39
  sealing of open pneumothorax, 40
  splinting of chest wall, 39–40
Thoracostomy tube drainage, 41–46, 54
Thoracotomy, emergency, 57–62
  compound rib fracture and major chest wall defect, 59–60
  esophageal perforation, 61
  intrathoracic foreign bodies, 61–62
  intrathoracic hemorrhage, 57–58
  pericardial tamponade, 58–59
  rupture of larynx, trachea, and bronchi, 59
  ruptured aorta, 58
  ruptured diaphragm, 60–61
  thoraco-abdominal wounds, 60
Throat wounds, 112
Thrombosis
  acute arterial, 116
  acute massive, 119
  and traumatic aneurysm, 111
  venous, 118
    deep, 118–119
    iliofemoral, 119
    phlegmasia cerulea dolens, 119
    superficial, 118
Tibial fractures
  plateau, 212
  shaft, 212
  spine, 212
Tick paralysis, 343
Todd's paralysis, 341
Toe fractures, 216
Tongue-depressor test, 257

Tonometer, 284–285
Tourniquets, 108, 172
  in pulmonary edema, 68
Toxemia of pregnancy, seizures and, 156–157, 347
Toxicology. *See* Poisoning
Toxins, seizures and, 346
Trachea
  in infectious disease, 333–334
  rupture of, 57, 59
Tracheobronchial tree, 25, 26
Tracheostomy, 24–26, 35, 37–39, 339
  in maxillofacial injuries, 259–260
  for multiple rib fracture, 51–52
Traction
  head halter, 97, 218
  precautions with, 52, 197–199
  skeletal, 192–197
  skin, 190–192
Traction test, 256
Tranquilizers, 403–406
  intoxication with, 102
Transplant donors, 89
Trauma
  abdominal, 121–126
  in children, 168, 366
  ear, 292
  in genital injuries, 161–162
  ocular, 277–282
    blunt, 279–280
    chemical, 277–279
    sharp, 280–282
  pharynx and larynx, 297
  and psychiatric symptoms, 388
  sexual, 162–164
Traumatic aneurysm, 111–112
Traumatic asphyxia, 55
Trench foot, 114
Trichomoniasis, 164
Tubo-ovarian abscess, 158, 159

Ulcerative colitis, 318–320
Ulcers, 316
Ulna traction, 195
Ulnar nerve, 227
Unconsciousness, 99–106
  causes of faints, 63–64
  cervical fracture in, 89
  in children, 366–369
    common causes, 366–367
    emergency laboratory evaluation, 368
    supportive measures, 367–368

    treatment, 368
  and consent, 19
  differential considerations, 90–91
  differential diagnosis, 99–100
  emergency-room care, 100–106
  evaluation of, 87–91
  hospital admission, 101
  level of consciousness, 89–90
  in maxillofacial injuries, 253
  special problems, 99
  vital signs in, 89
  work-up, 100–101
Uremia, 103
Ureteral colic, 140–141
Uretheritis, 137–138
Urethra, 334
Urinary tract infection, 334
Urine retention, 141
Urological emergencies. *See* Genitourinary emergencies
Urological injuries, 135–137
  bladder, 136–137
  kidney, 135–136
  urethra, 137
Urticaria, 360
Uterus
  bleeding, 152–153
  concealed abruptio placentae, 153
  ectopic pregnancy, 153
  inversion, 155
  myoma, 152
  perforated, 153
  ruptured, 153

Vagina
  cancer, 151–152
  dysfunctional uterine bleeding, 152–153
  examination, in acute abdomen, 130
  hemorrhage, 145–153
  lacerations, 161
  postpartum, 150–151
  pregnancy, 146–150
  submucous myoma, 152
Vaginitis, nonspecific, 165
Varices, vulvar and vaginal, 162
Varicose veins, 120
Vascular emergencies
  complications, 115–120
  control hemorrhage, 108
  immediate management, 107–109
  mechanical injuries, 110–111

resuscitation, 108–109
types, 109–115
Vasospasm, 109–110
Venous thrombosis, 118–119
Ventilation. *See* Respiratory distress
Ventricle
fibrillation, 27, 81
in cardiopulmonary resuscitation, 72
tachycardia, 66, 78–79
Viral hepatitis, 322–323
Vision
loss of, 282–283
in maxillofacial injuries, 255–256
Vital signs, in neurosurgical emergencies, 88–89
Vomiting
in children, 362–364
induction in poisoning, 303
Vulva
hematoma, 162
lacerations, 161
varices, 162

Waiting area, 9
Waterhouse-Friderichsen syndrome, 354
Weakness, differential diagnosis of, 339–344
Weight loss, 380, 385
Weil's disease, 323
Wernicke's encephalopathy, 341
Wet lung, 26
Withdrawal syndrome, 404–405
Wounds, 171–182
abdominal, 121–126

abrasions, 176
animal bites, 172, 177
blunt trauma, 110–111
frostbite, 178
gas gangrene, 180
gunshot, 56, 252
human bites, 177–178
in infectious disease, 333
lacerations, 174–176
management of, 171–182
maxillofacial, 252–253
nonpenetrating, 50–55
abdominal, 123–126
penetrating, 55
abdominal, 45, 121–123
thorax, 45
vascular, 110
preliminary procedures, 171–174
puncture, 177
rabies prophylaxis, 180–181
stab, 55–56
tetanus prophylaxis, 179–180
thoraco-abdominal, 57, 60
thorax, 55
throat, 112
treatment, 178–182
types, 174–178
wrist, 112
Wringer injury of the hand, 235
Wrist
dislocations, 239
wounds, 112

Zygoma fractures, 263